Flower Essences and Vibrational Healing

by Gurudas

(Formerly titled Flower Essences)

Foreword by
Gabriel Cousens, M.D.

Cassandra Press

San Rafael, Ca

Cassandra Press
P.O. Box 868
San Rafael, CA. 94915

Printed in the United States of America

First printing 1983 by Brotherhood of Life

Revised and expanded edition 1989 by Cassandra Press

ISBN 0-945946-04-X

Library of Congress 88-63558

The use of the material described in this text is not meant to replace the services of a physician who should always be consulted for any condition requiring his or her aid.

"That which is looked upon by one generation as the apex of human knowledge is often considered an absurdity by the next, and that which is regarded as a superstition in one century, may form the basis of science for the following one."

Paracelsus

Front cover artwork by Catherine Andrews

Other books by Gurudas

Gem Elixirs and Vibrational Healing, Vol. I
Gem Elixirs and Vibrational Healing, Vol II
The Spiritual Properties of Herbs

Table of Contents

Foreword

For many reasons it was an absolute delight to read this transcript. If the information presented in this book is utilized appropriately, it has the potential to bring about a major evolutionary step in the application of vibrational medicine in the west, particularly in the healing science of flower essences. The direction of interest for many of us in holistic health seems to be away from the focus on the materialistic in health and toward a vibrational approach. As Dr. Bach pointed out years ago, materialism masks the real nature of disease. Because of this materialistic view, modern medicine deals with the symptoms and results of disease, not with the real causes. Flower essences are one of two major exceptions to materialistic science to be developed in the past several centuries; the other major exception is homeopathy.

This book is significant because it releases detailed information on how to maximize the use of flower essences right down to the practical basics of how to prepare, store, protect, use, and amplify them. With 112 flower essences, it gives the most detailed description of a flower essence ever put into print. Having used the Bach flower essences since 1974 and other newly developed flower essences since 1980, it was quite helpful to receive this information.

One question that may come up in many readers' minds about the information in this book is: what if I do not believe in channeling? Although there is a clear explanation of channeling and a historical review, including a partial list of important historical people who used channeled information as a resource such as Abraham Lincoln, Thomas Edison, and Franklin D. Roosevelt, some readers may still be wondering... must I accept this information on blind faith? The answer is no! One need not automatically accept any of it (and still receive a great deal of information from this offering made by the channeling, which comes from a voice who identifies himself as John). What is much more important than blind acceptance is the systematic exploration of the potential truth in what has been presented. This book should inspire people with an inquisitive New Age consciousness to explore the validity of this information in their healing work and, even more importantly, in their own personal healing and conscious growth.

We should also be aware that some of the apparently new insights presented in this budding field of vibrational medicine come from the ancient roots of recorded history. In India, the use of different vibrations of various gems for healing has been practiced for thousands of years. This is also true with sound and color therapies. Furthermore, although not widely understood in the west, there is a strong tradition in the Chinese Tao of using flowers for healing and conscious growth. The philosophical and scientific basis for vibrational healing that is presented in such conceptual detail in this book can be found in such ancient philosophies as the Vedas and Kashmir shavism, as well as in the Gospel according to John which says, "In the beginning was the Word"-the Word implying the primal sound vibration. This philosophical and scientific basis can also be found in Einstein's theory of relativity and in the last thirty to fifty years of quantum physics. Because of this new understanding, many modern physicists are now saying that all creation, including the material world, is just different levels of vibrating energy.

The vibrational healing approach offered in this book presents a detail and theory which can allow us as scientists to elevate the field of flower essence healing into a very conscious science as well as an art. The discussion of applying the living vibrations of plants to balance the different vibrational bodies, chakras, and nadis creates the framework for some very interesting areas of research. The discussion on miasms, which until now has been in the domain of homeopathy, opens up a whole new area of flower essence usage and exploration. The findings of this research may reveal a quite exciting and profound step in achieving total health for us as individuals as well as for the whole planet.

But before we get carried away with these new potentialities for flower essences, quartz crystals, pyramid technologies and the like, we must not forget the even deeper message of this book. John states: "... but none must supplement the content and nature or even be as given as the higher priority then to know that God is within you. These things that are given forth are teachings, then as applied teachings, then as to stimulate more that each and everyone of thee may as make progressions and evolve toward that which ye already are which is God's love which is within thee, which begets harmony and peace." On a deeper level this book is concerned with the evolvement of our awareness. Only with this heightened awareness are we able to heal ourselves, and then by our own harmonious beingness we can fully participate in the healing of others.

The flower essence healing system utilizes the bond between plants and humans to help all of us evolve into higher consciousness. Although most of us are at least vaguely aware of this bond from our own experience of being in the presence of plants and from books like *The Secret Life of Plants* in which the authors mention that the mental hospitals in Russia use gardens to stimulate mental harmony in patients, the awareness and use of this bond of friendship with our flower friends is explained here at a new level of specificity. It also implies that the more conscious we become, the better use that we as healers will be able to make of our partnership with our plant friends.

Although we often misperceive disease as something that happens on the physical plane, the true cause of disease comes from a conflict between the mind and the soul. While vibrational therapies such as flower essences can help overcome these problems, even stimulating healing of physical diseases, inner tranquility and calmness to prevent and overcome the real causes of diseases can only be obtained through spiritual practices such as meditation.

If we do not understand and put into practice the deeper message of this book, we will become just another group with an interesting healing system. To develop this system to its highest, we ourselves must become healed on every level. As John so eloquently states, "... for in closing on these things, all these affairs are but tools to bring harmony which is an expression of God's love. But it is only love itself that is God." To experience oneself as completely healed is to revel in the ecstasy of being that love. Then, as the flower essences are tinctures of liquid consciousness that heal by inspirational rather than causal force, so we too, by our state of love, by being our human essence, will spontaneously inspire others to heal themselves.

Gabriel Cousens, M.D.

Preface

The material presented in this book has been trance channeled through Kevin Ryerson and Jon Fox. Ryerson is a professional psychic and trance channel with over thirteen years experience in the field of parapsychology. Since the age of five, Ryerson has experienced psychic phenomena such as seeing future events in his dreams. During his teenage years he studied the Edgar Cayce material, which stimulated his spiritual and psychic unfoldment. After further growth experiences with his psychic and clairvoyant abilities, he developed his own trance state at the age of twenty-one. He received his formal training in this field through the University of Life in Phoenix, Arizona. This school, which was established by Dr. Richard Ireland in 1960, trains people in psychic development.

Ryerson enters a deep state of meditation called trance channeling, which allows his consciousness to be temporarily set aside, giving time for other evolved souls to speak through him. Ryerson has been doing this work full time since 1976, and during this period he has trained numerous people to become trance channels. He travels about the United States and Canada conducting seminars and private readings with various medical, scientific, and spiritual researchers. Ryerson's work is similar to that of Jane Roberts and her guide Seth who channeled information to her. Ryerson's work is also similar to Edgar Cayce who received most of his information from his higher self.

Much of the new information in this revised edition was provided by Jon C. Fox, a channel in California. Fox has become increasingly respected for his ability to accurately research a wide variety of technical subjects. He began his channeling career eight years ago as a conscious channel. In recent years, he has expanded his gift to include trance channeling, because that often makes it easier to present technical information.

While almost finishing a master's degree in political science and being in law school for a year, I have also for some years been involved in various spiritual practices. This interest stimulated three trips to India in the early 1970's. Since 1976 I have worked with flower essences and homeopathic remedies, first as a student and then, since 1978, in my own private practice for several years. This work also includes giving advice relating to herbs, nutrition, gem elixirs, and bath therapies. Since 1978 I have also taught classes on different natural healing topics. In 1983 I founded and managed Pegasus Products for four years. This company produces and distributes about 700 different flower essences and gem elixirs. These products are prepared according to the principles described in this book.

In the summer of 1979, I learned of a psychic surgeon from the Philippines, and with my keen interest in this form of healing, I visited him. In the middle of the session, several of my guides appeared, and they stated that my healing research would improve if I worked with a good trance channel. A few days later, a friend returned from San Diego describing Ryerson's work, and I was interested. I borrowed several tapes of Ryerson's public talks in trance and after listening to the voice of John, one of Ryerson's guides, and hearing the information that was being discussed, I felt there might be a deep connection here. After a period of meditation, I called Ryerson and in October, 1979 he visited San Francisco. From that period for five years, we did numerous research readings. This present book on flower essences is the first in a series of volumes on various forms of spiritual and natural healing topics.

The nature of channeled teaching is such that to produce much information many questions must be asked. If one were to just sit back and listen, a fair amount of information would be presented, but it would usually not match what can be given if the inquirer comes prepared with many questions and a good background and training in the field of inquiry.

Fortunately, I have an inquiring mind, an academic back-ground that demands objective information, a natural gift for asking questions to beget specific information, and a fair degree of training in several holistic health modalities. Channeled teaching is a slow, time consuming process in which a certain amount of information is discussed, which I gradually assimilate. Then I return to discuss new information and to sometimes ask additional questions to expand on previously discussed material.

The main focalizer for Ryerson's work is John. To many who work with Ryerson, John appears to be John the Apostle, the disciple of Jesus and author of the Book of Revelation. In the Bible, John 21:20-23, Jesus asked John to stay behind in service;[1] for the last 2,000 years John has inspired many people, including Leonardo Da Vinci, on inspirational and trance channeling levels. John, who is the most universal of Ryerson's guides, has full access to all the information and wisdom from Atlantis and Lemuria. Atlantis and Lemuria were two ancient land masses and civilizations. Lemuria covered much of the Pacific Ocean, while its colony Atlantis covered much of the Atlantic Ocean. Carl Jung would call this the collective consciousness of the planet.[2] With this ability Ryerson, in trance, discusses highly technical issues on any subject including advanced concepts in physics, building specific machines, complex medical questions, or philosophical and spiritual truths.

One reason why John is allowed to render so much technical information in such detail is because people are now ready and willing to receive this new material. As a society we have reached a state of conscious and technological development so that, while some of the information John shares may seem radical at times, many have the capacity to assimilate and apply it.

Hilarion is the main guide who works though Fox. Hilarion focalizes the fifth ray, which consists of technical and scientific information. Some may be aware that Hilarion has recently been the source of an entire series of channeled books from the Marcus press in Toronto. Hilarion has provided inspirational guidance and technical advice to many people for thousands of years.

1 F. C. Eiselen, Edwin Lewis, and D. G. Downer, ed., *The Abington Bible Commentary* (Garden City, NY: Doubleday & Co. 1979), p. 1092.
2 Carl Jung, *Man and His Symbols* (New York: Doubleday & Co., 1969).

Introduction

This revised and expanded edition contains much new material on how specific flower essences can be used with plants, animals, astrology, and the twelve rays. While most of the changes in this text have been placed where the individual flower essences are presented, thoughout the book new points have been added and expanded upon. Several new flower essences have also been included.

The information presented in this book has been divided into several sections. Initially there is a review of the general principles and historical uses of flower essences in various ancient civilizations. There is a discussion of Dr. Bach's life and the relationship of the Bach flowers to this new work. (Edward Bach was an English physician who lived early this century. His research and life have inspired many people over the years.) New techniques are offered in preparing, storing, and protecting flower essences. The storage and protection of flower essences is certainly an important issue with so many environmental pollutants now present. Techniques involving the use of quartz crystals, pyramids, and orgone energy are also described. The book includes an extensive discussion on how flower essences actually work in our physical and subtle bodies.

There is a discussion on the relationship between flower essences, homeopathic remedies, and gem elixirs. This includes how these three forms of vibrational therapies work differently in people, how they can interfere with each other if taken at or near the same time, and how flower essences affect the miasms. In homeopathy, the miasms are considered to be the root cause or primary factor in all chronic diseases.

Of the hundreds of hours of channeled information that Kevin Ryerson has shared with me in the last three years, one of the most important teachings is that there are two and soon three new inherited miasms. These are the radiation miasm, the petrochemical miasm, and within eight years the heavy metal miasm. Having used homeopathic remedies and flower essences since 1976, I feel it accurate to state that homeopaths and people using flower essences have almost no understanding of these new miasms and little comprehension of how these factors can block the well chosen remedy from working. The relevancy of flower essences here is that they can have a profound effect on eradicating all the miasms.

Advice will be given to the practitioner and patient in using flower essences. This includes depicting various amplification and diagnostic techniques. There is also material on how flower essences can best be utilized in bath therapies.

Section 2 lists the information to be given with each flower essence. The twenty points covered with each flower essence help the reader estimate the range of clinical effectiveness for these new remedies. Just over 100 new remedies will then be presented. In addition, charts will be presented to help the reader assimilate this new material.

The final section involves looking at future developments in the application of flower essences. Vibrational remedies such as flower essences will become increasingly popular in the coming years. New diagnostic equipment will soon make it easier to test and prove the clinical validity of these remedies.

The data presented in this book is not meant to be the final word. It is my sincere wish that this book stimulate greater awareness, understanding, and clinical research of these remedies. It is only a matter of time before others publish books on this system of natural healing.

Most objective observers will agree that a good deal of valuable new information has been provided in this text concerning the clinical use of various flower essences. It is the channeled guidance that not all the clinical information on these remedies is to be provided here. Part of our work and responsibility in this learning process is to expand, on our own, an understanding of how these healing agents can be utilized in mind, body, and spirit.

After working with this channeled information for three years and being able to test and prove many different modalities in the clinical setting of my own private practice and that of associates including various physicians, I am confident that the test of time will prove the accuracy of the information presented in this book. I have seen others get similar positive results with this work. In time, I hope to complete a book of case reports and double blind studies demonstrating how flower essences have been used.

Most of the information in this text was channeled through Kevin Ryerson from January, 1980 to September, 1982. Important blocks of information were channeled to a study group that met for one year starting in January, 1980. The rest of the information comes from my own private research, including private readings I had with Ryerson and Fox. Most of the new material in the revised edition of this book was channeled through Fox from Hilarion in my research with them in 1987 and 1988. In various sections of the book, the actual questions asked with the verbatim responses are included so that the reader will comprehend how the information has been obtained.

During one of the readings the question was raised as to how this research differs from magic or sympathetic magic. The channeled answer was as follows:

"You are developing this as a belief system, and if people do not believe that a helicopter can fly, they will not develop it. But if you believe in heavier-than-air flight, eventually you will develop something. Indeed, it all starts out with specific thought, then a creative idea, then literally pulling it out of the ethers.[1] It is different from magic in that you are taking a point of research and building case studies and the fact that the properties already exist in the flowers. We are bringing them to you on a general 'raw data' basis, and you are making them more specific through your researches and applications. Most of science, in its early stage, came from what was originally accused of being magic. The system we are giving is being channeled, a bit synthesized from various cultures, but it is a restoration of the system."

With a few exceptions, commonly known and used plants and trees are presented in this text. While these are primarily flowers common in the west, others normally found in tropical countries will be presented in the future. In the channelings, it was explained why certain flowers were chosen.

"The reason we are sticking to the popular forms of flowers is to give a broad sense of knowledge that is applicable for many practitioners, not only on the more esoteric levels, but for lay practitioners also. You are getting a large body of raw data that can be refined down to a specifically closed system for the more orthodox researchers. With the entire body of knowledge people get what they need and a tightly closed, scientifically researched system will eventually be evolved by and for those of that kind of mind. Some of the problems with esoteric systems is that they can get so complex that the lay person is discouraged but, at the same time, due to the fact that your societies are very exacting, it is wise to have a specific body of knowledge for scientific researchers."

This book is presented in the tradition of the empirical school of thought. Two main traditions have dominated western medical history. While practitioners did not necessarily clearly follow one of these schools, this philosophical schism has generally been present in western medicine.[2]

The rationalists see the human body as a material or mechanical vehicle, and seeks to understand the causes and treatment of disease in an analytical fashion. They put labels on the disease process and tend to treat diseases, not people.

In the empirical tradition, reliance is placed more on experience, observation, and the individuality of each person. There is general recognition of each person as a spiritual being with a life force connecting him or her to the spiritual realms or forces of the soul. In this belief system, there is more openness to working with intuition and to testing the validity of channeled teachings. In these days, increasing numbers of people are accepting channeled teachings as a reliable source of information. This trend will certainly continue in the coming years.

1 The seven ethers are seven dimensional states that vibrate at a speed faster than the speed of light. Many scientists in the 1800's believed in this concept, and today scientists are again studying this principle. Some speculate that there are eight ethers and dimensional states. Other esoteric terms are defined in the esoteric glossary in the back of this book.

Alice A. Bailey, *The Soul and Its Mechanism* (New York: Lucis Publishing Co., 1981).

Dr. Guenther Wachsmuth, *Etheric Formative Forces in Cosmos, Earth, and Man* (Spring Valley, NY: Anthroposophical Press, 1932).

Alice A. Bailey, *Telepathy* (New York: Lucis Publishing Co. 1980), p.167.

Pat Flanagan, *Pyramid Power* (Marina del Rey, CA: DeVorss & Co. 1976), p.106-168.

James Trefil, "Nothing May Turn Out to Be the Key to the Universe," *Smithsonian*, XII (December,1981), 143-149.

2 Harris Coulter, *Divided Legacy: A History of the Schism in Medical Thought*, Volume III, (Washington, DC: Wehawken Book Co.,1973).

Section I

Chapter I

General Principles and Historical Use of Flower Essences

In this first chapter, John describes the fall of humanity to the earth plane and the rise and fall of several ancient civilizations. It is important to understand this material because using flower essences originated in these ancient periods. The inhabitants of Lemuria were completely self-contained, being in harmony with each other and with the harmonics of nature. All communication occurred on the level of the mind through telepathy, and only in the latter stages of Lemuria did the ability to form sounds and speech develop.[1] The destruction of Lemuria took place when there was the desire for knowledge of the material world that was out of balance with the forces of nature. Atlanteans lacked the Lemurians' intuitive understanding of nature; indeed, the focus there was on advanced technologies much like what has developed in America.

There are many books that describe the ancient Lemurian and Atlantean civilizations. The most detailed are the series of books by James Churchward on Lemuria, (or Mu, as it is sometimes called)[2] and the book *Edgar Cayce on Atlantis.*[3] Rudolf Steiner, in his book *Cosmic Memory: Atlantis and Lemuria*, probably has the broadest vision of these ancient cultures.[4] Many of the teachings and cultural experiences from these ancient civilizations are still relevant today. For instance, flower essences were extensively used in Lemuria and Atlantis.

Q John, will you now give a discourse on the history of using flower essences in various ancient cultures and describe the principles and dimensions of this system?

"You would find that first there was the Great Creator or the first Great Spirit who created all things within the universe through natural laws and events. The flow of evolution was of such a nature so as to bring forth balance and harmony within all the planes of existence.

"Then there was the creation of souls to go forth and create diversity as amongst that one original creation. Those souls, having moved close to this plane as such with the abilities of projecting through the time flows, saw the diverse potential and alternative realities that souls could bring forth upon this plane. It was not in the original plan that there would be as the fall of spirit onto this plane, for souls were to remain in the angelic state, which is the natural order of things. Even without the intervention of these souls certain animal, mineral, and plant forms developed according to the natural dynamics of the dimensions as they manifested on this plane."

Ages ago humanity fell into this plane basically from curiosity and pride. Individual souls got too close to the physical plane, and gradually they got attached to the workings and designs of the earth plane. Many felt they could reshape the environment, including the many animal, plant, and mineral forms, in manners superior to that created by God. John has stated that this was the first great karmic action or error.[5]

While it was not part of the original plan for souls to fall to this plane, it was indeed originally ordained that many mineral, plant, and animal forms would become established on the earth. The earth was to be a park or Garden of Eden which many souls from above could look down upon to see, admire, and be taught. When many souls decided to take physical bodies in the earth plane this was allowed to happen. We are all born with free will, for it is not God's wish that we follow His laws as slaves or servants.

"You would find that the plants and all systems of evolution extending forth from the simple amino acids and rising up first from the sea floor and then extending onto the land is symbolic of the gradual evolution of the spirit itself and the spirit of mankind. You would then find that a spirit entered the earth plane and raised up the body physical from the lower primates into the humanoid form which you now bear. So in turn did they become specifically localized or stabilized in the current human physical form. Therefore, you would find that being specifically localized therein is where the thought forms of the body physical and various plant forms began to integrate according to the peculiar needs of the spirit. Up until those time periods, evolution was but a natural force guided by degrees of intelligence, but not a specific intelligence shaping plant life according to its needs. The body physical became as the pattern for many plant forms within the Garden of Eden that was indeed Lemuria, and gave a forebearance to healing properties for the needs of those physical bodies according to the intelligence that inhabited them of the spirit therein.

"In this evolutionary plan, flowers were and are the very essence and the highest concentration of life force in the plant. They are the crowning experience of the plants' growth. They are a combination of the etheric properties and at the height of the life force, so they are often used in the fertility portions of the plant's growth."

When many souls fell and got trapped on the earth plane, God manifested His spirit here in a specific intelligent pattern to shape and guide these souls. Part of the plan was to establish a specific relationship between the many plant forms and the humanoid form. With this development, these plants were gradually used as an enhancement for growth in mind, body, and spirit.

The fall from spirit that John described above is quite similar to creation myths in many cultures.[6] For instance, the first three chapters of Genesis in the Bible, *The Book of Enoch*,[7] and the *Nag Hammadi Library*,[8] the ancient scrolls recently found in Egypt, all tell a similar story.

"Continuing on this path of evolution, the natural rapport between the plant, animal, and human forms would have ultimately dictated, independently of spirit, an evolution paralleling the doctrine of signature. There still would have been, therefore, a sympathetic anatomical structure between the plant, animal, and human forms. With acts of consciousness, however, spirit brought forth the beginning patterns of the doctrine of signature millions of years before the fall from spirit. This was to assure that there would be the proper anatomical form corresponding with various human internal organs for the eventual rise of homo sapiens. The medicinal properties of those particular plant forms, however, did not necessarily arise until after the incarnation of spirit onto this plane. Botanically, certain plant forms can be traced back many eons before the time periods of Lemuria, and their anatomy reflects the doctrine of signature, but their medicinal properties would not have been the same. Other plant forms developed specifically in Lemuria through manners of hybridization and thought projection became the unique species they now are, but their traceable botanical ancestors existed before that time.

"Thus, there are two correlated factions in the development of plant forms. One is as before the fall or incarnation onto this plane; the souls' force, moving speculatively with the environment, set such species in development. Then there was applied evolution from the level of the incarnate state. This was, of course, Lemuria where the medicinal properties became activated by the very presence of spirit being incarnate in the physical form, completing the cycle of the doctrine of signature. This then became part of conscious reality. This was applicable to the human form because before Lemuria the human form did not exist. The doctrine of signature, in part, existed philosophically for many developing plant forms, but it is a philosophical point of view that cannot necessarily exist independently of human consciousness."

Before humanity fell onto the earth plane it was understood on the angelic planes that this fall from spirit would take place, so many plant forms were shaped in relationship to what was understood would become the developing shape of people on the physical and subtle anatomical levels. This is the doctrine of signature—there is a relationship between the anatomy of people and the shape, color, and texture of many plants. In this relationship lie many clues as to how these plants can be used in healing and conscious growth.

This entire process of development was, in part, conscious speculation, because the fall from spirit had not yet actually taken place. In early Lemuria, as the actual anatomical shape of people developed, the doctrine of signature was then extended to its second stage. Then, the medicinal properties of plants could be shaped to more perfectly match and harmonize with the physical forms of people. To achieve this second more sophisticated state, it was necessary that souls incarnate onto this physical plane. With this development it became possible to use many plant forms in healing and conscious evolution. While there was some help in this process from various angelic forces, this second state was primarily accomplished by individual souls through meditation and mental projection of the mind's energy to shape these various plant forms.

Traditionally it has been said that the doctrine of signature originated with Paracelsus in the 1500's.[9] He was a prominent alchemist who is credited with a number of original discoveries in science and medicine. I am attempting to give a more complete picture of the historical background of this doctrine.

Q Will you now describe how flower essences were used in Lemuria?

"In the time period of Lemuria approximately 500,000 years ago, there was that which we now know as the sciences of horticulture and agriculture of the content wherein all gardening, all horticulture, and all botanical techniques were accomplished on the level of the mind. Herein is where there was an extended development of the doctrine of signature wherein plant growths of a similar nature to the anatomy of man can have as a forebearance and impact upon specific portions of the anatomy according to basic principles of shape, color, and texture. All the Lemurians were gardeners upon the levels of the mind and this was the Garden of Eden. Each of the plants and all the herbs of the field were given unto service to mankind.

"In those days, beings were androgynous; they were divided into neither male nor female. Lemuria indeed is as the time period wherein man and woman had not yet been separated in the physical form. In this anatomical form, the properties of the individuals were and had higher degrees of spiritual impact, higher degrees of evolvement of society, and higher properties in social and spiritual consciousness."

While it may sound strange to some that John speaks of our ancestors as having lived in an androgynous state, many respected authorities have stated the same thing. For instance, Madame Blavatsky in her magnum opus, *The Secret Doctrine*,[10] Rudolf Steiner in *Cosmic Memory: Atlantis and Lemuria*,[11] W. Scott-Elliott in *The Story of Atlantis and The Lost Lemuria*,[12] and a number of books written by Alice A. Bailey with her guide, the Tibetan master Djwhal Khul,[13] describe this physical state as an historical fact. The androgynous or hermaphroditic state is a common theme in alchemical symbolism.[14] Even today it is a fact that people are born in this hermaphroditic state.[15] One has only to look up the term hermaphroditism in the *Index Medicus*[16] in most reference libraries to see how the medical profession continues to treat people in this physical state.

Many flower essences in Lemuria were specifically used to shape and mold the human form. In the second part of this book where the individual flower essences are discussed, some information will be given to show how specific flower essences were used concerning the androgynous state. But the channeled guidance is that most information in this area concerns more advanced technologies that shall be fully discussed in future volumes.

In the gradual transition from Lemuria to Atlantis it was realized that for humanity to evolve spiritually, it was necessary for the human race to be divided into two sexes because people were too self-contained. With the division of the sexes, marriage and raising children occurred as a shared responsibility. Individuals were then, through this greater sharing and responsibility, able to learn more lessons in life for their greater spiritual evolution.

"Individuals in Lemuria lived and saw things on luminous levels,[17] even as there are those today who observe the contents of the human aura, or those who seek to heal through acupuncture, or those who study the significance of Kirlian photography.[18] These resources were always available to the Lemurians. They had the capacity to see on luminous levels whereas ye see light reflected off various surfaces and those illuminations constitute information upon which ye function. So in turn was it with the Lemurians that seeing luminosity and the aura dynamics of solidly physical objects, they were able to perceive extra properties.

"These properties that were seen were the healing beneficial effects upon the individual human forms. It came about that as an individual having an aura, as ye in turn still do, approached specific blooms, he did not have to physically ingest any portion of the fruit, leaf, bloom, or root. So sensitive were the Lemurians that by only approaching the bloom they would observe radical alterations within the structure of the aura, the bloom and the transference of energy. This became as clues in Lemurian society to understanding the principles of energy healing stored within flower essences.

"These healing properties evolved from cohabitation on the planet of both the human personality and the human spirit, they being the evolutionary force as discoursed upon earlier. In this substance, the basic balance was and is that there is a cosympathetic bond or empathy between the human form and plant life, even as there is compatibility or cosympathetic bond between all life forms. The Lemurians had the ability to logically detect this bond; therefore, they could organize it into a complete system of healing and medical practice. They generally used flower essences to evolve in spiritual consciousness. It was not critical to healing their physical forms, for little disease was found amongst them. When consciousness proceeds the material follows therein."

Although a great error occurred when souls ages ago attempted to alter God's plan for the development of mineral, animal, and plant life on earth, this was not the case with the Lemurians' extended development of the doctrine of signature by their deliberate shaping of individual plants and flower essences to better assimilate their medicinal and spiritual values. They merely added details to God's plan.

It is really a matter of working with, not against, the evolutionary plan as established by God. Once it was understood that many souls would fall to this physical plane, a plan was manifested from the higher planes so many souls could learn their lessons and gradually reach a state of evolved consciousness in which they could, on their own, make a choice that there was no longer any need to return to this physical plane. As shall be pointed out in this and future books, releasing the spiritual and medicinal properties stored in flowers is one of the great keys to unfolding God's plan on the earth plane.

"You would find that the essence of healing and conscious growth was the most predominant thought in the Lemurian community. Healing was considered harmony. There was a symbiotic link placed between the body physical, as a temple, and the outer world, which was the direct reflection of the individual's thought forms in those days. Through continuous meditations various biochemical plant forms began to evolve. To heal the self, all the individual had to do was to have a basic knowledge of the anatomy of the physical body and its esoteric psychology. The person could then easily identify various plant structures on the basis of the doctrine of signature with the intended application of healing within the self. This began to be the essence of the foundation of the vibrational principles that ye term as healing with flower essences."

The Lemurians were for the most part content to live close to nature, so their intuitive and spiritual states of consciousness were highly developed. At least until the latter days of Lemuria, which were somewhat influenced by the Atlantean culture, there was no disease in that ancient civilization. The average life span in Lemuria was several thousand years. People left their physical body when on a soul level they felt enough life experiences had taken place in that particular incarnation. Flower essences were used primarily for spiritual growth and for regeneration of physical body tissue.

Q Will you now explain how flower essences were used in Atlantis?

"Flower essences began to be used as a system of medicine in Atlantis for herein is where diseases like those orthodox physicians study had their origins.

Then the blooms were put on water so the flowers could be as exposed to the pranic forces of the rising sun. There had been the fall from grace within the physical in the Garden of Eden or in Lemuria into the Atlantean days. Because the Atlanteans were not properly in tune with nature many diseases developed for the first time on the planet. Flotation of the blooms on water was done in Atlantis because they did not have the sensitivity of their ancestors.

"Man in Atlantean days divided into three specific senses of social attitudes and studies of the origins and predominance of society. There were those who were purely spiritual, those of the priesthood, integrated between science or the material and the spiritual, and those who were purely materialistic and studied only the material and the various patterns of the material seeking the origins of life, having forgotten their own foundations. These are the foundations that led to the necessary homeopathic systems of science, the divisions into allopathic medicines, and of those who practiced more on the spiritual path. Those who traveled the spiritual path apart from homeopathic and allopathic medicines were those who were purely spiritual and used more the accord of flower essences. Those of the priesthood were homeopathic for they traveled the patterns between the spiritual and the material. Those of the material accord were allopathic.

"There was a concentration or heightened usage of flower essences in Egypt not only because of Atlantean influence but as a historical point of social force because there was a gathering of critical bodies of information in Egypt for the preservation in the pyramidal forms within the capacity of the hall of records.[19] The reason for the heightened usage was not because there was a peculiar civilization developed or even a higher degree of development of flower essence usage than in the Atlantean period, but because there was a gathering of the body of knowledge for the express purpose of preservation. It was more an historical quirk than heightened research."

In Atlantis, they focused on and achieved a high degree of technological advancement, far beyond what we have achieved today. Presently, people who want to protect the environment and live what could be called a more natural life style, have this belief system often to an important degree from having spent many lives in Lemuria. In contrast, people interested in the continued development of more advanced technologies from space travel to atomic energy, often do so partly from the influence of past Atlantean lives. The stresses of life in Atlantis led to new physical, emotional, and mental diseases. The average life span in early Atlantis approximately 150,000 years ago was 800 years, but by the collapse of Atlantis about 12,000 B.C., the average life span had fallen to around 200 years.

In early Atlantis, natural or holistic healing was the predominant system of medical practice. Gradually, new and then radical healing techniques like what we now call allopathic or orthodox medicine developed. Many in the holistic schools were against these materialistic teachings, so certain members of this new system were persecuted by the authorities. It is an interesting karmic pattern that certain individuals from that early period of Atlantis have again reincarnated as natural healers and this time they have trouble with the established orthodox medical profession and the law. These people attacked others for their teachings, so now they in turn have similar problems for merely following their own beliefs.

"When the fall from spirit took place, there became ingested into the system of society unique beings known as elves, devas, and various beings of light who have come to be known mythologically as fairies. Working as a collective conscious-ness, they in many ways manifested the original angelic order or commandment to be in the Divine creating and inspiring new life forms, yet not to fall into the physical and attempt to manipulate. Their influence progressed from the minerals, to the plants, to even, for a time, being considered demigods in certain nature cul-tures as reflected in the Greek mythos. The Lemurians and nature spirits coexisted, and many times the Lemurians became these nature forces.

"When Lemuria was destroyed many inhabitants of that civilization rejected the described three paths of Atlantis and chose to remain to complete systems of study in the spirit. They desired to continue manifesting that which was known as the ethereal or aural bodies that were developed for travels in the earth plane along the lines of astral projection.[20]

"These are souls or human forms or human personalities that have become pro-gressive with their elements to the level of luminosity and partake and blend to-tally with the environment and nature. Nature spirits are as appealed to by various religious, philosophical, and spiritual societies. Do not worship these souls, but communicate with them as they are thy brothers and sisters. Dialogue with such beings should not be so much for appeal only to their nature of that which may be as given but also that which you may receive from learning the lessons they have learned by living totally in harmony with nature upon the levels of the etheric, still as incarnate and encased with the human form. These beings have now become unique principals in the application of flower essences.

"Even as ye have thy specific level of three dimensional existence, so in turn is their reality based upon the vibrations emitted constantly on the molecular level of various essences and the flowers they tend to. Even as ye could not survive in time without thy agriculture to feed the body physical, so in turn can they not maintain their level of existence without the essence of certain plant structures. As ye study horticulture and agriculture to survive as a community, so in turn do they study the patterns and intelligent energies of plant life for their own learning.

"You would tend well to these intelligences as ye shall encounter, for they are sympathetic with thee and ye in turn with them for ye are all souls. Even as ye have different races in thy own humanoid forms, so in turn they are but souls dwelling in another dimensional state, not unlike thy own, but slightly different in vibration. It could even be said that ye enter into a period of negotiations with these individuals to tend after their industries, which are healing and are designed to create a proper manifestation of balance in the entire environment. Their concerns with the pollutions of the environment are great; thus, you will find that people studying the biochemical states shall eventually turn to those who are continu-ously maintaining the environment, perhaps for the greatest source of healing. These are the things that you are beginning to study; these are things that you must begin to undertake."

Q Why do devas need the essences of certain plants to maintain their level of exis-tence?

"As ye draw in oxygen from thy atmosphere, so in turn the devas in their exis-tence are electromagnetic beings in same. Even as ye draw nutritional elements from the energy of the sun for thy physical bodies, so in turn the nutritional ele-ments relevant in the perspective of the devic beings concern the aspects of their needs from the essences. The actual essence, of course, is the electromagnetic pattern of the plant form. Even as there are nutritional elements found in various plant forms that ye partake of for the physical body, so in turn are there various patterns of biomagnetic energies discharged by flowers and various plant forms. And the vitality of the life force increases about the area of the bloom. The biomagnetic properties of plants aid in maintaining the electromagnetic form of the devas."

There is a long tradition in western occult lore and mythology concerning the existence of nature spirits.[21] A classic in this field is the book by Arthur Conan Doyle, *The Coming of the Fairies*, with its interesting photos of these nature spirits.[22] The recent popularity of the Findhorn community in Scotland, which has provided detailed accounts of working with nature spirits to produce amazingly productive gardens and vegetables, shows the continuing interest in this field.[23]

Ages ago in the original fall from spirit and during Lemuria many evolved souls made a conscious choice not to incarnate upon this plane. The number of those nature spirits dramatically increased with the physical destruction of Lemuria. Many souls who had lived physical lives in Lemuria had not yet evolved to a point in which they could permanently return to the higher planes. They settled into the devic realm, which is an ethereal dimension faster than the speed of light. To continue residing in this dimension and to maintain their ethereal bodies, it was necessary for them to assimilate vibrational energies emitted by various plants and trees and their flowers. Specific nature spirit orders, which formed only after the destruction of Lemuria, attached themselves to various plants and trees.

In early Atlantis, the existence of these nature spirits was rediscovered by the priesthood. Entire fields were organized with various gems placed in specific locations to enhance through meditation and telepathy a better communication with the leaders of the various devic orders. In those days alliances were formed with the devic orders to sustain the environment. In the coming years, this sort of telepathic communication and cooperation, which is already taking place in communities such as Findhorn in Scotland, will become more common. As John has pointed out, such communication is not worship or any form of magic; it is communication with souls similar to ourselves who happen to exist in a dimensional state slightly more vibrational than ours. As we shall see in chapter V, nature spirits play a role in the process of assimilating the energy from flower essences into our system.

Today, a fair number of people have what is called a 'green thumb'. These are people who have a keen aptitude and affinity for nature and gardening. Most of these people have this innate ability, to an important degree, because they are now working on inspirational levels with souls they were close to in Lemuria. These old Lemurian souls, in turn, as members of the various devic kingdoms, seek again to work with these individuals. Indeed, many of these gardeners will tell you about the various fairies and devas in nature, but, of course, this acknowledgement will depend on how open they sense you are to this topic.

"As you begin to work with the specialized system of knowledge, as would be applicable to thy own peculiar system of culture in western systems of thought, you will find that there has been a gradual evolution of these properties and it is wise that ye know their foundations and their executions, in that they are a spiritual body of knowledge, as well as a specifically applied body of knowledge for healing. You would find that the content of the individual attitude of he who would desire to work within the said structure, must be cleansed and have the proper aspect of projection of attitude upon the level of mind, body, and spirit. For herein you would find that you work strongly with the vibrational principle, and in this way and in this system of thought the individual must be cleansed to be able to properly apply the flower essences. The foundation of the systems of mechanisms that make up the ability of the flower essences to heal the invididuals' bodies is that there is a sympathetic attunement between the body physical of humanity and individual flower essences."

Q You refer to the western culture in using flower essences. Does this mean that other flower essences and principles will be described later for people from non-western countries?

"No, all can equally use and apply these remedies. It is only that the bulk of information is going to extend through western academic systems of thought in its clinical approach.

"Flower essences have in these days a unique educational principle that the more individuals as men and women become reeducated to the subtleties of their existence and to the subtleties of their consciousness, then the impact the flower essences can have upon healing is increased. The original structure in using flower essences was based upon lackings in the psychological make up of the individual. Through positive reinforcement of the psycho-spiritual dynamics of the individual, they in turn serve the greater whole in penetrating their healing to the level of physical properties. Flower essences have impact upon the physiology and physical healing in general, independent of the psychological structure of the individual. To use them it is wise to enhance them with creative visualization and various cleansing techniques perhaps amplified through various crystals and other forms of healing. These have as tendencies to amplify and magnify the properties of each flower essence.

"The purpose of flower essences are upon several levels. Many individuals receive them as though they are a medicine that would work, and indeed they do work, independently of any evolved state of consciousness. But also they are tinctures of liquid consciousness and stored within them is an evolutionary force, indeed the life force itself, shaped to a particular pattern. As there is the partaking of the essences, they become an evolutionary force in the consciousness of the individual, affecting not only the individual's free will, but becoming a progressive element that may stimulate inspiration and eventual change. They are not the causal force, but they are the inspiration that may inspire the causal force, the free will of the individual, to cause further development of his own consciousness.

"These then are the actual sources of physiological and anatomical change. These even slight inspirations can as cause radical changes within the physical substance of the individual. Flower essences can be organized into various sciences and can be applied to portions of the anatomy causing physical change and inspiration. Above all they are as a liquid tincture of consciousness that can be considered educational for the psycho-spiritual dynamics of the individual. For even in thy psychologies, it is necessary to educate the individual to the sources of neurotic and hypersensitive behavioral patterns found perhaps in the sexualities as explored in orthodox psychologies. Thus, in turn, are flower essences, when applied correctly, an educational process to rediscover the sources and principles of thy own true behavioral patterns, which are as spirits and as beings of light. As thy sciences organize into various levels as though the personality is biological, so in turn upon levels of holistic principles, flower essences are a system of organized vibrational tinctures that may accomplish similar principles but on the level of spiritual healing. In this system of thought, healing comes from levels within the self and is activated upon the levels of the soul and then is reflected into the body physical. For what you are doing is activating ancient doorways to levels of consciousness that were held within the structures of the Garden of Eden from the Lemurian days and their science of mind, body, and spirit."

1 Rudolf Steiner, *Cosmic Memory: Atlantis and Lemuria* (New York: Harper & Row, 1981).

2 James Churchward, *The Children of Mu, The Cosmic Forces of Mu, The Lost Continent of Mu, The Sacred Symbols of Mu, The Second Book of the Cosmic Forces of Mu.* Most are currently out of print.

3 Hugh Lynn Cayce ed., *Edgar Cayce on Atlantis* (New York: Warner Books, 1968).

4 Rudolf Steiner, *Cosmic Memory: Atlantis and Lemuria* (New York: Harper & Row, 1981).

5 Mary Ann Woodward ed., *Edgar Cayce's Story of Karma* (New York: Berkley Books, 1972).
Rudolf Steiner, *Karmic Relationships*, Vol. I (Spring Valley, NY: Anthroposophical Press, 1981).
Reincarnation and Immortality (Blauvelt, NY: Multimedia, 1970).

6 David Maclagan, *Creation Myths* (New York: Thames & Hudson, 1977).
Raymond Van Over ed., *Sun Songs: Creation Myths From Around the World* (Bergenfield, NJ: New American Library, 1980).

7 R. H. Charles ed., *The Book of the Secrets of Enoch* (Mokelumne Hill, CA: Health Research, 1964).
Richard Laurence trans., *The Book of Enoch the Prophet* (San Diego: Wizards Bookshelf, 1972).

8 James Robinson ed., *The Nag Hammadi Library* (New York, Harper & Row, 1977).

9 Arthur E. Waite ed., *The Hermetical and Alchemical Writings of Paracelsus*, Vol. II (Boulder, CO: Shambhala Publications, 1976), p. 304-305.

10 Helena Blavatsky, *The Secret Doctrine*, Vol. 2 (Wheaton, IL: The Theosophical Publishing House, 1980), p. 197.

11 Rudolf Steiner, *Cosmic Memory: Atlantis and Lemuria* (New York: Harper & Row, 1981), p. 87-99.

12 W. Scott-Elliot, *The Story of Atlantis and the Lost Lemuria* (London: The Theosophical Publishing House, 1968), p. 89-92.

13 Alice A. Bailey, *A Compilation on Sex* (New York: Lucis Publishing Co., 1980), p. 16, 65, 140, 147.

14 Titus Burkardt, *Alchemy* (Baltimore: Penguin Books, 1971).
F. S. Taylor, *The Alchemists* (Frogmore, St. Albans, England: Paladin, 1976).

15 June Singer, *Androgyny: Toward A New Theory of Sexuality* (New York: Doubleday & Co., 1976).

16 This monthly publication is a bibliographic listing of references to articles from 2,600 of the world's biomedical journals.

17 The Lemurian science of luminosity is an extensive subject with many advanced technologies for healing and conscious growth.
18 Oscar Bagnall, *The Origin and Properties of the Human Aura* (Secaucus, NJ: University Books, 1970).
Daniel Rubin and Stanley Krippner ed., *The Kirlian Aura* (New York: Doubleday & Co., 1974).
Walter J. Kilner, *The Human Aura* (York Beach, ME: Samuel Weiser, Inc., 1975).
19 The hall of records referred to here is the same one that Edgar Cayce often mentioned in his channelings. In other readings, John has made some interesting comments on this. Originally, before Atlantis collapsed into the Atlantic Ocean from moral decay approximately 12,000 B.C., many in the priesthood understood that there would soon be this massive destruction with the ancient teachings of Atlantis being lost for many ages. About 144,000 individuals gradually migrated to Egypt to preserve many of these teachings by building the pyramids at Gizeh as well as to build a hall of records. Time capsules are, on occasion, established today so it should not be surprising that a technologically advanced civilization would do the same thing thousands of years ago.

This ancient soul group of 144,000 people later reincarnated in Israel several thousand years ago as members of the Essene community. Jesus, as a member of this soul group, assisted in the building of these pyramids and the hall of records. In that incarnation he was known as Hermes Trismegistus who is today considered to be the founder of alchemy. According to alchemical history, Hermes Trismegistus is supposed to have lived in Egypt in some distant past.

John elsewhere reports that recently some members of the Egyptian government and the society that Edgar Cayce established have found the entrance to this hall. Some of them suspect that this may be the hall of records that Cayce spoke of, and it is now only a matter of time before the hall is entered.
20 Robert Monroe, *Journeys Out of the Body* (New York: Anchor Books, 1977).
21 Alice A. Bailey, *Letters on Occult Meditation* (New York: Lucis Publishing Co., 1973).
A Treatise on Cosmic Fire (New York: Lucis Publishing Co., 1977).
22 Sir Arthur Conan Doyle, *The Coming of the Fairies* (York Beach, ME: Samuel Weiser, Inc., 1972).
23 Findhorn Community, *The Findhorn Garden* (New York: Harper & Row, 1972).
Paul Hawken, *The Magic of Findhorn* (New York: Bantam Books, 1974).

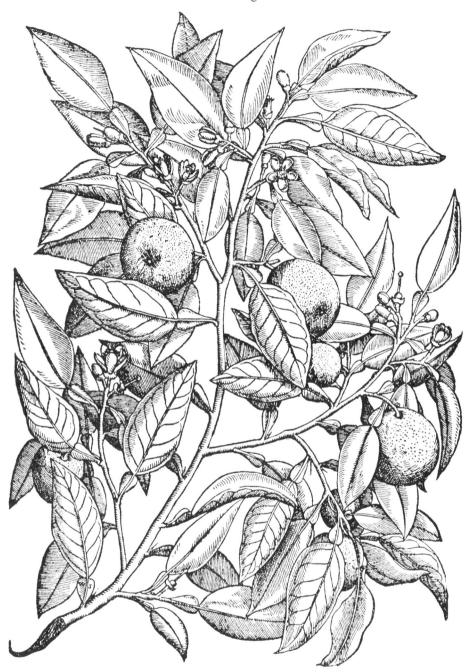

Orange

Chapter II

Dr. Bach and the Bach Flowers

Bach is one of many people who has worked with flower essences over the ages. With his genius and deep dedication to humanity he reintroduced the ancient system of using flower essences in healing and conscious growth. His work with flower essences was done from 1928 to 1936.

Bach was born in England in 1886 near Birmingham. Even as a youth he was guided by great powers of concentration, intuition, and sensitivity to the needs of those around him. He had a deep love of nature, and he often wandered about the English countryside. During his years in London as a physician, he rarely spent time in the countryside or in the London parks because he felt it would be difficult to readjust to the conditions of city life. Bach felt he might get distracted from his medical research.[1]

From 1914 until the end of 1918 Bach practiced orthodox medicine. Then, from 1919 until he left London in 1930 he was a homeopathic practitioner. His increased understanding of health and disease inspired him to convert to homeopathy. During these years he did much original research in these two different fields of medicine. He gave lectures and wrote articles in medical journals on his research,[2] so many orthodox and then homeopathic doctors held him in the highest regard. As a pathologist and bacteriologist he developed vaccines from intestinal bacteria that helped many people suffering from chronic diseases. He also discovered that doses were more beneficial if only repeated when the improvements resulting from a previously given dose had ceased. As a homeopath he expanded this work to develop what are still known as the Bach nosodes.[3] Nosodes are homeopathic remedies prepared from toxins such as viruses. He isolated, homeopathically prepared, and used these same organisms from the intestinal tract with excellent clinical results. Many homeopaths still use the Bach nosodes. With these new homeopathic remedies he was also able to use oral vaccines instead of injections, which he so disliked.

In the fall of 1928, Bach visited Wales where he acquired two wild flowers, the impatiens and mimulus. He homeopathically prepared and clinically used each with excellent results. He soon understood that there was great healing power in flowers, and gradually, with his keen intuition, he developed the sun and boiling methods of preparing flower essences.

In 1930, Bach quit his busy homeopathic practice and research (he even burned his papers) to live in the English countryside to develop a new healing system. When Bach made up his mind, he was not one for half measures. Indeed, in recent years I have met two people who were acquainted with Bach, and both commented on his strong will and determination to conduct his research.

An interesting point here is that in channeled guidance, it has been noted that Bach was, in part, influenced by the spiritual researcher Rudolf Steiner. Steiner visited England several times in the early 1920's and during these visits gave lectures before several groups of physicians. At that time Steiner spoke briefly of the great healing value in flowers that would someday be discovered.

From 1930 to 1936, Bach lived in several parts of rural England, and he discovered thirty-five more flower essences. That, combined with the three he discovered before leaving London, brought the total number to thirty-eight. There is also the rescue remedy, which is a combination of five remedies from the thirty-eight individual essences.

In prescribing these flower essences, he gradually determined the principles involved in preparing and clinically using these natural remedies. He became so sensitized that upon tasting a flower or just holding it in his hand, he intuited clear impressions of its effect on people. In this research, Bach used his keen intuition and traditional scientific methodology.

In 1930, Bach wrote *Heal Thyself*,[4] a booklet all natural healers would do well to read. In this booklet, Bach discusses the reasons for the problems with modern medicine, the real cause and cure of disease, and the philosophy of true healing. Bach understood that the underlying moods or states of mind that different types of people experience are a key cause of most diseases. He was years ahead of his time in perceiving the relationship of stress to disease. Bach realized that in all true healing there is the materialization of spiritual forces from the higher realms and from one's higher self for a cleansing of mind, body, and emotions.

Bach wanted to develop a simple natural healing system that all could use. He did not want it limited to the medical profession. In 1932, he wrote a booklet, *The Twelve Healers and Other Remedies*,[5] in which he described the newly discovered flower essences. During these years of research and discovery, Bach reached such a state of consciousness that he became a channel for healing people just by putting his hands on them. He even did this by astral projecting to them some miles away. Patients later told him of these nighttime visits and how they then felt much better.[6]

In November, 1936, Bach quietly passed away in his sleep. Bach did not feel he had discovered all the flower essences that could be used in healing and conscious growth. If he had lived longer, gradually new flower essences would have been presented.

Q Can you explain exactly how Bach deciphered how to use the different flower essences?

"Empirically, frankly. The man was a scientist and a classically driven genius. He was a man after simplicity, but he was still a scientist. Thus it was his motivation and inspiration in this work. He preserved enough of his scientific training to treat it empirically using observation and insight, and to document it scientifically. Bach established the clinical criteria that are currently being used in flower essence research. The fact that he prescribed the essences clinically is one of his main contributions to the historical perspective of flower essences."

In many ways, the Bach flowers symbolize how the system of healing with flower essences will develop now and in the future. There are interesting similarities between the Bach flowers and many of the new flower essences now being introduced. The Bach flowers consist of shrubs such as gorse and cerato, and certain wild flowers such as mimulus and impatiens. Many of the new flower essences come from these same categories.

Almost half the Bach flowers come from trees. This trend will continue as the flowers from trees are often especially valuable. With the Bach flowers we have cherry plum, crab apple, olive, walnut, and several types of chestnut. As will be seen in this and future books most of the fruit and nut tree flowers are particularly important.

The Bach system, moreover, includes the wild rose, rosa canina. Roses are a separate and complete system of healing and conscious growth in themselves, and will become extremely important in the future. The use of the Bach flower, crab apple, in baths further exemplifies how many flower essences can be utilized.

It is not essential that plants grow in their native habitat or even in the same climatic conditions to be used as an essence. This is illustrated by the use of cerato and scleranthus in the Bach system. Cerato is native to the mountains of Tibet and West China, while scleranthus originated in Australia. Cerato was a commonly cultivated garden flower in England and the United States from the 1930's to the 1950's. Bach made it into an essence in someone's garden.[7] This, in addition, symbolizes that flower essences can be made from cultivated plants. It is not essential that the plants grow in the wild; however, organic growing methods are necessary.

It is certainly wise to gradually determine the exact species to use in the different botanical groupings, as Bach did. And on occasion, as with the chestnut, there are some new essences in which several related species or varieties of the same plant have special value.

Bach was quite astute in making the bud of horse chestnut into a flower essence. The buds of all flower essences are especially valuable for the unborn during pregnancy and the newborn in the early months of life. There is certainly much room for research here. Finally, with the rescue remedy we see the first of many combination remedies with different flower essences fused together for specific imbalances.

Q Why is there very little literature on how the thirty-eight Bach flowers influence the physical body and spiritual nature in people?

"This is because there has not been much publication of case studies. Many flower essences do work primarily on the physical body or on more ethereal levels. It so happens that the Bach flowers tend to focus more on the mental and emotional states, although in time research will indeed prove that some of them are effective in various physical and spiritual activities. Of course, by implication in the Bach flower literature, and when people actually take such remedies and experience mental and emotional purification, there is often physical and spiritual enhancement."

In my years of treating people with the Bach flowers, I have certainly seen people undergo very positive physical and spiritual purification. Indeed, while many of the sixteen points discussed with each new flower essence in this text have never been considered with the Bach flowers, they will be as more research takes place.

The Bach flowers have been used by thousands of people for over fifty years. This natural healing system as currently practiced is one of the more evolved systems of healing using nothing but energy in a preserved form to heal the individual. Surely, with thousands of flowering plants and trees, most would agree that many other flowers can be used in this type of healing. It is only a matter of time before many new flower essences are accepted and widely used.

1 Nora Weeks, *The Medical Discoveries of Edward Bach: Physician* (Saffron Walden, England: The C. W. Daniel Co. Ltd., 1976).
2 Edward Bach, M.D., "The Relation of Vaccine Therapy to Homeopathy," *British Homeopathy Journal*, X (April, 1920), 67-81.
_____. "A Clinical Comparison Between the Actions of Vaccines and Homeopathic Remedies," *British Homeopathic Journal*, XI (January, 1921), 21-44.
3 John Patterson, M.D., "The Role of the Bowel Flora in Chronic Disease," *British Homeopathic Journal*, XXXIX (January, 1949), 3-26.
A. C. Gordon Ross, M.D., "The Bowel Nosodes," *British Homeopathic Journal*, LXII (January, 1973), 42-44.
4 Edward Bach, M.D., *Heal Thyself* (Saffron Walden, England: The C. W. Daniel Co. Ltd., 1976).
5 Edward Bach, M.D., *The Twelve Healers and Other Remedies* (Saffron Walden, England: The C. W. Daniel Co. Ltd., 1975).
6 Nora Weeks, *The Medical Discoveries of Edward Bach: Physician* (Saffron Walden, England: The C. W. Daniel Co. Ltd., 1976), p. 43, 107.
7 Ibid., p. 68.

Chapter III

Preparing Flower Essences

The preparation of flower essences requires several items. First, a clear bowl, preferably made of glass or quartz, is needed. Quartz is best, but it is more expensive. The bowl should hold around twelve ounces of water, but the amount can vary according to individual preferences. The bowl should be plain with no designs on it; otherwise, a pattern could vibrationally influence a flower essence. Also needed are storage bottles, funnels, and labels to put on the bottles. It is best that the bottles and funnels also be made of glass or quartz. These items should be new and cleaned when initially used. Sterilize these articles by placing them in hot water, preferably in an enamel or glass pot, for around ten minutes. If using a metal pot, it should be made of copper or stainless steel. Never use aluminum pots because they are highly toxic.[1] If using a pendulum, it is easy to tell exactly when these articles have been cleansed.[2]

The final item needed to prepare flower essences is wax bags. They preserve dried flowers to later prepare recipes or homeopathic remedies. Wax bags are the best item to use because they are strictly organic. If you do store the flowers this way, it is essential to first carefully dry them in the sun or by a heater, otherwise they will develop molds within a few days.

Q Should distilled water or local spring water be used to prepare flower essences?

"Use local spring water if you can locate a pure spring that flows continuously and that is unblemished by pollutants. Because there are so many pollutants in your society, it is difficult to find such a spring. Distilled water is usually the purest water to obtain; thus, it is generally the best for most people to use.

"It is also helpful to wear boji stone and star sapphire when preparing flower essences. Boji stone attunes one to nature, and star sapphire opens the higher spiritual properties."

Q What is the minimum amount of brandy that must be in a mother essence bottle to protect the flower essence? (The mother essence bottle is the original bottle that the flower essence goes into.)

"Except for a few flower essences with an intense life force, 25% is usually sufficient."

Q Are certain brandies better than others?

"Yes, the more processed the less effective."

Many involved in this work feel that Korbel brandy, produced in Guerneville, California, is the purest brandy available. There are probably several other brandies with a similar organic content. While there has been a tradition of filling half the essence bottle with brandy, this usually is not essential for brandy to fulfill its purpose of preserving and protecting the flower essence. However, there are some flower essences in which the life force is so intense that it is important to fill half the essence bottle with brandy. Otherwise, it is possible that viruses and bacteria could gradually form in the bottle. This could happen with lotus, papaya, mango, all roses, and others that predominantly affect the crown chakra. This problem will not automatically occur, but it is best to be safe. It is already understood that leaving the Bach flowers under the sun too long can sometimes cause this problem to develop.

It is best to prepare flower essences on a cloudless day, early in the morning, preferably in the spring or summer when the sun is strongest. If you start preparing the essence later than early in the morning or if there are some clouds in the sky, the essence can still be made, but the flowers should be on the water longer than three hours if that is possible. Usually the flowers should be on the water for three hours.

As long as the essence goes under a copper pyramid for at least two hours, the quality of the essence is maintained. If the sun is unusually intense do not leave the flowers on the water for more than three hours. When the temperature gets into the high 80's, the water starts to evaporate.

Try choosing an area where the flowers are growing abundantly, so you can pick flowers from different parts of the plant or plants. The flowers can be growing wild, but they can also be cultivated if grown under organic conditions.

Always start the process by entering a quiet meditative state. Sit quietly by the plant to tune into its vibrations and that of the nature spirits associated with this plant.

Q I do not have verbal or telepathic communication with the nature spirits. Does this affect my ability to prepare flower essences? And can you explain how to develop a more coherent communication with these forces?

"First, these forces do not automatically flee from the essence, even though you have not established a full dialogue with them. With continuous abuse, disrespect, and perhaps a lack of communication, however, they would as begin to flee, and there would be the dropping in the individual's ability to prepare flower essences. Be conscious of the existence of the fields of energy and life about flower essences, for the structure of flower essences is a pattern through which the life force flows to produce healing. Thy communication in a dialogue needs to be sensitive to the fields of light and life about these essences, for herein is the dimensional state upon which the devic forces exist. As you work with plant structures placing flowers on the water, be in communication with these intelligences as though they were present with thee even though you may not see them with the physical eye. Eventually you will evolve, with the ability of the physical eyes, to see those energies or nature spirits. This increases your communication with them as forms of intelligence and acknowledges their existence. This comes as direct conversation or dialogue upon telepathic levels. But remember, never pray to devas, pray only to God. Communicate with them as co-workers, explaining what ye do, asking their permission in same."

Explain to the nature spirits exactly what you are doing, so they will understand and help in the process of transferring the life force of the flower into the water. In picking flowers you are literally stepping into someone's territory. If you want to walk across someone's private property, it is courteous to first ask permission. There are some occasions when for some reason it is not wise to pick flowers from a given plant, and you may be telepathically warned by the devas. I once did receive such a warning when the plant looked quite healthy. I later learned that a plant virus was in that plant.

It is important to realize that the devas are not dancing around in the water during this process. As carefully discussed in chapter V, flower essences function in a vibrational frequency similar to the level upon which the devas exist. It is essential to understand that preparing flower essences is not just a mechanical process. The individual's consciousness is vitally important in this technique.

Q Can flower essences be contaminated by thoughts from the individual preparing them?

"Yes, to a degree. But if the essence was put under a copper pyramid with quartz crystals around it, most of these issues would be solved."

Q In traditional alchemy, the main factor is not picking the plant, but gathering the plant's essence. Usually when you pick a plant its essence returns to the earth. How true is this, and can you suggest a way to control this when picking flowers to prepare essences?

"This in many ways depends on the collector's consciousness. The essence returning to the earth is as the principle of fertilization. It has traditionally been believed that after plants were picked the critical element or essence immediately returned to earth. The trauma of the picking in its own right, as you would term it, shocks the plant, disturbing its harmony with the universe. Removing flowers from the plant with a silver instrument or piece of quartz stabilizes the life force of the flowers. If the flowers are immediately placed on the conducting fluids or water, this facilitates balancing and receiving the life force, for the essence does not immediately return to the ground."

Q Is it true that the stage of a flower's development influences when to pick flowers to prepare an essence?

"Preferably prepare an essence in the maturity of the bloom. There are slightly different effects if the flower is still maturing or if it is reaching the end of its cycle, but both carry the basic properties. Preparing it just before full maturity generates slightly heightened properties."

When you feel properly attuned to a plant's vibration note the time and carefully pick the flowers and put them on top of the water in the bowl. One technique is to cut and handle the flowers with a leaf taken from that same plant to avoid touching the flowers or water. You can also use a quartz crystal or silver to sever the flowers. These techniques ease the plant's shock.

It is best to cover the full surface of the water with flowers; however, it is not essential to do this if there are not enough flowers. Again, once the prepared flower essence is put under the copper pyramid for two hours it is enhanced to full quality. If there are not enough flowers to cover the water surface, you could use a rock or dirt to tilt the bowl, so there would be less water surface to cover with flowers. If you have many flowers available, including several plants to choose from, pick the healthiest looking flowers on different parts of the plant to place on the water.

Try to place the bowl with the flowers close to the plant where the flowers came from. This may not be possible because occasionally a shadow blocks the sun. At times it may be wise to place the bowl on an elevated surface because of stray animals. In such instances place the bowl only on a natural surface such as wood and not on metals or cement. Usually this entire process requires just a few minutes to place the flowers on the water and a few minutes three hours later to bottle the liquid and store the flowers.

Before pouring the water from the bowl into the storage bottles, first from a slight distance, fill up to half of each bottle with brandy, which is a natural preservative. By doing this first, the vibration of the flower essence will not permeate the brandy bottle where it could enter other storage bottles being prepared then or in the future. Next, carefully remove the flowers from the water, perhaps using a leaf from the same plant so as to not touch the water. It is wise to use the leaf to remove insects that may have gotten into the water. When done, the water looks crystal clear and is often full of small, sparkling bubbles. Then pour the water into the bottles using a funnel. If you are preparing several flower essences together, be sure to briefly put your hands under water each time that you put the flowers on the water and later when you bottle the essence in the stock bottles, otherwise the vibrations from the different essences will intermingle. Remember to label the storage bottles. If you are making several flower essences together, label the bottles and perhaps the bowls used in the process to avoid any confusion.

Q Can you discuss the feasibility of making flower essences at night for night-blooming flowers?

"Night blooming flowers can be prepared as flower essences in the evening or under the sun. When such an essence is prepared under the sun, it tends to represent the properties of the conscious mind. If prepared under the moon, it tends to represent the properties of the subconscious mind. The yang or male properties are emphasized when it is made under the sun, while the yin or female attributes of the essence are underscored when it is made under the moon. Three to four hours under the moon are sufficient, and slightly enhanced properties are obtained when such essences are prepared under a full moon."

Q To reuse a bowl when making a flower essence, I boil it in water and then dry it. Are there superior ways of removing the vibrations of the essence from a used bowl?

"The quickest way is a very efficient way. Take some crushed quartz crystals and put them in very clean linen that has no synthetics in it. Then briefly dip the quartz and bowl in pure distilled water or pure spring water and dry the bowl. To cleanse the quartz just dip it in distilled water again. You can clean many of your tools with this technique."

Q When preparing different flower essences on the same day, can several bowls be boiled together for around ten minutes so they are all sufficiently cleansed, or is it better to boil each one separately?

"Several bowls can be boiled together for cleansing purposes. The water removes the flower essence vibration from each bowl. It is important that new water be poured into the pot each time new bowls or funnels are cleansed. And magnets can be placed around the pot for a few seconds each time new bowls are boiled. Before initially cleansing bowls or funnels in this manner, boil just the pot for ten minutes to cleanse it. Then remove that water and pour in fresh water with the bowls or funnels. If someone prepares many flower essences, it is best that one pot be set aside for just this purpose."

Q Are the bottles, bowls, and funnels that come from manufacturers ready to be used, or do they need to be initially cleansed.

"Placing them under a copper pyramid for thirty minutes to two hours would be wise with any new supplies. These items should not touch each other while under the pyramid."

Q What if someone uses a plastic funnel, instead of a glass funnel, to pour the essence liquid into storage bottles?

"While it is best to not use petrochemicals with vibrational remedies such as flower essences, this is not a rigid rule. Putting the bottles under a copper pyramid for two hours negates the plastic's influence."

Quartz crystals and copper pyramids involve important new technologies in cleansing and enhancing flower essences. These principles are discussed in chapter IX.

Q Is the boiling method of preparing flower essences just an alternative technique to use in bad weather, or does it have some special value with specific plants?

"While it is an alternative method to use when there is not enough sun, it also has special value with some essences. It especially activates the properties of essences that primarily influence the physical body. The sun method is usually best, however, because it releases more life force from the sun. This is important because flower essences are vibrational energy patterns that usually affect the psyche and soul forces."

The boiling method requires the same items needed to prepare flower essences by the sun method, but filter paper or non-synthetic linen such as a handkerchief made of cotton are also required. Try picking the flowers early in the morning, especially if there is some sun. Take the boiling pot with you, with the lid covering it to keep out any dust or dirt. As described in the sun method of preparation, first sit by the plant for a few minutes to attune to its vibration, and then carefully pick the flowers.

Q Traditionally it has been stated that in the boiling method one should add twigs and leaves from the same plant to the boiling pot. Just how valuable is this technique?

"This is only a slight enhancement. It is better to add seeds from the same plant in the sun or boiling methods. There is more life force in the seeds and they contain the entire genetic pattern of the twigs and leaves."

Partially put the liquid essence into the pot which should have some pure water in it, to ease the shock when the flowers are picked. Put the lid back on the pot and quickly return to where you can boil the contents. Fill the pot with more pure water and then boil it at medium temperature for half an hour with the lid off the top. During the boiling, you can stir the water with a twig from the same plant, but this procedure is not crucial to the process.

After half an hour, put the pot outside for another half hour to allow the pot to cool. Then with a twig or leaf from the same plant remove the pot's contents and let the water sit awhile to allow the sediment to settle to the bottom of the pot. Then carefully pour the water into a jar or bottle with non-synthetic filter paper or linen on top. You may have to repeat this process several times to separate the water from the sediment. When done, you may want to leave the liquid in the sun for a while, if there is any, to further energize the essence. Finally, label the storage bottles and fill up to half their volume with brandy and then fill them with the essence liquid.

Q Is there any difference in the quality of an essence if it is prepared outside its native habitat?

"Such an essence would be only slightly weakened. If placed under a copper pyramid for awhile, it would be fully energized."

Q Would an essence be weakened if it was prepared from a fruit or nut tree that did not produce any fruit or nuts because it was grown in a cold climate outside its native habitat?

"This would have almost no impact, and again, using the pyramid procedures solves this question."

Q Can flower essences be prepared from a plant growing in an urban environment without danger from pollutants, provided people follow the purification procedures you have outlined?

"Yes, it is merely a matter of putting essences through proper purification procedures. If there is a choice, it is usually best to prepare flower essences in a rural environment, but today, even in rural areas, there will usually be pesticides or radiation in the air. The purification techniques we have given are quite important, and it is wise to always use them when preparing flower essences."

Q Is there any difference in clinical effects from making a flower essence of a grafted dwarf variety in contrast to the original or natural species plant or tree? Many fruit and nut trees have been hybridized.

"The life force increases with dwarf trees if they are several generations removed from the original mutation or grafting. They then would be natural again and the initial shock from the graft would have passed. Many roses important to this work have been hybridized in the last ten to several hundred years."

It is also important to understand that fully opened flowers should not be mixed with buds when making flower essences. Buds work more on the fetus and the newborn, and they are aligned with certain advanced principles of tissue regeneration and genetic engineering. Bud essences are a unique system within this healing work.

While discussing the apricot flower essence, an interesting point developed. Flowers facing the east side of the tree toward the rising sun are the most potent, while flowers facing the west side opposite the rising sun are the least potent. Flowers obtained from the top of the tree treat emotional imbalances that the specific tree or bush alleviates, and flowers taken from the bottom of the tree or bush stabilizes the person. To be rigorous in this work, these principles can be applied to many trees and bushes, not just the apricot essence, but it is not crucial to do this with all essences.

Q With the sun method of preparation what, if any, physical properties from the flower are transferred in a diluted form into the water? Is it merely an etheric imprint or are some oils transferred in this process?

"It is merely an etheric imprint; nothing physical gets transferred. It is nothing that can be seen under a regular microscope. If you took a Kirlian photograph,[3] or possibly just an infrared picture immediately after removing the flower from the bowl, you would see a ghost-like imprint of the flower with small trailings of light connected to the water. In this work, you are working strictly with the ethereal vibration of the plant, the intelligence of it. The sun upon striking the water melds into the water the life force of the flower, and this is transferred to people when they assimilate these vibrational essences."

Stock bottles are prepared from the above described mother essence. They usually contain several drops from the mother essence, brandy, which is a natural preservative, and some pure water. It is wise to add seven drops whether the size of the stock bottle is several drams or several ounces because flower essences work partly from the influence of the seven dimensions. If less than seven drops are added to the stock bottle, it still works, as has been done in the past, but this amount enhances flower essences' clinical effectiveness.

Preparing flower essences into homeopathic potencies has been done by increasing numbers of people in recent years. The procedures for doing this are about the same as in traditional homeopathy.[4]

The mother tincture in homeopathy is roughly equivalent to the mother essence in flower essences. They are different partly because the homeopathic mother tincture contains elements of the original physical element, while the flower essence does not. Each represents the first state of the dilution and potentization of the original physical substance. As in homeopathy, the vehicles used in potentizing a flower essence can be a form of sugar such as sac lac tablets or pure alcohol. A vehicle is an inert substance having no therapeutic value. It is used in the preparation of mother tinctures and homeopathic remedies. In homeopathy, dispensing alcohol is used, and while it is also a good vehicle to use with flower essences, it may be difficult to obtain if one is not a physician or pharmacist. Vodka or brandy can be used.

Homeopathic remedies are prepared by two main processes of dilution and potentization. In the decimal scale, take nine drops of alcohol to one drop of the mother tincture and mix them together to get 1x. Repeat this process with nine drops of alcohol to one drop from the 1x to get 2x. This same procedure is repeated in the centesimal scale except here take ninety-nine drops of alcohol to one drop from the mother tincture and mix them to get 1c. Again take ninety-nine drops of alcohol and one drop from 1c to get 2c. This procedure is the same with sac lac tablets except that, instead of using alcohol, use one, nine, or ninety-nine sac lac tablets.

With either of these two processes the dilution can continue with flower essences, as it does with homeopathic remedies, to 100,000 dilutions and even more. With each level of dilution, you must succuss or shake the resulting mixture. In homeopathy, there is disagreement as to how many times to shake the preparation, but most agree that a succussion of fifteen to twenty times per dilution is sufficient. This shaking with each stage of dilution releases the pure energy stored in the atoms of the original physical substance. Increased dilution and succussion increases the power or potency of the resulting remedy.

Some feel there should be an interval of one to seven days with each stage of dilution and succussion. The practitioner should wait at least one to two days between each level of dilution or potentization.

Preparing flower essences is a simple process that usually does not take too much time. The problem can be in locating certain plants and trees to prepare the essence. After preparing over 300 flower essences, I find that I always enjoy the process because it brings me closer to nature.

1 Dr. Le Hunte-Cooper, *The Danger of Food Contamination by Aluminum* (London: John Bale Sons and Danielson Ltd., 1932).
H. Tomlinson, *Aluminum Utensils and Disease* (London: L. N. Fowler & Co., 1967).
2 See chapter X for information on using the pendulum.
3 Oscar Bagnall, *The Origin and Properties of the Human Aura* (Secaucus, NJ: University Books, 1970).
Walter Kilner, *The Human Aura* (York Beach, ME: Samuel Weiser, Inc., 1975).
4 Dr. K. P. Muzumda, *Pharmaceutical Science in Homeopathy and Pharmacodynamics* (New Delhi: B. Jain Publishers, 1974).
Margery Blackie, M.D., *The Patient Not the Cure* (London: Macdonald and Janes, 1976), p. 213-225.
Wm. Boericke, M.D., *A Compend of the Principles of Homeopathy* (Mokelumne Hill, CA: Health Research, 1971), p. 99-108.

Chapter IV

Storage, Protection, and Cleansing of Flower Essences

Flower essences are vibrational remedies; consequently, they are quite sensitive to environmental pollutants. It is wise to take special precautions during their storage. Before storing the essences, first wash the area with distilled water using organic linen such as a cotton handkerchief. After cleaning the area, leave it empty for several days prior to use.

Keep a pyramid, quartz crystals, gold, silver, or copper in the storage area. Any of these can also be put in the storage space in the brief period before putting in the essence bottles. Depending on the number of bottles being stored, you could also put small pieces of quartz by the four corners of the storage area.

Do not usually leave flower essences in the kitchen where they can be negatively influenced by odors such as caffeine or camphor. Never leave them under the sun because extreme heat can damage flower essences. Essences exposed to extreme cold would not be damaged if they are carefully thawed under a pyramid for about two hours. After the water thaws, 62 degrees F. is the best storage temperature for flower essences. Never leave essences near toxic metals such as aluminum or lead.

"Blue is the best colored bottle to store flower essences in because it promotes healing. Blue is a neutral and stabilizing color."

Q Will background pollutants such as radiation or petrochemicals damage flower essences, especially when they are stored for long periods?

"If protected with pyramids, crystalline structures, and other forces described, these factors pose no dangers."

Q How often should people cleanse mother essence bottles, stock bottles, and homeopathically prepared flower essences?

"Stock bottles and homeopathically prepared flower essences should be purified once every thirty to ninety days. Wipe the bottles with sea salt using pure linen and distilled water. It is beneficial to put the bottles under a pyramid for thirty minutes to twenty-four hours, but just putting them by quartz crystals also enhances them.

"Mother essence bottles should be cleansed quarterly, although if stored properly, once a year would be sufficient. This, of course, depends on the needs and concerns of the practitioner. Each time mother essence or storage bottles are opened they should be wiped with sea salt using pure linen and put under a pyramid for two hours. This requirement is not necessary with stock bottles. Stored flower essences should not touch each other because the different essences gradually merge over ten to twenty years. Over several years, this process begins to take effect.

Thus, if stored flower essences are touching each other, put the bottles under a pyramid every two years for twenty-four hours and wipe the bottles with sea salt."

Q Should flower essences prepared into homeopathic potencies be cleansed more often than traditional homeopathic remedies?

"In part, as such, for total enhancement. This is because ye are dealing with levels of consciousness. Consequently, greater care should be given by the individual because the essences work more directly with the subtle anatomies, therefore more closely to the levels directly enhancing the personality. Surely the personality, which is the closest essence of the being to the spirit, requires greater meticulous care than even perhaps the body physical.

"Certain mother essence bottles stored for long periods should have 50% brandy in the bottle. The roses, lotus, papaya, mango, and other essences that affect the crown chakra and the higher spiritual center exemplify this pattern. This is because the life force is so strong in these essences that viruses or bacteria may form in the bottle. If these mother essences had only 25% brandy in them the problem would rarely occur but this is a good preventative measure. One drop of pure alcohol could be added to such bottles for increased protection."

While seeds or leaves can be added to the liquid when preparing flower essences, only the pure liquid should be in storage bottles; otherwise, the seeds or leaves make it easier for viruses or bacteria to form in them.

With all these suggestions what counts is the concern of each individual. To leave flower essences under the sun or by toxic substances invites trouble, but otherwise most of the above described procedures are not essential. These procedures are offered as aids, especially when flower essences are stored for long periods of time. Just being in a clear conscious state is usually sufficient.

Chapter V

How Flower Essences, Homeopathic Remedies, and Gems Work in People

Exactly how flower essences and other vibrational remedies work in people is a complex process that has never been fully explained. Dr. Roberts, a prominent homeopathic physician, even stated that it will never be possible to understand how homeopathic remedies assist the vital force to conquer disease.[1] While the complete process is not described in this text, much information is presented.

Q Would you describe how vibrational remedies work in people?

"When a flower essence, homeopathic remedy, or gem elixir is ingested or used as a salve they follow a similar specific path through the physical and subtle bodies. They initially are assimilated into the circulatory system.[2] Next, the remedy settles mid-way between the circulatory and nervous systems. An electromagnetic current is created here by the polarity of these two systems. There is an intimate connection between these two systems in relation to the life force and consciousness that modern science does not yet understand.[3] The life force works more through the blood, and consciousness works more through the brain and nervous system. These two systems contain quartz-like properties and an electromagnetic current. The blood cells, especially the red and white blood cells, contain more quartz-like properties, and the nervous system contains more an electromagnetic current. The life force and consciousness use these properties to enter and stimulate the physical body.

"From midway between the nervous and circulatory systems the remedy usually moves directly to the meridians. There is a direct link with the nervous, circulatory, and meridian systems partly because ages ago the meridians were originally used to create these two parts of the physical body. Consequently, anything that influences one of these systems has a direct impact on the other two areas. The meridians use the passageway between the nervous and circulatory systems to feed the life force into the body, almost extending directly to the molecular level. The meridians are the interface or doorway between the physical and ethereal properties of the body.

"From the meridians, the remedy's life force enters the various subtle bodies, the chakras, or returns directly to the physical body to the cellular level through several portals midway between the nervous and circulatory systems. Its path is determined by the type of remedy and the person's constitution.

"The three main portals for the remedy's life force to reenter the physical body are the etheric body and ethereal fluidium, the chakras, and the skin with its silica or crystalline properties.[4] The ethereal fluidium is the part of the etheric body, which surrounds the physical body, that brings the life force into the individual cells. Hair, with its crystalline properties, is a carrier of the life force; it is not a portal. Specific parts of the physical body are portals for the life force of a vibrational remedy only because they are associated with different chakras or meridians. The pineal gland, for instance, is directly associated with the crown chakra. The life force of a vibrational remedy usually gravitates toward one portal, but it may reenter the physical body through several portals. For example, vibrational remedies with crystalline properties gravitate toward the skin.

"When the life force leaves and reenters the physical body, it always passes through the etheric body. This body is not necessarily considered a portal, however, if it is not in some way especially affected by the process."

Q When a remedy's life force returns to the physical body, does it go directly to the injured area or must it first pass midway between the nervous and circulatory systems?

"After passing through one of the described portals the life force always passes midway between the nervous and circulatory systems. Then it enters the cellular level and imbalanced areas of the physical body.

"This entire process takes place instantaneously, but it usually takes awhile to experience the results. In a similar fashion, if you get punched in the face, it may take several days to feel swelling or soreness."

Q Would you expand on your comment that there are quartz-like properties in the body?

"There are various quartz-like crystalline structures in the physical and subtle bodies that augment the impact of vibrational remedies. In the physical body, these areas include: cell salts, fatty tissue, lymphs, red and white cells, thymus, and the pineal gland. These crystalline structures are a complete system in the body but are not yet properly isolated and understood by modern medicine. Quartz is increasingly being used in medicine. For instance, in the last few years, it has become common for liquid quartz to be used to fill cleansed cavities.

"Crystalline structures work on sympathetic resonancy. There is an attunement between crystalline properties in the physical and subtle bodies, the ethers, and many vibrational remedies, notably flower essences and gems. These properties in the body magnify the life force of vibrational remedies to a recognizable level to be assimilated. These crystalline properties are relay points for most ethereal energies to penetrate the physical body. This allows for a balanced distribution of various energies at correct frequencies, which stimulates the discharge of toxicity to create health. In a similar fashion, vibrations of radio-wave frequency strike a crystal in a radio. The crystal resonates with the high frequency in such a way as to absorb it, passing along the audio frequencies which are perceivable by the body.

"When vibrational remedies are amplified, their life force reaches the imbalanced parts of the body faster and in a more stable state. The remedies may cleanse the aura and subtle bodies so those imbalances will no longer contribute to ill health. If this sounds strange, remember scientists have many times proven that subtle energies such as ultrasonics and microwaves can cause sickness. Why cannot other subtle energies produce health?

"The internal working of the ethers, which are forces that travel slightly faster than the speed of light, amplify energy that passes through a crystalline pattern. When the life force of vibrational remedies passes through a crystalline pattern, there is a slight amplification from a temporary expansion of mass that transpires as the energy approaches the speed of light. The property of amplification creates more stability in energy. The crystalline pattern also stores electromagnetic energy and amplifies thought projections.

"The pineal gland is a crystalline structure that receives information from the soul, higher self, and subtle bodies, particularly the astral body. The subtle bodies often act as filters for teachings from the soul and higher self. From the pineal gland information travels to the right portion of the brain. If there is a need to alert the conscious mind to this higher information, it passes through the right brain in the form of dreams. Then the left brain analyzes it to see if the information can be grasped. This often occurs with clear dreams that offer messages. From the left brain information travels through the neurological system, specifically passing through two critical reflex points-the medulla oblongata and the coccyx. There is a constant state of resonancy along the spinal column between the medulla oblongata and the coccyx; properties of the pineal gland resonate between these two points. Then the information travels to other parts of the body through the meridians and crystalline structures already described. The life force of vibrational remedies activates this entire procedure. This is a key process the soul uses to manifest karma in the physical body."

Q Why is there constant resonancy between the medulla oblongata and coccyx?
"First, these are two reflex points by which the body's responses are processed. Pulling back from a sudden shock exemplifies this. This area is in a continuous state of stimulation; therefore, it amplifies ethereal energy associated with the pineal gland. It also translates energy from the subtle bodies into the physical body, especially the nervous system. The kundalini energy is augmented by this constant stimulation."

Q What happens when toxins are pushed out of the body by vibrational remedies?
"Toxins are pushed to the outer limits of the aura for purification. Some toxins are pushed into the ethers where they are purified, while others are pulled back into the body by the mind. The mind does this because vibrational remedies only temporarily stabilize the physical and subtle bodies until there is a cleansing of consciousness and a release of emotional attachments and mental misconceptions.

"All energy is secondary to the energy of the ethers. The ethers exist and flow in a perfect state of harmony with time and nature. Toxins in the body do not share this harmony in their chemical composition and molecular structure. This makes them unstable and easier to transform.

"Study the patterns of sand placed on the bottom of the ocean. If your hand disturbed the sand, the water would immediately become clouded. This symbolizes toxins traveling into the aura. Just as ethers affect toxins in the aura, after awhile water currents restore sand to its original pattern and the water is purified and stabilized.

"The physical body is a flow of energy in the flow of time-past, present, and future. Existence of disease means the physical body is dwelling out of synchronicity with the time flow, which crystallizes karma. Being in proper synchronicity with time means you are in perfect health."

Q Will you explain why nature spirits influence flower essences?

"First, nature spirits do not rush about each person activating flower essences. In the same way that there are different wave lengths for sound, light, and other energy patterns, there are different wavelengths in the life force or ether fields. Nature spirits exist in a spectrum or frequency of life force similar to that which flower essences function upon. This sympathetic resonancy creates a background effect amplifying flower essences. As electromagnetic beings of pure consciousness they especially amplify the nervous system, which is notably electromagnetic in its operation. Nature spirits also occupy strata of energy that is associated with the subtle bodies. Nature spirits have less influence on flower essences prepared in the lower homeopathic potencies. At lM or higher they are again closely resonant to flower essences."

Q Do nature spirits have similar impact on homeopathic remedies and gems?

"No, because they work on different spectrums of the life force. But nature spirits and gemstones do share an attunement. Historically, in Atlantis and Lemuria, certain gemstones were used for telepathic communication with nature spirits."

Q Why do certain substances block vibrational remedies from working?

"Certain toxicities block the passageway of the remedy's life force through the physical and subtle bodies. Stress, a lack of B vitamins, and a weak spinal column, especially in the coccyx or medulla oblongata, weaken the nervous system. Heavy metals in the system or a lack of iron weakens the circulatory system. It has long been understood by some that aluminum in the body is highly toxic[5] and that it usually interferes with the action of homeopathic remedies.[6] Steroids block the nervous system, muscular system, spleen chakra, and heart chakra. Other chemicals block various parts of the passageway of vibrational remedies life force.

"Camphor and caffeine lodge in the etheric body and occasionally in the emotional and mental bodies. They sometimes irritate, but do not fully penetrate, the astral body. These four bodies have a special connection with the nervous system. While both substances interfere with the circulatory and nervous systems, camphor notably blocks the nervous system. Caffeine overstimulates the nervous system causing a constriction in the meridians and circulatory system.

"Alcohol interferes with the astral and mental bodies. Other substances that can block vibrational remedies include: a poor diet, mints, menthol, thymol, odor of garlic, and strong perfume, especially if it contains aluminum and other synthetics. The odor of garlic can block the throat chakra, the abdomen, and the base of the spine. Mints sometimes weaken the entire process; they do not notably affect particular areas. With a few people sulphur interferes with vibrational remedies because it interacts with ammonia in the skin. This only happens when a deficiency of iron in the blood weakens the magnetic properties in the ethereal fluidium.

"While these substances can block flower essences and gems, they are usually more of an irritant. The problem is greatest with homeopathic remedies because they are so imprinted within the physical body. When flower essences and gems are prepared into homeopathic potencies, these substances present greater problems if the homeopathic potencies below lM are used.

"Biofeedback, correct diet, creative visualization, herbs, hypnosis, meditation, and massage, including chiropractic and osteopathic adjustments ease these blockages. Fasting removes caffeine from the body. These modalities seal the healing pattern of vibrational remedies."

Q Is it possible to scientifically prove that vibrational remedies work this way with people?

"Sophisticated medical devices can be used to monitor different parts of the body, including the meridians. This demonstrates that remedies affect specific parts of the body."

Q Will you explain how flower essences, homeopathic remedies, and gems work differently in people?

"When the pattern of flower essences travels to the meridians from midway between the circulatory and nervous systems, its main effect is more on ethereal parts of the body such as the psyche. At the same time, when flower essences primarily affect the physical body, more of the life force moves directly back into the physical body from the meridians. Homeopathic remedies and gems generally affect the physical body; therefore, most of their life force also moves into the physical body from the meridians. When these remedies affect the emotions or psyche, however, some of their life force goes from the meridians into the subtle anatomies, aura, and chakras, rather than primarily into the physical body."

The material presented in this chapter is some of the most fascinating in this book. A number of other issues will be discussed in the future concerning how vibrational remedies work in people. This is a complex topic.

1 Herbert Roberts, M.D., *The Principles and Art of Cure By Homeopathy* (Saffron Walden, England: The C. W. Daniel Co. Ltd., 1976), p. 44.

2 Rudolf Steiner, *The Etherisation of the Blood* (London: Rudolf Steiner Press, 1971).
The Occult Significance of the Blood (London: Rudolf Steiner Press, 1967).

3 Alice A. Bailey, *Esoteric Healing* (New York: Lucis Publishing Co., 1980), p. 46, 106, 142, 165, 240, 337, 628.
The Soul and Its Mechanisms (New York: Lucis Publishing Co., 1974), p. 103, 104, 112-113.

4 Rudolf Steiner, *Spiritual Science and Medicine* (London: Rudolf Steiner Press, 1975).
_____ and Ita Wegman, M.D., *Fundamentals of Therapy* (London: Rudolf Steiner Press, 1967).

5 Gary Null, "Aluminum: Friend or Foe?" *Bestways*, X (October, 1982), 60-65.
David Ulmer, M.D., "Toxicity From Aluminum Antacids," *The New England Journal of Medicine*, Vol. 294 No. 4, (January 22, 1976), 218-219.

6 H. Tomlinson, M.D., *Aluminum Utensils and Disease* (London: L. N. Fowler, 1967).

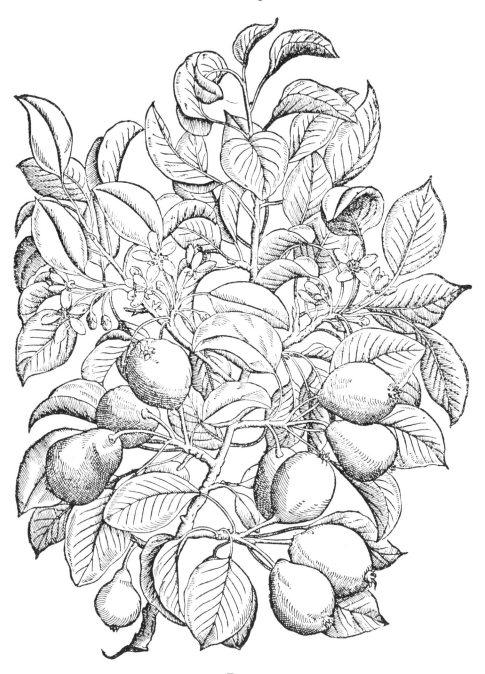

Pear

Chapter VI

The Relationship of Flower Essences to Homeopathy, Herbs, and Gems

Many people use other therapies with flower essences, so it is important to discuss the relationship of several of these modalities. This can avoid certain problems and improve clinical results with these remedies. The primary focus will be on vibrational therapies because there is not yet a proper understanding of the principles of these healing systems.

Q Will you explain the difference between flower essences and homeopathic remedies?

"Homeopathic remedies usually come from denser inorganic material, while flower essences have a much higher concentration of life force. Homeopathic remedies often vibrationally duplicate the physical disease in a person to push that imbalance out of the body. Homeopathy integrates into the subtle bodies but still functions upon the vibrational level of the molecular structure. Homeopathy is a bridge between traditional medicine and vibrational medicine.

"In contrast, flower essences adjust the flow of consciousness and karma that create the disease state. They influence the subtle bodies and ethereal properties of the anatomy and then gradually influence the physical body. The fact that flower essences come from flowers, which are the most concentrated area of the life force in plants, is one key reason why there is more life force in flower essences than in other forms of vibrational medicine."

Q What is the relationship of gem elixirs to flower essences and homeopathic remedies?

"Gemstones function between flower essences and homeopathic remedies. When a physical gemstone is ingested after being crushed, it is closer to homeopathy and notably influences the physical body with medicinal, nutritional, and antibiotic properties. When a gem is prepared into an elixir, however, using the sun in a method similar to preparing flower esences, that remedy functions slightly closer to flower essences and is more ethereal in its properties.

"With either method of preparation gems influence specific organs in the physical body, while homeopathic remedies have a wider impact on the entire physical body. Gems carry the pattern of a crystalline structure, which focuses the physical body's mineral and crystalline structures on the biomolecular level; therefore, gems work more closely with the biomolecular structure to integrate the life force into the body. Gems function between the other two systems of vibrational medicine because they have a stronger impact on the ethereal fluidium. Flower essences come from the living vehicle that holds the pattern of consciousness, while gems amplify consciousness.

"The most efficient way to experience the effects of flower essences is through baths because they are more ethereal in their effects and bathing makes it easier for nature spirits to assist in the process of assimilating the life force. Ingestion is best with homeopathic remedies because they work more directly on the physical body. Either method is superior with gems, but there is a slightly increased impact with ingestion."

Q Why can people take a number of flower essences together but only one or a few homeopathic remedies at the same time?

"Flower essences work in realms of consciousness and are self-adjusting, so they can be assimilated at the same time in a coordinated fashion. The body selectively applies the various essences. Flower essences work more in ethereal areas and less directly in the physical body, as with homeopathic remedies, so it is easier to assimilate many flower essences at once. With the broad sweeping social changes and changes in consciousness in recent years many now have an expanded and more complex subtle anatomy, so they can assimilate greater numbers of flower essences.

"It is harder to take too many homeopathic remedies together because of the increased stress placed on the physical body from the greater number of pollutants in society today. Because homeopathic remedies work directly upon the physical and cellular levels and are less self-adjusting, too many remedies taken at once would tend to overstimulate the release of toxins from the system. This would often cause sharp aggravations and a healing crisis that many people would find disruptive.

"Gems, when prepared as elixirs have some of the self-adjusting properties of flower essences. When prepared into low homeopathic potencies up to 1M, they lose some of their self-adjusting activities and are closer to homeopathic preparations. In the higher homeopathic potencies, from 1M and higher, gem elixirs have a higher degree of self-adjusting properties. Generally, gemstones ground up and ingested have less self-adjusting properties than gem elixirs."

Q What is the relationship of herbs to vibrational remedies?

"Herbs have nutrient and medical properties, so they augment the body and repel invading toxins. Individual herbs and vibrational remedies that influence the same diseases and body elements can be given in unison to support each other. For instance, the herb chamomile and a flower essence made from chamomile could be taken together."

I have recently completed a book *The Spiritual Properties of Herbs*. This is the first in a series of books that explains how herbs effect us consciously. The relationship of herbs to flower essences is described in more detail in that text.

Q Can flower essences, homeopathic remedies, and gems be taken at the same time without interfering with each other?

"Usually no, unless a skilled practitioner prescribes them in unison. It is also best to not be treated by two or more people at the same time with vibrational remedies. They may not of themselves cause an interference effect but the by-products of their activities may stimulate such effects. To illustrate, a flower essence may release emotional tensions causing a physiological change that could interfere with homeopathic or gem remedies.

"Some flower essences are so ethereal and universal that they do not interfere with other vibrational remedies. These include: cherry, larkspur, lilac, lotus, mango, papaya, yarrow, and all roses. Flower essences sprayed over the house or put into clothes will not interfere with gem or homeopathic remedies. Homeopathic remedies, flower essences and gems prepared into homeopathic potencies at 1M and higher or in the neutral homeopathic potencies—6x, 6c, 12x, 12c, 200x, 200c, and 10MM—interfere less with each other. When prepared at stock bottle level or in homeopathic potencies below 1M there is a greater chance for an interference effect. Gem elixirs prepared into elixirs with the sun are slightly less apt to interfere with other vibrational remedies than are gems ground up for ingestion. It is especially important to remember these guidelines when vibrational combination remedies are taken.

"Meditation, chanting, and creative visualization together with these remedies lessens the chance of them interfering with each other. These practices particularly enhance the properties of homeopathic remedies and gems to thoroughly integrate into the body's biomolecular properties, so flower essences can be used with no interference.

"The main problem occurs when clients are treated by two different people or when they also take vibrational remedies on their own. In such cases, if this procedure continues, it is best to stop the treatment because it is difficult to be of assistance in such cases and disruptive aggravations could occur.

"There is a special meditation that can be done when taking vibrational remedies, so they will not interfere with each other. Sit on the floor or ground with the palms turned upward and the spinal column straight. The lotus position in hatha yoga exemplifies this. The head should be tilted slightly upward, and you *must* be aligned with true or magnetic north. Then visualize light from the center of the heart spiraling out to each of the seven main chakras, arriving at the base and crown chakras simultaneously. With this visualization do deep rhythmical breathing. Then concentrate on sending light to the imbalanced chakras and diseased areas of the body. These blocks in consciousness can be predetermined through diagnostic techniques such as pulse testing or use of the pendulum.

"This exercise should be done upon rising and before sleep for at least three days when taking different vibrational remedies. If this meditation is practiced when only taking one vibrational remedy, its effects are amplified.

"In using these remedies, it is sometimes wise to initially use homeopathic remedies or gem elixirs to alleviate chronic physical problems, before using flower essences. This is one reason why the Bach flowers often take so long to effectively treat certain physical problems. The interference of physical problems can block flower essences from properly influencing the ethereal realms of consciousness.[1] Since many new flower essences work prominently or exclusively on the physical body, however, this principle is no longer as applicable as when only the Bach flowers were available. The Bach flowers usually have greater impacts on the psyche and personality, rather than on the physical body."

Q Will you give further information on the effects of flower essences when they are used in various homeopathic potencies?
"Preparing flower essences into homeopathic potencies always releases more energy and gets closer to the basic energy and life force pattern within each flower. Whether or not it is wise to use flower essences homeopathically prepared depends,

in part, on the individual's consciousness. Some people may not feel comfortable working with homeopathic principles because they lack training or experience.

"Flower essences are slightly less self-adjusting when prepared into homeopathic potencies below 1M. This is because, generally speaking, the closer to a stock bottle or mother essence level that a flower essence is, the more physical are its effects. Flower essences at the homeopathic potency of 1M and above are again fully self-adjusting partly because they are then especially ethereal in their effects."

Q What happens when you take too much or too little of a flower essence, gem elixir, or homeopathic remedy?

"If one takes too much of a flower essence, the effects are cancelled because they are self-adjusting and work on realms of consciousness. If one takes too little of a flower essence, its properties are properly amplified and assimilated because the ethereal digestive tract is activated. This refers to the crystalline structures in the body that were previously discussed. These structures are similar to the digestive enzymes that break down and assimilate various nutrients.

"If one takes too much of a gem elixir, there could be a mild healing crisis similar to what occurs with homeopathic remedies. This would rarely become a major problem, however, because gems maintain sufficient self-adjusting properties. When one takes too little of a gem, its effects may be too weak to cleanse or assist the system. The crystalline structures of the body are then only slightly activated with gem elixirs because there is less life force in gems than in flower essences, and gems primarily influence the physical body. The more ethereal vibrational remedies usually have greater impacts on the crystalline structures in the body.

"If you take too much of a homeopathic remedy, numerous complications and problems can develop. If you take too little of a homeopathic remedy, the crystalline parts of the body are only slightly activated; thus, there tends to be little or no cleansing from that remedy. The crystalline structures are not sufficiently activated because there is usually not sufficient life force in homeopathic remedies, and they work so closely to the physical body."

Q Why are there different types of aggravations with flower essences, homeopathic remedies, and gems?

"First, flower essences do not negatively affect people. What some call negative influences are really healing crises. As ingrained emotions are released, points of confrontation may be experienced. This sometimes creates illusions that the essence negatively affects the person. If some emotional problems are too difficult to face, the essence only gradually influences the individual. As previously stated, flower essences work on levels of consciousness, so they are self-adjusting and do not violate the individual's free will. If there is an emotional blockage that should not be released at a particular time, the flower essence will usually cancel itself in that part of the person's consciousness.

"However, there is not a 100% guarantee that extreme emotional states will never be created as flower essences release emotional blockages. When people do experience aggravations with these essences, it is often because it is important to their psychological rigidity and paranoia that the remedy not work. People should have enough common sense to understand that if extreme emotional reactions result from taking a flower essence that substance should probably be discontinued at least for a while. The client and, to a lesser extent, the practitioner should take some responsibility in this process. Expert psychological counseling can be crucial in some instances.

"There can be abuses in this process even with positive personality changes. If a person gains a great deal of confidence, that individual may become loud and obnoxious. You cannot blame the essence for such a response; it is the consciousness of the individual. Certain personality flaws were not properly treated in a therapeutic setting.

"Flower essences gradually heal within the capacity and limitation of the individual to create stable changes in mind, body, and spirit. This is why the results with flower essences tend not to be instantaneous.

"Sometimes when taking flower essences there is a sensation of negative energy attacking you. Released emotional tensions or physical toxins can trigger a concentration of orgone in the emotional chakra that your system cannot always easily handle. The released energy travels out the crown chakra through the kundalini processes three to four feet into the aura and back into the emotional chakra. This is partly why there is a sensation of energy entering you. Demons and devils attacking you are usually your own emotional negativity. In addition, this sensation sometimes causes nausea, and it generally increases the white blood cells. This process is about the same, or more intense, with homeopathic remedies and gems.

"Homeopathic remedies and gems work more closely to the physical body and have less life force than flower essences, so there is an increased chance of aggravations occurring. If the wrong homeopathic remedy or gem elixir is given, the aggravation can at times be intense. Such a problem is more likely to occur with homeopathic remedies than with gem elixirs. If the wrong flower essence is prescribed, it will almost always pass right through a person. Greater clinical skill is needed to prescribe homeopathic remedies than is the case with flower essences and gem elixirs."

Q In homeopathy, the clinical effects of many remedies have been discovered by conducting provings. A group of healthy people over a period of weeks ingest a homeopathic remedy or a placebo. The subjects who ingest the homeopathic remedy gradually develop symptoms that are carefully recorded in a diary and discussed or reviewed by an attending physician. The participants are not told if they have been ingesting the remedy or a placebo. The logic of this is that symptoms created under such conditions can also be treated by the same remedies when people become ill. Can these tests be conducted with flower essences to increase our understanding of their clinical effects?

"Yes, the tests could be conducted the same way they have traditionally been conducted with homeopathic remedies. This would be another way to validate the clinical value of new flower essences. However, one difference would be that with flower essences the initial symptoms that manifest would usually be shifts in the consciousness and personality and then, depending on the physical effects of the essence, changes in the physical body. For certain homeopathic remedies the same results could occur, but generally speaking because they have more of a direct effect on the physical body, the initial symptoms tend to manifest there. These provings can also be conducted with gems.

"These provings are positive in their own right because by bringing to the surface symptoms, they often reveal dormant patterns within the individual that could ultimately lead to disease. Symptoms that result from provings with flower essences are usually mild, and they usually last only three to eight hours after the essence is ingested. While any potencies can be used to manifest symptoms during provings, 10MM and the mother tincture or stock bottle levels are best. There is a slight pattern for symptoms to be harsher when the remedy is below 1M and to be milder in the potencies at 1M and higher. Again, this is because there are greater self-adjusting properties in the higher potencies."

As originally stated by Dr. Hahnemann, the founder of homeopathy in modern times, miasms are the root of all chronic diseases and can be a contributing factor in some acute problems.[2] They are the vibrational foundation of genetically inherited diseases in the body, which are passed on from generation to generation. These miasmatic traits include viruses or bacteria that lie dormant in the cells for many years or entire generations in a delicately balanced symbiosis.[3] They occasionally flare up, which leads to chronic or acute illnesses, trauma, stress, and old age. As individuals age their vitality weakens, which allows miasms to penetrate the physical body from the subtle anatomies.

The relevancy of flower essences here is they often have a profound effect on eradicating various miasms from peoples' systems. In section 2 of this text, the impact individual flower essences have on the miasms is depicted.

It is essential that holistic health practitioners understand the profound impact miasms have on chronic diseases. Underlying miasms contribute to making one susceptible to various acute illnesses. What usually happens today is that the client is treated with natural remedies, yet the underlying miasmatic problems are not even considered or examined. The overt symptoms are treated, but the underlying cause is not confronted. Today, only a few homeopaths consider the miasms in their clinical practice. Effectively treating the miasms is essential if the holistic health movement is to reach its full potential of restoring people to health in mind, body, and spirit.

"Miasms are stored in the subtle bodies, especially in the etheric, emotional, mental, and, to a lesser extent, astral bodies. Some miasms are passed on to the next generation genetically by inhabiting the molecular level of the physical body, which is the genetic code. A miasm is not necessarily a disease; it is the potential for a disease. Indeed, miasms are a crystallized pattern of karma. The merger of the soul's forces and ethereal properties determine when a miasm will arise in the physical body to become an active disease. This happens only when the miasm's ethereal pattern projects into the physical body from the subtle bodies. Miasms may lie dormant in the subtle bodies and aura for long periods of time. They are organized in the subtle bodies, and gradually, through the biomagnetic fields about the physical body, miasms penetrate the molecular level, then the cellular level (individual cells), and finally the physical body.

"There is a general misconception in homeopathic circles that miasms represent the imbalanced pattern that blocks the person's vitality and the life force of a vibrational remedy. This observation is not wrong; it is just incomplete. Miasms are not just darkness or tainted energy; they are more the lack of light or life force-the one true energy. It is the void or lack of life force that is the miasm. The imbalanced pattern and blockage is the void and lack of life force. The life force is the causal element that arranges the pattern correctly; thus, healing occurs when the life force penetrates into the void. Many times, individuals remove blockages but still do not permit the light or life force to enter, thus recreating the circumstances.

"There are three types of miasms, including planetary, inherited, and acquired miasms. Planetary miasms are stored in the collective consciousness of the planet and in the ethers. They may penetrate the physical body, but are not stored there. Inherited miasms are stored in the cellular memory of individuals. Acquired miasms are acute or infectious diseases or petrochemical toxicity acquired during a given lifetime. After the acute phase of an illness, these acquired miasmatic traits settle into the subtle bodies and the molecular and cellular levels where they ultimately may cause other problems. These three levels of miasms can aggravate the body, preparing the system for more miasms to develop."

Hahnemann stated that there are three inherited miasms: psora, syphilitic, and sycotic. Most homeopaths today accept this principle. With the psora miasm, one manifests an imbalance in the rhythmic functions of the body, general mental and physical irritation, numerous skin disorders, congestive states, and deformities in the bone structure.[4] Such people are usually tired and mentally alert but often anxious, timid, and perhaps sad or depressed.[5] Hahnemann said psora is the mother of all disease.

The syphilitic miasm, which is partly caused by syphilis, has a destructive effect on all tissues, especially bones. Imbalances in the elimination functions often lead to ulcers. Cardiac and neurological symptoms abound. Meningitis exemplifies this trend. Such people are easily upset, sentimental, irritable, and suspicious.[6]

The sycotic miasm, which is partly caused by gonorrhea, produces disordered assimilation leading to deposits, congestion, and tumor formation. Disorders often occur in the pelvic and sexual areas, skin, digestive, respiratory, and urinary tracts. Rheumatism of the small joints is another problem with this miasm. These people tend to be fearful, nervous, and morally degenerate.[7]

In the 1880's a debate developed in homeopathic circles concerning whether or not tuberculosis was a fourth inherited miasm.[8] Many today consider this to be true, and the channeled guidance agrees. With this miasm one is prone to respiratory, circulatory, urinary, and digestive problems. Mental illness and cancer also develop. Chilliness and weight loss likewise occur.[9] Such individuals cannot make decisions or face the realities of life in a stable fashion. They have a lively imagination, an artistic sense, and a flight from material reality.[10]

One of the most important pieces of new information that I have learned in the channeling is that there are now two, and soon three, new inherited miasms. Except in a few instances,[11] this is not understood in homeopathic circles. These new miasms are the radiation and petrochemical miasms, and the heavy metal miasm by 1990 if present environmental trends continue.

"The radiation miasm is associated with the massive increase in background radiation, especially since World War II. It contributes to premature aging, slower cell division, deterioration of the endocrine system, weakening of bone tissues, anemia, arthritis, hair loss, allergies, bacterial inflammations especially in the brain, deterioration of the muscular system, and cancer, especially leukemia and skin cancer. Skin disorders such as lupus, rashes, and loss of skin elasticity occur. Individuals are furthermore subject to hardening of the arteries and the full spectrum of heart diseases. Females are prone to miscarriage and excessive menstrual bleeding, while men experience sterility or a drop in the sperm count.

"The petrochemical miasm is caused by the major increase in petroleum-based and chemical products in society. Some of the problems caused by this miasm include: fluid retention, diabetes, hair loss, infertility, impotence, miscarriages, premature greying of the hair, muscle degenerative diseases, skin blemishes, and thickening of the skin's tissues. Metabolic imbalances that cause excessive storage of fatty tissue may occur. It is harder to resist stress and psychoses, especially classical schizophrenia and autism. Leukemia and cancer of the skin and lymphs also occur. It is also harder to assimilate vitamin K, circulatory disorders result, and endocrine system imbalances develop.

"At the present time, the heavy metal miasm is cross-indexed with other miasms. For instance, radioactive isotopes often latch onto heavy metals. The contents of this miasm include lead, mercury, radium, arsenic, sulphuric acid, carbon, aluminum, and fluoride. The symptom picture of this developing miasm includes allergies especially from petrochemicals, excessive hair loss, excessive fluid retention, inability to assimilate calcium, and susceptibility to viral inflammations. It is taking longer for this problem to become an inherited miasm for the planet because these minerals have existed in minute degrees in people and in the water and atmosphere for thousands of years. Consequently, a tolerance has developed. This tolerance, however, is for elements that have traditionally existed in the water. The growing prevalence of these pollutants, especially in the atmosphere is a key factor in this problem becoming an inherited miasm."

Conditions causing these three new miasms are very recent in their development. It is only in recent years that people have been excessively exposed to these pollutants. One has only to read in the daily papers about nuclear accidents, toxic waste dump problems and mass evacuations, or the debate over unleaded gasoline to sense the great concern over these issues.[12]

Most homeopathic research was conducted in the 1800's and early 1900's when these problems did not exist or were of little consequence. Homeopaths and practitioners using flower essences have little understanding of these problems partly because they rarely recognized these issues as problems. In addition, except for an occasional recognition that chemical drugs can interfere with homeopathic remedies, there is no real understanding that these toxicities play a major role in blocking most vibrational medicines from working properly. This is one of the main reasons why clinical results with homeopathic remedies are not the same now as they were before these pollutants became so common.

When I used to treat people, I and several associates who have incorporated some of these concepts, constantly found that these new miasms exist in a high percentage of clients. It should be realized that the well-chosen vibrational remedy will not properly work until these problems are dealt with. In our complex society, people typically have several of the old and new miasms in their system.

Planetary miasms were first discussed in 1953, in *Esoteric Healing*, by Alice A. Bailey,[13] but this concept has had no real influence in homeopathic circles. The three planetary miasms are cancer, syphilis, and tuberculosis. Syphilis and tuberculosis have settled into the cellular level of individuals to also become inherited miasms, but this has not yet happened with cancer. It remains stored in the planetary collective consciousness and ethers, not in the cellular memory of individuals. When someone has the gonorrhea, heavy metal, petrochemical, or tubercular miasms, they are more susceptible to developing cancer. While some homeopaths consider cancer a separate miasm, most who study the issue consider it a combination of one or more miasms.[14]

In recent years, some homeopaths have accepted the fact that miasms can also be acquired by numerous infectious illnesses, especially the childhood diseases. This view was first presented by Dr. Taylor in 1933.[15] These infectious toxins settle into the cells as acquired miasms where they often remain dormant for many years before producing symptoms that seemingly have nothing to do with the original infection.[16]

In 1969, United States scientists working at the National Institute of Health discovered that a rare brain disease that killed about 200 youths a year was caused by measles that these people had had years ago.[17] Today, it is widely understood in orthodox medical circles that many chronic degenerative diseases are caused by slow or unapparent viral infections.[18] Extensive medical research is now being conducted to discover which acute infections tend to relate to which degenerative diseases many years later.[19] The relationship of measles to multiple sclerosis is one such example. Slow viruses and acquired miasms are related. It is only a matter of time before orthodox medical practitioners and classical homeopaths discover this.[20] As with inherited miasms, difficult cases are relieved when acquired miasms are isolated and treated.

Q What percentage of the United States population now has the seven inherited miasms?

"At this time, 35 to 42 percent of the populace have the syphilitic, psora, and gonorrhea miasms, and 27 to 32 percent have the tubercular miasm. Concerning the developing new miasms, 10 to 15 percent have the heavy metal miasm, but in the next generation that percentage could rise to 46. Presently, 23 percent have the radiation miasm, but in the next generation that could rise to 48 percent. Currently, about 11 percent have the petrochemical miasm, but that figure could rise to 23, 37, or 42 percent in the next generation."

There is one other category of miasms to consider—the remedy miasm. A remedy miasm can occur if someone takes too many doses of a remedy. The vibration of a remedy can attach itself to the individual, and there can be problems releasing this vibrational frequency. It is easier for this problem to occur at high homeopathic potencies—200x or 200c and higher. This is one reason why only a few doses are prescribed for homeopathic remedies at high potencies. Remedy miasms can be considered a subcategory of acquired miasms in that both develop during a given lifetime.

Q Can flower essences cause remedy miasms?

"Constant exposure to a flower essence creates, not so much a remedy miasm, but a change in the individual's consciousness. When the actions of a flower essence release emotional tensions, this can sometimes seem to be associated with remedy miasms. Some very sensitive or spiritually aware people sometimes seem to experience remedy miasms with flower essences because such people are almost pure consciousness and usually less in need of physical treatment. Consequently, the subtle bodies are usually temporarily aligned, and the properties of flower essences are almost immediately activated into the consciousness and physical body."

Q Explain how flower essences affect the miasms, and contrast this with homeopathic remedies.

"Flower essences do not so much directly abate miasms; they merely create a clear state of consciousness that then affects the personality, physical body, and genetic code to entirely eliminate miasms from the physical and subtle bodies. Flower essences that notably influence the crown chakra and subtle bodies weaken all the miasms. When discussing individual flower essences only a few miasms are mentioned because they are the ones especially affected.

"In treating the miasms with flower essences, first isolate the main diseases caused by different miasms. Then combine several flower essences together to form one remedy to treat various miasms. In fact, combination remedies consisting of flower essences, homeopathic remedies, gem elixirs, and sometimes herbs can be prescribed to eradicate the various miasms. This gradually releases the miasms from the genetic code and subtle bodies, so they can be discharged from the system. This procedure, however, requires skillful treatment.

"Homeopathic remedies attempt to duplicate in the physical body a vibrational frequency similar to the miasm to expel it. It is easier to create a remedy miasm by taking too much of a homeopathic remedy than with other vibrational remedies because they work more directly in the physical body. With homeopathic remedies, and to a lesser extent with gem elixirs, remedy miasms do not necessarily disappear right away once you stop taking them."

Q How do gems affect the miasms?
"Gems function along similar lines and principles as homeopathy, but also integrate more closely to the level of the subtle anatomies, not unlike the properties and activities of flower essences. Gems balance the physical body and subtle anatomies more than homeopathic remedies, so they weaken the miasms slightly more than homeopathic remedies."

Q Speak on the miasms in relation to mankind's spiritual growth.
"The miasms collectively reflect peoples' wish to return to spirit in that diseases arise from blockages in accepting and acknowledging being Divine. This, of course, may lead to various levels of stress that may activate the miasms and create disease. Miasms crystallize mankind's struggle toward spiritual evolution. First there is the need to rise above base sexuality, which includes overcoming syphilis and gonorrhea. Next, there is the use of breath to draw upward and overcome tuberculosis. Finally, there is the need or attempt to overcome and master the environment. Thus, there is now the radiation, petrochemical, and soon the heavy metal miasms. The psora miasm helps mankind understand the universal laws of God. Miasms reflect blockages in conscious growth that mankind has not yet overcome."

More information could be presented here on the miasms, especially the new ones, but to do so would go beyond the scope of this book. There is much information on the miasms in traditional homeopathic literature,[21] in the two gem therapy books I have written, and in *Esoteric Healing* by Alice A. Bailey. Hopefully, in time, holistic health practitioners will jointly use flower essences, homeopathic remedies, and gem elixirs. For toxicity to be cleansed from the body's cellular level, vibrational medicine or spiritual healing must be used. Only then can all miasms be eradicated and true health prevail.

1 Aubrey Westlake, M.D., *The Pattern of Health* (Boulder, CO: Shambhala Publications, 1974), p. 14-15.

2 Wm. Boericke, M.D., *A Compendium of the Principles of Homeopathy* (Mokelumne Hill, CA: Health Research, 1971), p. 73-74.

3 Aubrey Westlake, M.D., "Miasms," *Psionic Medicine*, I (Winter, 1969), 71-72.

4 T. D. Ross, M.D., "Miasmatic Thoughts," *British Homeopathic Journal*, LI (April, 1962), 71-83.

5 George W. Mackenzie, M.D., "The Principles of Psora," *British Homeopathic Journal*, XXVIII (October, 1936), 392-415.

6 A. C. Gordon Ross, M.D., "Chronic Disease," *British Homeopathic Journal*, LI (April, 1962), 85.

7 Ibid., 85.

8 T. D. Ross, M.D., "Miasmatic Thoughts," *British Homeopathic Journal*, LI (April, 1962), 72, 78.

9 Aubrey Westlake, M.D., "Miasms," *Psionic Medicine*, I (Winter, 1969), 21-22.

10 Victor Bott, M.D., *Anthroposophical Medicine* (London: Rudolf Steiner Press, 1978), p. 108-110.

Dr. Fortier-Bernoville, "The Tuberculinique States and Hahnemann's Psora," *British Homeopathic Journal*, XXVIII (October, 1936), 358-391.

11 Aubrey Westlake, M.D., *The Pattern of Health* (Boulder, CO: Shambhala Publications, 1974), p. 145.

12 _____. "The Contribution of Psionic Medicine to Hahnemann's Miasmic Theory," *Psionic Medicine*, XI (Winter, 1974), 24-25.

13 Alice A. Bailey, *Esoteric Healing* (New York: Lucis Publishing, 1980), p. 221-242.

14 T. D. Ross, M.D., "Miasmatic Thoughts," *British Homeopathic Journal*, LI (April, 1962), 75-76.

Aubrey Westlake, M.D., "Miasms," *Psionic Medicine*, I (Winter, 1969), 22.

15 Dr. Tyler, "Hahnemann's Conception of Chronic Disease, As Caused By Parasitic Micro-Organisms," *British Homeopathic Journal*, XXIII (January, 1933), 1-56.

16 Aubrey Westlake, M.D., "Miasms," *Psionic Medicine*, I (Winter, 1969), 16.

_____. "The Contribution of Psionic Medicine to Hahnemann's Miasmic Theory," *Psionic Medicine*, XI (Winter, 1974), 26.

17 "Miasms and Smoldering Virus," *Psionic Medicine*, I (Winter, 1969), 23.

18 Aubrey Westlake, M.D., "The Contribution of Psionic Medicine to Hahnemann's Miasmic Theory," *Psionic Medicine*, XI (Winter, 1974), 27-31.

19 John Holland, "Slow, Inapparent and Recurrent Viruses," *Scientific American*, CCXXX (February, 1974), 32-40.

20 Aubrey Westlake, M.D., "The Contribution of Psionic Medicine to Hahnemann's Miasmic Theory," *Psionic Medicine*, XI (Winter, 1974), 27-31.

21 Herbert Roberts, M.D., *The Principles and Art of Cure by Homeopathy* (Saffron Walden, England: Health Science Press, 1976).

J. H. Allen, M.D., *Chronic Miasms* (Calcutta, India: C. Ringer & Co., n.d.).

Samuel Hahnemann, M.D., *The Chronic Diseases-Theoretical Part* (New Delhi, India: B. Jain Publishers, 1976).

Chapter VII

Advice to the Practitioner and Client

Since flower essences are a vibrational therapy, it is wise for the practitioner to have an understanding and respect for these remedies. Flower essences represent the life force shaped into a particular pattern; they are an educational principle that attunes people to their natural harmonics with nature.

Q When working with flower essences, is it best to develop a sacred feeling and acknowledge the life force that is within them from the heart rather than have a mental understanding and analytical approach?

"In part, it is wise to employ the clinical analytical approach and respect the essences. Otherwise, you may approach levels of worship, which is unwise. To approach levels of worship approaches systems of magic. Again, these are not magic, these are communication with levels of intelligence upon a telepathic level according to natural principles. It is wise, however, to have a degree of sensitivity within the personality as to the import of levels of intelligence that ye work with. Development of sensitivity within the personality draws each of you closer together until eventually you become one unity."

Q Do practitioners' positive or negative thoughts influence the effect flower essences have on clients?

"While the practitioners' attitudes have little effect on flower essences, they can influence the client. This is the critical element. Practitioners should seek to balance themselves in their own accord by constant purification to dwell in the light. They should remove themselves from improper motives and cultivate love for the client."

Q Is there any limitation on applying flower essences from a client's lack of consciousness?

"These remedies are as applicable to all individuals because in their continuous application there is the ability for all to be totally susceptible to them."

Q Would it be wise to use other methods for some people to first raise their consciousness?

"Who would have the wisdom to discriminate? It says, 'Cast not thy pearls before swine,' yet also, 'Ye are thy brother's keeper.' "[1]

Q In prescribing flower essences, how can practitioners explain that this is not simply a potion but is a process of teaching people to create greater balance in their lives? What factors in people open them to receive this form of treatment if they are not amenable to it?

"To decide whether an individual is receptive or not, explain the basic laws upon which flower essences work. Describe the laws of vibrational medicine and the levels of intelligence that work through flower essences. It is not essential to mention the devas to everyone. Explain the importance of the subtle bodies in vibrational healing.

"You may also depict the relationship between flower essences and homeopathy. Comment that homeopathy has existed for around 170 years, is today quite popular in Europe and India, and is now recognized as nonprescription medicine in America. Describe flower essences as a spiritual form of treatment. They are an educational process that awakens people to spiritual realities. Explain to them, for instance, natural healing abilities, like laying on of hands, and document some case histories such as in Christian Science. Finally, discuss the extensive literature on psychosomatic illness and the involvement of stress in many forms of sickness. This way you can be clinical and also satisfy their conscious objectivity. Tell them, just as attitudes are important in any form of psycho-spiritual form of disease, so are individual's spiritual attitudes important in healing with these particular remedies. People can enhance the effect of these essences through positive thinking and creative visualization because they work on levels of consciousness."

Q What is the best way to explain how flower essences work to more materialistic people?

"With those of the materialistic accord, it is wise as to approach symptomatically the level of their experience perhaps to the levels of psychology. Even those of the materialistic accord can understand the mind's influence on the body physical, which can cause stress and disease. Incorporated with various mind-body therapies such as counseling, acupuncture, acupressure, and massage, this can be approached not only as therapy, but also as moving the person to greater sensitivity through a logical and psychologically principled application of the essences. With the materialistic individual, it is not so much the activities of the spiritual and philosophical inclination, as it is the adjustment of the attitudes in relation to principles of mind and body. This generates appeal within the individual that aids the process, for the process, unless entirely overridden by free will, still has impact independent of the individual's structure."

Q Is there an effect on the user of flower essences independent of his or her belief in them?

"If people believe flower essences will not affect them, they will still usually work in a fashion similar to the function of chemistry. Whether or not you believe in chemistry, take several drops of arsenic and you will probably be in a pine box the next day. In extreme cases, however, it is possible to override the effects of flower essences with a negative or materialistic belief system. There is the human factor because we are dealing with people."

Q Why do flower essences sometimes not work well with people who are very mental or materialistic?

"The mental force integrates the life force with the biomolecular and even the denser physical body, particularly into muscular tissues. When the mental force over-dominates the physical system, the neurological and muscular tissues experience stress. This interferes with the passageways by which flower essences penetrate from the physical system to the subtle anatomies, eventually focusing the flow of the life force to create healing in the body physical and ethereal dimensions of people. The first stages of flower essences are not so much directed toward the particular behavioral pattern desired to be altered. Flower essences must first address the issue of the imbalance to much of the mental force and passageways that have become as blocked from this process. Generally, the individual, in addressing too much the mental body, is also the materialist. This is why again there is appeal to mind-body principles. These align the individual both intellectually and logically to receive flower essences."

As discussed in Chapter V, flower essences work through certain parts of the physical and subtle bodies. When these passageways are obstructed by an overactive mind and mental body, the effectiveness of flower essences is weakened. Practitioners using flower essences should take special note of this issue, but a person must be an extremely closed materialist or intellectual rationalist for flower essences not to work. The typical questions or reservations a person might have when first learning about flower essences will not block them from working.

Q When prescribing flower essences to conscious people would it be wise to tell them about the devas?

"Generally, yes, but this is not crucial. Philosophically, there is the content that using these essences graduates people more closely to the kindred nature of man's spirit. The devas are, of course, as a terminology used as consciousness running through various accords of light or the greater powers in same. Philosophically they draw ye closer to the natural elements realigning people with their environment."

Q What if you gave flower essences to someone who was unconscious?

"Then the subconscious acts as the mental factor. Actually, a person in a sleep state is usually quite responsive to flower essences."

Q Why do practitioners have different preferences and get different clinical results with various flower essences?

"All essences in their own right have varying heightened qualities. Their clinical application is influenced by the personal preferences and prejudices of practitioners and by the type of people they treat. Various cultures and geographical locations also influence the applicability of flower essences. To illustrate, the dietary needs of people in Africa differ from those native to northern climates. All these patterns explain why practitioners get different results with flower essences. Future scientific studies will validate the authenticity of each flower essence and resolve seeming discrepancies."

Q Should we recommend the dosages as outlined by Dr. Bach?

"Generally, yes. The traditional dosages suggested are fairly reliable. However, it is best to take flower essences at the stock bottle level and not the further diluted dosage bottle level. The further reduction of a flower essence preparation to the dosage bottle level causes a reduction of approximately 65% in the clinical effectiveness of the resulting preparation. This sharp drop in clinical effectiveness is partly lessened if the preparation is placed inside a properly constructed pyramid for one or two hours.

"When merging individual flower essences, gem elixirs, or homeopathic remedies together in a combination, drops from individual stock bottles can be taken at the same time, but the recommended technique, for greater amplification, is to pour equal amounts from each stock bottle into a new or carefully cleansed bottle. Then briefly shake the bottle with the new combination and, if possible, place it under a pyramid for one or two hours before using it. This helps unify the individual preparations into a new combination, and they remain at the stock bottle level. After each stock bottle is opened, briefly put your hands under running water to prevent the liquid remaining in each stock bottle from merging with each other. And do not open the bottles at the same time while making a new combination. It is also wise to consider adding lotus, pineapple, jamesonite, or quartz (clear) to all vibrational combinations. These preparations always greatly amplify such combinations, they remove blockages, and they further unify the individual constituents of such combinations. Wallflower flower essence amplifies other essences but does not unify the remedies or remove blockages in a new combination. While diamond does not unify or amplify a combination, it does remove blockages that will interfere with the combination's effectiveness.

"It is sometimes wise to store opened flower essences in a cold area such as a refrigerator, especially if you are taking the preparation beyond a few days. If possible, do not touch the glass dropper to your tongue to prevent any bacteria from getting into the preparation. If diluting the flower essences below the stock bottle level to the dosage bottle always add at least 50% brandy and pure water to the bottle. These procedures are even more relevant during the hot summer months, in tropical areas, and with flower essences that naturally have an amplified life force such as lotus, all roses, papaya, mango, and many fruit, nut, and tropical trees, as well as others that strongly effect the crown chakra."

The dosage bottle is traditionally filled with several to seven drops from the stock bottle. There is a slight amplification if seven drops are used. This is partly from the influence of the seven dimensions and seven ethers. Any bottles used to prepare a combination or a dosage preparation should be new, or at least be carefully cleansed. It is wise to label the bottle to avoid any confusion. Regarding John's statement that there is a sharp reduction in the clinical effectiveness of a dosage bottle, individuals questioning this are invited to confirm this by conducting tests on individual or combination preparations at the stock and dosage levels without being able to identify which is which during the tests.

Three or four doses a day are suggested with individual or combination flower essences. The doses should be taken early in the morning, before lunch and supper, and at night before bed. Generally, do not take flower essences or any vibrational remedies during a meal. In acute situations, flower essences can be taken more frequently, such as every quarter of an hour, until the person feels better.

Q Dr. Bach suggested keeping flower essences in your mouth for a minute to enhance their qualities. This principle is generally not stressed in homeopathy, so I wonder if this applies with all vibrational medicines?

"Yes, it does. This allows the remedies to be integrated with enzyme properties in the saliva that, in part, integrates it with normal enzyme properties. It is then quickly carried to the molecular structure by integrating it with normal physiological processes."

Flower essences are a vibrational form of therapy; consequently they work under certain laws of physics that are different from what one expects. To illustrate, with the occasional exception of hypersensitive people, it does not matter how many drops you take with each dose. It is the frequency of the doses that affect the person.

"To a degree, healing accelerates by prescribing flower essences more frequently, not by giving more with each dose. This is partly because the mind is the adjuster in its desire to accelerate the time flow. By taking the remedy more often, the mind focuses on it more often."

Q What is the effect, if any, when a person takes a large dose such as an entire bottle?

"Frankly it is your attachment to quantity and speed. One drop or an entire gallon usually affects you the same way. If there is attachment to the idea that more is better, then the recommended dosage could indeed be slightly raised. When flower essences are prepared into various homeopathic potencies, the dosage should be what has traditionally been suggested in homeopathy."

While there is a debate in homeopathy as to the correct dosage in various potencies, the following general guidelines are acceptable to most homeopaths: mother tincture to 6x or 6c—twenty to twenty-four doses, 12x or 12c—twelve doses, 30x or 30c—eight doses, lM—three doses, lOM—one or two doses, 50M to CM—one dose. These doses are usually taken once to several times a day. Each dose includes several drops, or one or two tablets or pillules. In acute cases, the frequency of dosage may be increased even to every hour, particularly if the potency is not higher than 30x or 30c. At lM and higher few homeopaths prescribe a remedy beyond the above stated guidelines.

Q Elsewhere you said except in certain acute cases homeopathic remedies should be given at least three hours apart or the separate doses tend to merge with each other. Is this also true with flower essences taken at the stock bottle or different homeopathic potency levels?

"Again, flower essences are self-adjusting. The three hour separation could apply but it would not be critical with flower essences. This principle is slightly more applicable to flower essences homeopathically prepared than to flower essences ingested at the stock bottle level. While homeopathic remedies harmonize with the biomolecular pattern integrating with the subtle bodies, they work more closely to the physical body than do flower essences. Therefore, their doses have implications of merging with each other at any level of potency."

Q You have also previously stated that some people become ill from handling homeopathic remedies over the years. Is this principle true with flower essences?

"No, again because flower essences are self-adjusting."

Q What advice would you offer for taking flower essences in combinations?

"Most people can now take six to eight flower essences together, and with the current level of consciousness some can take nine essences together. A few people meditating for some time can take twelve to fifteen essences together. Dr. Bach's suggestion to take only up to five essences together is generally no longer applicable because of progressions in consciousness since the 1930's. Note the radical sweeping social changes since that time, and today more people are involved in spiritual practices. This has caused a radical expansion and strengthening of the subtle bodies, so healing crises are less likely to occur with vibrational remedies. In addition, since 1951 many Atlantean souls have reincarnated and these therapies were commonly practiced in that civilization."

Q Is there any danger in using flower essences from plants that are toxic on the physical level?
"When flower essences are prepared by the sun method, on rare occasion some toxicities might, at the most, become allergies. With the boiling method of preparing flower essences, a fair amount of toxicity would be transferred to the flower essence; thus, as a general rule poisonous plants should not be prepared as flower essences and ingested at the stock bottle level of potency. But if a poisonous plant were prepared as a flower essence, with either method of preparation, and then raised to a homeopathic potency of at least 6c, there would be absolutely no danger. Poisonous plants prepared as flower essences often have highly beneficial effects. This principle has long been understood in homeopathy."

Q In our society, some people are so allergic to alcohol that the brandy in stock bottles would be disruptive. Is there a technique such people can utilize to ingest flower essences without experiencing the brandy?
"From the stock bottle continue to dilute the flower essence. Take an average of three drops to approximately one quart of distilled water. Then again take a few drops from that quart and put it in another quart of distilled water. This removes most physical traces of alcohol but does not lessen the potency of the flower essence. To prepare the essence into a homeopathic remedy succuss or shake each level of dilution. If you have diluted the essence once into some distilled water, shake that a set number of times before you dilute it further. To preserve the pattern even further put it under a pyramid or orgone device for approximately one hour. This removes most homeopathic traces of alcohol in the liquid. It is wise to store this liquid continuously under a pyramid or orgone device for one hour before the flower essence is ingested."

Q Do flower essences create permanent changes in people?
"They enhance the opportunities for changing the personality, but the human condition is not permanent. They create permanent healing if the person does not wander back into fields of negativity. If people are subject to extreme traumatization, normal psychological processes would usually restore the problem. It is often wise to enhance the healing process by also using other holistic remedies such as herbs, diet, creative visualization, meditation, other vibrational remedies, or counseling."

Q Can flower essences be taken indefinitely several times a day?

"Yes, there can be slight overamplification of the healing process, but since the essences are self-adjusting there would almost never be any problems. Eventually, you should be able to restore or maintain health mentally, physically, and emotionally without needing any natural remedies. Flower essences are aids toward that goal. Balancing your karma and keeping in touch with your higher self also aid in this process."

Moreover, there are the difficult to define spiritual awakenings that do indeed occur with flower essences. These are at times distinctly different from physical, emotional, and mental cleansings. It is often wise to discuss this issue with the client. John here gives some insights into this process.

"Bringing forth a particular pattern of the life force to the conscious levels of the individual creates choice and broader discrimination of those states of consciousness allowing for increased activity of free will. This allows the individual upon conscious levels to have choice in the behavioral patterns desired to be modified. This creates spiritual illumination in the sense that activities normally occurring in the subtle anatomies become almost a functional conscious property."

People respond quite differently to these essences. Some feel profound effects within seconds or minutes, while others experience subtle changes over the weeks, which clearly are associated with flower essences. Others cannot say they have specifically benefited from taking these remedies, yet there is agreement that certain positive changes are taking place. Most practitioners and clients benefit from using these vibrational remedies.

1 *Bible: King James Version* (New York: Thomas Nelson, Inc., 1972).

Chapter VIII

Bath Therapies

All flower essences can be used in baths. Simply put three to seven drops from a flower essence stock bottle into a bath, as has been done for years with the Bach flower crab apple. For advanced spiritual practices seven drops is superior because it helps you attune to the seven dimensions.

It is best, if possible, to take the baths in the morning before noon, because the life force is strongest with the rising of the sun. Stay in the tub for around thirty minutes. Cover as much of your body with water as is possible, and except for very young children, take these baths alone. Wait at least six hours between taking these baths; indeed, one a day or every several days is fine. The water temperature should be at body temperature or a bit warmer. If pregnant, the water temperature should not be hotter than just below body temperature, and never take warm baths after the fifth month of pregnancy. After the bath, lie down for a few minutes so the blood recirculates.

Q Can you now discuss the main principles involved in using flower essences in bathing?

"Water acts as a conductor of all electromagnetic energies. Bathing distributes the influence of the flower essence into the aura immediately and then into the subtle bodies. This bypasses the need to penetrate first into the physiology of the individual. The effects move directly into the activities of the aura, alleviating and activating karmic patterns within the capacity of the subtle anatomies. Bathing with flower essences is an attempt to distribute the properties of the essence with the conductive properties of water, its immediate and equal displacement throughout the water, and above all its continuous exposure to the individual while the person bathes. In fairly pure water or in distilled water, the properties of the essence are immediately and evenly dispensed.

"Try to use spring water or distilled water for the bath. If you must use city water, add a quarter cup of lemon juice because this cleanses the water. Next, the enamel in the tub should be thoroughly scrubbed, preferably with a mild abrasive-like action, possibly using baking soda or lemon juice. To potentize the water a bit more, especially if using city waters for the bath, leave some of the water under the sun or put it under a copper pyramid for about thirty minutes. In either case, add a small amount of lemon juice to the water. These techniques enhance the qualities of the water so that it can better receive vibrational essences.

"Before taking a bath or shower with flower essences, cleanse your body. Instead of just filling the tub with water, put five gallons of water into the tub. Then step into the tub and rinse your body with a pure sponge, preferably a clean linen or some substance like cotton with a form of crushed white, rose, or amethyst quartz. Use regular or homeopathically prepared quartz at 10MM or 30c. The crushed quartz, which stimulates the properties of flower essences, goes inside the pure linen. It could be wise to initially put only five gallons of water into the tub because this focuses the initial cleansing on the lower extremities where many toxic energies are stored. After five or ten minutes of such bathing add more water. In five gallons, or in a full tub, an average of three to seven drops of the flower essence is sufficient."

Q Would there be any difference in using a flower essence in a bath on the stock bottle level versus the homeopathic level?

"No, the influence would be about the same. Occasionally there would be a slight enhancing effect on the homeopathic level. With bathing, it is more a matter of just getting the energy of the essence into the water. Ingesting an accurately prescribed essence homeopathically prepared, however, is definitely superior to giving that same essence on the stock bottle level.

"Another technique is to place a few drops of oil from the plant that you are using as a flower essence into the water. Do this if there is only five gallons in the tub or if it is filled with water. Again, heat the water to around body temperature, and with this combination you have a system of aromatherapy and a direct immersion with the essence. No special technique is needed to combine the essence and oil together before putting them into the bath.

"An interesting showering technique is to take a pure piece of linen, soak it in lemon juice and powdered or small pieces of several varieties of quartz, then soak it in one or more of the essences that you want to bathe in. Place the quartz powder in the linen. Take the small metal device that goes on shower heads, open it and tuck in the linen or tie it to the shower head. As the water flows out, the lemon juice neutralizes the impurities in the water and the quartz amplifies the effects of the flower essence. Take this shower for twenty to thirty minutes."

Q How would the quartz be purified to reuse in future baths?

"Put the quartz in a bottle of distilled water, seal the bottle, and set that in some sea salt. Twenty-four hours in the distilled water and sea salt would be a sufficient cleansing. Or put the bottle under a copper pyramid for at least six hours, but the pyramid is not essential here."

Q Do these bathing and showering techniques differ from the ingestion method concerning the effects of the flower essence on the person?

"Bathing with flower essences is usually superior in clinical effects to ingestion, although ingestion is more convenient. A combination of ingestion and a quick shower under the same essence is just as effective as a full bath or shower with the essence. The baths are the equivalent of larger doses. This is because bathing dilutes and energizes the essence and spreads it over the entire skin surface. The skin is a natural assimilation point for the life force to enter the system through the pores, and the water brings you closer to the vibrational frequencies upon which the nature spirits reside."

Q Some people, rather than feeding the remedies orally to their children, because of their resistance to taking them, just flick the essence water onto their body. How effective is this method?

"This is a good method, but it is not superior to ingestion. A method similar to ingestion in its effectiveness would be massaging the soles of the feet because they are incredibly sensitive. Rubbing it on the palms of the hands or on the forehead is also excellent."

Q Would it be wise to hang a pyramid from your ceiling above the bathtub?

"It could be done, but do not make this a permanent structure because it could have negative effects. Pyramids tend to magnify whatever is put under them. If you enter a tub in a bad mood, that negativity could be amplified."

These bathing and showering techniques should prove quite effective for many people. Flower essences work if one just puts a few drops into a tub filled with water, but these extra purification techniques do indeed help. At the very least, clean a tub before taking a flower essence bath or shower.

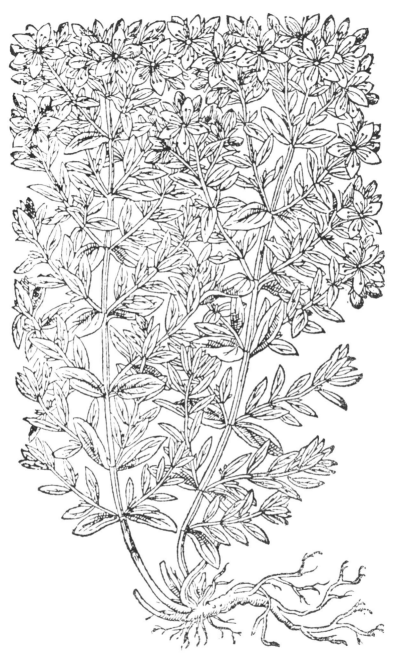

St. John's Wort

Chapter IX

Amplification Techniques

Various processes amplify the effects of flower essences. This includes related therapies such as creative visualization, meditation, nutrition, and psychotherapy. Some of these techniques are depicted in Chapter VII.

Q Explain how certain foods enhance the effects of flower essences?
"There are many techniques, but to keep it simple first fast on fruit juices and pure water. If the person has hypoglycemia drink vegetable juices and liquid tofu to keep some protein in the body. Black cherry juice is rich in iron, so it builds the blood and cleanses the liver. Carrot and papaya juices are also especially valuable. After fasting, and at least one day on water, the body is not so dependent on denser foods. Then a lighter diet—vegetarian and fruitarian foods—while utilizing flower essences allows their life force to more easily permeate the physical and subtle bodies. If done with care and moderation such a diet stabilizes a person emotionally. At the same time, flower essences work if people eat meat. These suggestions are offered merely as enhancements."

Q Can you speak on taking a flower essence and the same herb together?
"The flower essence enhances the assimilation of the herb's medical properties partly because the life force of that herb is already thoroughly integrated into the physical body. Taking the flower essence strengthens the ethereal fluidium for easier assimilation of the herb's properties. The flower essence is partly facilitated because part of its pattern is already assimilated into the physical body. Thus, when both are taken together, the life force in each is activated, but the herb receives greater benefits. Practitioners can always prescribe the same herb and flower essence together because the effects of each are always stimulated. When bathing with a particular flower essence, applying the oil of that same plant slightly enhances the properties of each."

Q Elsewhere you suggested a person should drink one glass of distilled water one hour after ingesting a homeopathic remedy and also drink other glasses of distilled water for the next few days. Is this true with flower essences?
"Yes, distilled water aids in the assimilation of flower essences and cleanses the body. This is likewise true with children."
Some homeopaths influenced by Dr. Voll from Germany have done this for awhile, but it is not understood that the liquid taken in coordination with the flower essence or homeopathic remedy must be distilled water. This removes toxins vibrational remedies release. Other liquids ingested then create biochemical reactions in the body that could interfere slightly with the toxins released in the system. Occasionally, a few days to a week after taking a

vibrational remedy, a client has told me he or she experienced pain in the kidneys. This is usually because released toxins have lodged there. Extra distilled water is generally sufficient to cleanse the kidneys. Or other kidney cleansing techniques can be used. This technique is more valuable with flower essences that markedly affect the physical body.

Q Are there any special meditation or visualization practices to execute with flower essences?
"Specific practices are not usually necessary. Use meditative practices and visualization exercises you feel attuned to. These align the chakras, which aids in the assimilation of flower essences."

Q How can flower essences be used with acupuncture?
"Acupuncture is but the life force flowing through the physical form of the needles. Acupuncture needles can be dipped into water infused with a flower essence. Moreover, having the flower essence bottle in the same room in which the treatment occurs slightly enhances the process. The bottle does not have to be open."

Q How important is it to shake a flower essence bottle to energize it before ingestion?
"This is an ideal enhancement because it activates the life force in the essence. Do this before each ingestion. This likewise attunes and personalizes the scope and range of the essence's vibration to the individual. This technique is equally valuable for a flower essence at stock bottle or homeopathic levels. Shaking the bottle around five times is sufficient."

Q In taking flower essences, does it matter if people live in the city or in the countryside?
"Flower essences educate you to the critical need to harmonize with nature. While a city environment is not that unhealthy, it can be further aligned with nature. Frank Lloyd Wright, Mayans, and Aztecs built cities that harmonized with nature. Natural healing systems work in metropolitan environments, but will be slowed somewhat because of extra tensions. Cities tend to block enhancing magnetic properties common in nature. This can be overcome with certain forms of architecture. If you live under a dome or pyramid, flower essences work faster. Boxes or rectangular structures weaken energy by their very shape. Organic substances such as wood and higher metals such as gold, silver, and copper are also quite suitable. Flower essences put you in touch with nature in concrete city environments.
"Older structures are better because they are more likely to consist of natural material such as wood, and the architecture is less cubical and harsh in angular structures. This is why cities can sometimes be fairly psychic areas.
"The vibration of flower essences can even saturate clothes. Add a few drops of a flower essence to water you are washing clothes in or to water-based items such as paint. You can also treat carpets, draperies and numerous substances using an atomizer. Then your environment becomes more natural.
"Put two or three drops of the essence into distilled or spring water also adding sea salt and some rose water or castile soap. Leave the clothes in for thirty minutes to two hours. The vibrational effect of the essence lasts indefinitely unless there is

a noticeable shift in the individual's consciousness. It helps to rewash the clothes and place them under a pyramid briefly because when the clothes are cleansed and worn, detergents and dirt gradually permeate them. Without this occasional cleansing, the flower essence would be directed toward this problem rather than augmenting the individual's consciousness."

The relationship of geometric patterns or shapes to consciousness is a very complex subject. Each geometric pattern has therapeutic power with the pyramid being the most important. Pyramidal shaped churches are a vestige of the ancient wisdom that different shapes influence health and conscious growth. John has previously stated that in the coming age entire cities will be built using pyramidal and dome shapes and crystalline material as was done in ancient Lemuria and Atlantis.

The best material to use in constructing a pyramid is gold and then silver, but because these are expensive, copper, the third best metal, is usually suggested. Other metals and even wood can be used, but they would not work so well. Aluminum or plastic should never be used because they are toxic to health. The base angles of the pyramid should be 62 degrees. There is some debate in the literature on this because the Egyptian Cheops pyramid is 51 degrees at its base angles.[1] The channeled guidance is that 62 degrees is superior because the pyramid someone builds is much smaller. One angle of the pyramid should be pointed toward magnetic north. This properly aligns the pyramid with the earth's magnetic energies. The actual size of the pyramid can generally vary depending on preference and what is to go under it; however, a base of eight inches as a minimum is best. In constructing a pyramid, if glue is used, only a natural non-chemical glue such as silica glue should be used. The pyramid can be fully enclosed or be skeletal in design. [See figure 1.]

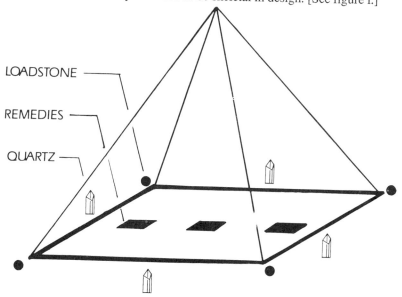

LOADSTONE

REMEDIES

QUARTZ

FIGURE 1

In esoteric literature on Atlantis, there is often reference to the extensive use of quartz crystals.[2] Quartz crystal is a crystalline form of the element silica. It exists in various colors such as pink, red, white, black, yellow, and purple. White or clear quartz is the purest and most powerful kind.[3] For this work use quartz that is clear, geometrically proportioned, and one-pointed, instead of several small clusters. Place quartz by the pyramid's four sides. Small pieces of lodestone may be placed by the four angles of the pyramid in the shape of a horseshoe. It is best that only the positive and negative lodestones face each other. While it is wise to use lodestone, if one does not, the quartz pieces should be placed by the angles instead of along the four sides.

Pyramids, quartz crystals, and to a lesser extent lodestones, amplify thought and regenerate what they come into contact with. This is particularly so with any form of vibrational remedies. A fully enclosed pyramid is slightly better than the skeletal pyramid. The difference is minor, especially if lodestone and quartz are placed at the angles of the pyramid.

On the bottom of the pyramid place a sheet of magnetized rubber, which can be bought in some industrial shops. It is best if both sides of the sheet are magnetized, but if only one side is magnetized it should be facing upwards toward the pyramid. You could also place a copper sheet above or below the magnetized rubber.

Q What if two magnetized rubber pieces are magnetized only on one side and face opposite each other, so they are magnetized on the top and bottom?

"This would not necessarily improve efficiency because of the insulation between the magnetic fields in the two pieces."

You can put the quartz or lodestone on small sheets of copper or natural wood. While it definitely helps to add these various items to the pyramid, they are not essential. Each item, however, enhances the purification of the remedies that are placed inside the pyramid. Using the pyramid with quartz crystals and lodestone around it, as depicted in figure 1, is a powerful way to amplify flower essences.

"Mother essence bottles should go under the pyramid for two hours and stock bottles for thirty minutes, if quartz and lodestone are used. If neither is used, this time should be doubled. If only one of them is used, the time under the pyramid should be increased by approximately 25-35%.

"Mother essence bottles do not have to go inside the pyramid immediately after being prepared, but they should not be opened before going under the pyramid. If they are opened, leave them under the pyramid for three, not two, hours.

"The bottles should never touch each other while under the pyramid. If they do, the vibrations from each bottle intermix. If two bottles touch each other, they *must* separately be under the pyramid for twenty four hours to negate the influence of the other remedy. If three or more bottles touch each other while under the pyramid, they *must* be thrown out. If bottles touch each other while being removed from the pyramid, they would be slightly weakened. In other words, when around the pyramid, flower essence bottles should not touch each other.

"Place bottles under the pyramid in the morning before noon when the life force is strongest, but this is not a crucial point. One or more small pieces of quartz can be placed in between several bottles under the pyramid. While remedies are under the pyramid, do not walk over the pyramid because it should not be disturbed in any way.

✓ "A gold, silver, or copper pyramid never needs to be cleansed because of its innate shape and pattern. Each time one or more remedies have been under a pyramid the quartz crystals must be replaced with a new set or wait fifteen minutes before reusing them so they get recharged. The validity of this can easily be tested with a pendulum. For fifteen minutes after remedies have been removed from a pyramid, the pendulum will read negative over the quartz pieces and then the swing is positive.

✓ "Every three months the quartz crystals need to be cleansed by being placed in pure sea salt under the pyramid for thirty minutes to two hours. Or they can be put under the pyramid for thirty minutes to two hours separately and then in sea salt outside the pyramid for thirty minutes. Paper bags can be used but glass is superior. If several quartz crystals are in the same bag or glass, they should not touch each other. As a crystalline structure sea salt removes toxicities from quartz. Sea salt should only be bought in a health food store because commercial salt often contains aluminum, which should never be used to cleanse anything. The labels on bulk sea salt bags usually state what, if anything, has been added to the sea salt. One can also follow the American Indian tradition of cleansing quartz in the sun or in the ground, especially in mud for a few hours.

✓"The lodestones need to be cleansed every three to six months. Put them under the pyramid for thirty minutes to two hours. Fresh lodestones could, during this cleansing, be placed on the four corners of the pyramid in a horseshoe shape.

✓"Each side of the magnetized rubber should be cleansed every three months. Put the pyramid in the center of the magnetized rubber with quartz crystals on the four corners for fifteen to twenty minutes."

Q Can you suggest a device to amplify flower essences that incorporates orgone energy?

"Take a natural or organic linen such as cotton preferably naturally grown rather than from an animal. The inorganic material is crushed quartz or a plate glass of quartz crystal. Plate glass of quartz crystal should be 1/8 to 1/4 inch thick. If crushed quartz is used, use silicon glue to bind it or sew it into the linen or cotton in a form of padding. Silicon glue and quartz crystal plate glass or crushed quartz can be purchased in certain industrial shops. It is important to use silicon glue in this process because it is the only glue available that has no synthetic chemicals.

"The device should be pyramidal shaped with 51 degree angles. The higher vibrational elements of gold, silver, or copper can be used as the outer layer of the device. Depending on personal preference a quartz plate can also be the outer layer. There are seven layers, including quartz and linen for each layer. The inner layer must always be quartz to intensify the orgone in the center chamber. This increases the amplification of the remedies and prevents DOR (deadly orgone radiation) from forming. The base of the device should be a quartz plate or one of the three metals.

"This device generates only clean or pure orgone. No DOR is generated because quartz and organic material is used, and no metals with a lower vibration are used. Dense metals especially gather DOR over the months. DOR is created when orgone devices over-amplify natural background radiation and radiation from nuclear reactors and nuclear testing. Consequently, the device needs little cleansing for protection from DOR, but it does need cleansing because of the effects of vibrational remedies placed in it.

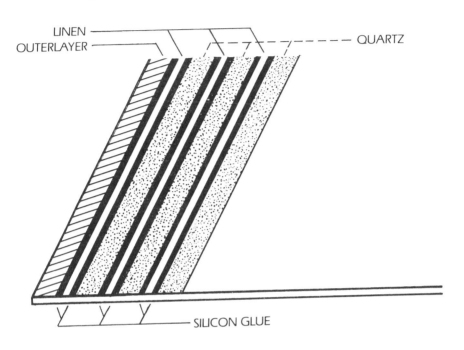

LINEN

OUTERLAYER

QUARTZ

SILICON GLUE

FIGURE 2

"The device could be constructed so the different layers can slide into slots and be pulled out easily to be cleansed. Wipe each layer and the base with sea salt or seal them in sea salt for at least two or three hours with twenty-four hours being ideal. The layers of linen or cotton can be replaced with each cleansing. If the outer layer is quartz, cleanse the device every three or four months. If one of the metals is the outer layer, cleanse it every sixty days, otherwise, over several years low levels of DOR could develop.

"Any remedies can be placed in this device if they do not touch each other. Usually, leave remedies in the device for three hours. While the pyramid or orgone device can be used, the orgone apparatus has slightly superior effects."

The various modalities suggested in this chapter enhance the life force. Anything that does this stimulates the effects of flower essences. These amplification techniques are not essential, but clinical results improve with their use.

1 Greg Nielsen and Max Toth, *Pyramid Power* (New York: Warner Books, 1976), p. 140-141.
2 Hugh Lynn Cayce, ed., *Edgar Cayce on Atlantis* (New York: Warner Books, 1968), p. 62.
3 George Kunz, *The Curious Lore of Precious Stones* (New York: Dover Publications, 1971).

Chapter X

Diagnostic Procedures

Determine which flower essences to prescribe through various procedures common in holistic health. For instance, medical astrology can determine which areas of the physical body and psyche are unhealthy. Then prescribe essences that apply in these types of imbalances.

"Study the various psychological states attributed to each essence as empirically tested by Dr. Bach. And use these methods to discover how the new flower essences can be applied. At times, rely upon your own intuition using the pendulum, muscle testing, and kinesiology. If specific organs or meridians are not functioning properly, you may put certain flower essences into the aura's field or over the pulse of the person and do a pulse test. A well chosen essence causes subtle improvements in the pulse that a skilled practitioner could detect.

"The doctrine of signature, which has been discussed previously, can be applied here. To illustrate, walnut, in part, looks like the brain. Walnut essence stimulates neurological tissues, especially in the brain."

With many flower essences presented in this book, the test point has been described. The test point is the area in the body in which there is a physiological response with measurable results either through the body's functions or with diagnostic instruments. This enables one to determine which essence to prescribe. Press a particular test point and have someone hold out his or her arm to see how well they resist your pressing down that arm. Then the person holds a particular essence that either works well in that part of the body or that heals specific imbalances the person may have. You could also place the flower essence next to the afflicted organ or by a particular chakra point and again muscle test the person. Press the arm down and if the remedy is well chosen the arm would now be more resistant to this pressure. This procedure and variations of it are commonly practiced in America today.[1]

The pendulum can be utilized effectively to determine which flower essence or essences an individual needs. In working with a pendulum, you should already understand what the different pendulum movements mean before using it in diagnostic work. For instance, run the pendulum along a person's body and at a particular point of imbalance the pendulum gives a distinctly different response. Generally the pendulum swings clockwise, while over the area of disturbance it swings counterclockwise. Different people get different pendulum responses, so this is something the practitioner needs to carefully analyze.

Instead of using a pendulum for direct body application, it could be used with witnesses from a client. A witness is hair, saliva, or blood. Other witnesses such as a signature or a photo could be used, but this is recommended only for the skilled practitioner. The witness attunes the healer to the energy pattern of the patient.

Lists of flower essences arranged according to different psychological states and diseases can be used. After talking to the client to discover the main problems, check these lists. Put the person's witness on top of each list and if you get a positive pendulum swing, check the essences in that list to see if any are needed. I have, over the years, seen several people use this method quite effectively.

It is wise to cleanse a pendulum in pure sea salt, under a pyramid, or under the sun for half an hour every one or two months. Two or three of these cleansing techniques can be utilized together.[2]

Q Some feel the practitioner interferes with diagnosing flower essences more than with other vibrational remedies. Is this true, and if so, why?

"This tends to occasionally happen with healers also involved in spiritual practices because the essences are so attuned to realigning the consciousness. Thus, at times the personal prejudices of one's consciousness may interfere. There can be too close a merger of the consciousness of the healer and the flower essence. Clarity of thought by the practitioner concerning principles of diagnosis can solve this problem. Traditional practices such as meditation, creative visualization, and chanting aid in attaining this clarity. This problem occurs less often with homeopathic remedies and gem elixirs because they work closer to the principles of traditional medicine. There is then less interference with the practitioner's consciousness."

Q Can you discuss using flower essences in the traditional patient-client interview?

"This involves the skilled practitioner's sensitivities. There are no new principles to depict beyond what is commonly understood in this field. The healer should carefully listen to the patient's complaints to also involve the patient in the process. These procedures are already well documented."

More could be said about these various diagnostic practices, but that would be beyond the focus of this book. Many diagnostic techniques are available, and numerous books are in print that describe these procedures.

1 John Diamond, *Behavioral Kinesiology* (Los Angeles: Regent House, 1981).
John Thie, *Touch For Health* (Marina del Rey, CA: DeVorss & Co., 1973).
2 Tom Graves, *The Diviner's Handbook* (New York: Warner Books, 1977).
Francis Hitching, *Dowsing the Psi Connection* (New York: Anchor Press, 1978).
Aubrey Westlake, M.D., *The Pattern of Health* (Boulder, CO: Shambhala Publications, 1974).

Section II

Chapter 1

Information To Be Discussed
With Each Flower Essence

One hundred and twelve flower essences will be described in detail. These mostly common plants and trees have been divided into two groups. One section lists flower essences predominantly affecting the physical body, while flower essences in the other section mostly influence the psychological and spiritual nature. Some flower essences exclusively influence one of these two areas, but most have at least some impact on both areas. In most instances, male and female flower essences can be used interchangeably. In the few cases in which it is best that people use only the male or female prepared flower essence, this is stated.

Initially some botanical information is presented on each flower essence. This generally includes a listing of the native locale of the plant or tree, the exact Latin name of the species that is best to use, and a description of the flowers. Obviously, much more botanical information could be presented, but that information is readily available from many sources.

Usually, one species has superior properties, but in a few cases such as with maple any species is sufficient. The reason for this is as follows:

"In the course of evolution certain species have kept a common ancestry because they have not drifted too far apart. Thus, they are not too divided and separate vibrationally or in their genetic structure. The life force in these plants and trees remains similar because that same life force was not exerted to create so many new and different species. This close association is why the properties of these flower essences are similar."

In a number of instances such as with comfrey and dandelion, there is only one species in existence. In other cases such as with jasmine and star jasmine, two botanically different plants can be used interchangeably as flower essences. This is because of the following reason:

"While these plants or trees now appear botanically different, they originally separated from a single common ancestry. Vibrationally they continue to have similar properties. There are still some subtle differences in their clinical effects, however, that researchers can discover."

There is generally a brief commentary on the traditional medical use of each plant or tree when such information is available. This may include its use as an herb, homeopathic remedy, or essential oil. Not too much information is provided here because this information is available elsewhere.

Many plants and trees were formed in ancient Lemuria and Atlantis through the use of meditation and creative visualization to learn specific lessons for conscious growth, to help shape the body, and to manifest healing in mind, body, and spirit. It is wise to understand the historical origin and karmic pattern of flower essences because they usually still have similar effects on people. For instance, there was a highly charged emotional debate in Atlantis about the development and use of orange as a fruit and flower essence. Thus a pattern developed in which orange flower essence calms highly charged emotional states. This pattern was repeated a few years ago when Anita Bryant and the homosexual community had an intense emotional debate over the value of homosexuality. Anita Bryant was then a public figure partly because she represented Florida orange growers in the media.

The shape, color, texture, odor, taste, and nutrient qualities of many plants and trees are associated with the human body. This relationship is known as the doctrine of signature. This is another issue discussed with many flower essences.

Plants from the United States Southwest desert regions such as saguaro must have a degree of self-confidence and self-reliance to survive in such harsh climatic conditions. These same qualities are transferred to the flower essence. Conical or bell-shaped flowers when prepared as flower essences usually release information from the higher self by stimulating the mental body and left brain. Petunia exemplifies this pattern. With many plants and trees such as amaranthus and khat, the signature lies specifically in their innate medical properties. In such instances, the medical effects on the physical level, such as when the flower is used herbally, are usually transferred to the flower essence as part of the plant's signature.

As discussed in chapter I, this relationship exists because many plants and trees were formed before and during the existence of Lemuria and Atlantis to enhance spiritual growth and to stimulate mental, physical, and emotional cleansing. Consequently, the karmic origin of many plants and trees and their signature is often related. These plants and trees were originally created with the understanding that through the doctrine of signature they could be used to treat people.

Although the internal human form has changed considerably since early Lemuria, the doctrine of signature is still usually applicable for many flower essences. Bathing with flower essences is always wise because the metabolism is so purified that the body approaches the purity and consciousness attained in early Lemuria, which makes it easier to assimilate the life force from flower essences.

Occasionally, fruits and nuts offer clues concerning the clinical value of flower essence. When these trees originally developed, their fruits and nuts contained many healing and spiritual properties. During the course of evolution these properties were gradually transferred to the flowers. Even today, however, eating the fruit or nuts of many trees often has properties similar to, but milder than, the tree's flower essence.

The effect of flower essences on the physical body, including the cellular level, diseases, miasms, and nutrients are also considered. The anatomic level of the physical body consists of specific groupings of cellular tissue that genetically form into a specific organ such as the heart. The cellular level refers to the physical body, but on the level of each individual cell such as the individual neurological cells. The terms molecular and biomolecular refer to chemical activity on the subatomic level within each cell that organize into structures such as DNA and RNA to become genetic tissue. The term genetic refers to a specific function upon the cellular level. Cell mitosis or cell division is the dividing point between the cellular and molecular levels. The word biomagnetic refers to patterns and fields of magnetic energy that are generated as a by-product of molecular activity. This released energy extends out and becomes part of the aura. Mitogenic energy is the plasma-like quality that exists between the molecular and biomagnetic states.

Flower essences aid in assimilating nutrients, almost in a homeopathic fashion, partly because various nutrients exist in plants and trees. In such instances, this would be part of the flower essence's signature. Flower essences often profoundly affect many obscure trace minerals that western medicine is gradually coming to appreciate as having great value for the body to function properly. Except in a few cases, this information is not discussed in this text. To illustrate, chamomile flower essence enhances the assimilation of gold partly because traces of gold exist in this plant. Too little gold in the body is associated with most neurological diseases. This is why Edgar Cayce said gold is a good remedy for treating multiple sclerosis.[1]

As discussed in chapter VI, the miasms contribute to causing all chronic and many acute diseases. While many flower essences influence most miasms, only the miasms notably affected are mentioned with individual flower essences.

While reference is made to some devic orders with individual flower essences, most of this data will not be discussed in this text. Usually, nature spirits from specific devic orders attach themselves to different plants and trees. This understanding enhances the preparation and sometimes the clinical effectiveness of flower essences.

In many instances using flower essences externally as a salve, ointment, spray, or mouthwash is recommended. It is usually best to mix flower essences with essential oils because of their ethereal nature, but if used as a spray or mouthwash, pure or distilled water is generally sufficient. Even when the external use of a flower essence is not suggested, it can be rubbed over the body as a supportive therapy. On the other hand, when it is recommended to externally apply a flower essence, ingestion is still usually superior. The few exceptions involve flower essences that are notably effective in direct body treatment such as in acupuncture, massage, or chiropractic manipulation.

Rub the flower essence over the afflicted area, directly upon pressure points associated with specific internal organs, or over organs associated with different meridians and chakras. Externally applying flower essences is almost always a mild tonic and is especially valuable in acute problems. In addition, rubbing a flower essence over the palms, forehead, or medulla oblongata usually enhances spiritual growth.

Specific or general test points are usually recommended with each individual flower essence. A test point is a particular part of the body to which individual flower essences are attuned. If an essence eases heart problems then the heart might also be the test point for that essence. When specific test points do not exist for flower essences, general muscle testing can usually be done.

When a particular area is pressed, a person's outstretched arm will initially weaken rapidly when you press it down, if the person needs treatment in that area of the anatomy. If the person then holds the flower essence you are considering for prescription, the individual may sharply resist when you again press the arm down. This suggests that that remedy would ease the problem. If the arm still noticeably weakens when the person holds the flower essence, then that remedy will probably not be of much aid. It is easier to do this testing when a flower essence is a liquid, not a powder or a tablet. Many people today do this form of diagnosis.[2]

When the test point is a chakra or meridian, press an area in the physical body associated with these ethereal elements. For instance, if the test point is the heart chakra, use the heart as the focal point in the physical body. The chakras, and to a lesser extent the meridians, are often test points because they are often associated with high concentrations of nerve endings in the body. The medulla oblongata is often a test point because so much life force enters the physical body here.

Other areas which are considered with each flower essence include: chakras, meridians, nadis, subtle bodies, psychological and spiritual influences. Most flower essences affect people, at least to some degree, psychologically and spiritually. Again, this is because they work on realms of consciousness.

The meridians are passageways for the life force to enter the body. They lie between the etheric and physical bodies and have a direct association with the circulatory and nervous systems. The meridians connect the different acupuncture points in the body. As with the miasms, most flower essences influence the meridians, but the meridians are not mentioned unless particular flower essences especially influence them.

Chakras are centers of energy situated in the subtle anatomy. Spiritual information and life force is channeled into the body through the chakras. In traditional esoteric literature it is generally stated that there are seven chakras. In a few instances, twelve chakras are described.[3] These other five main chakras are on the two hands, on the two feet, and the medulla oblongata coordinated with the midbrain. Others consider the five chakras above the seventh chakra by the head region to be the next five most important chakras. In this text, when there is reference to the eighth to twelfth chakras the five chakras above the head are being referred to. My book *Gem Elixirs and Vibrational Healing,* Vol I has detailed information on these chakras not found in this text.

Unfortunately, only a few understand that there are just over 360 chakras in the human body. The exact number varies according to various ancient religious traditions. These many chakras are described in great technical detail in some of the ancient religious scriptures of India such as in some of the Upanishads and in ancient Egyptian, Mayan, and Atlantean texts. Although this information could be trance channeled, because it has existed in some of the Indian scriptures for thousands of years, it would be better if it were translated into several western languages. Alice A. Bailey[4] and several others have described some of these minor chakras.[5] Conscious people in the west are certainly ready for this new material. Practitioners of acupuncture, jin shin jyutsu, and shiatsu will find this new information especially helpful in their work. While the influence of the flower essences on minor chakras is described in some instances, most of this material will be discussed in a future text.

There has been much confusion in the literature concerning the organs associated with the seven main chakras.[6] This is because there are many minor chakras, and because there are two different chakra systems in the east and west. When these two chakra systems merge a new chakra system is created. For people in the west, the seven organs associated with the seven main chakras include: the testicles or ovaries for the first chakra, the spleen for the second chakra, the stomach or abdomen for the third chakra, the heart for the fourth chakra, the thyroid for the fifth chakra, the pituitary for the sixth chakra, and the pineal for the seventh chakra. People in the east have these organs associated with the seven main chakras: the coccyx for the first chakra, the testicles or ovaries for the second chakra, the stomach or abdomen for the third chakra, the thymus for the fourth chakra, the thyroid for the fifth chakra, the pituitary for the sixth chakra, and the pineal for the seventh chakra. It should not be surprising that people from different races have different organs associated with the seven main chakras.

"When people draw from eastern and western spiritual traditions or when individuals basically reach elevated states of consciousness, several parts of the body are activated in association with each of the seven main chakras. This activation may also occur when one moves between eastern and western cultures. These parts of the body function in polarity to balance the individual; the polarities created are as follows: the coccyx and testicles or ovaries represent the first chakra; the adrenals and pancreas represent the second chakra; the spleen and stomach or abdomen represent the third chakra; the thymus and heart represent the fourth chakra; and the thyroid and parasympathetic represent the fifth chakra. The pituitary and medulla oblongata represent the sixth chakra when the seventh chakra has not yet opened. When the seventh chakra is opened then the sixth chakra in the body is represented by a polarity between the pituitary and pineal glands. The seventh chakra is represented by the pineal gland and the left and right brain. To have a full awakening there must be a balanced trine of mind, body, and spirit."

Q Where exactly are the chakras located in the body? There is a debate in the literature concerning this issue.[7]

"They are focused in the neurological ganglions along the spine extending to the organs they are associated with. In their farthest extensions, the chakras extend to the front and back of the body. In addition, the chakras are oval, not circular in shape."

Unfortunately, the information available on how the seven chakras affect people is somewhat incomplete. Therefore, some information from the channeling will be presented.

"Proper stimulation of the first chakra eases all lower extremity diseases, particularly in the thighs' muscular tissue and circulation in the feet. Thus, this chakra enhances energy that enters the body through the feet, minor chakras in the feet are activated, and massage therapies associated with the feet are helped. This chakra eases diseases associated with disorientation, subtle or hidden fears, and diseases associated with the adrenals, particularly heart disease, stress, and anxiety.

"Opening this chakra releases past life talents to stabilize a person and develop strength of character. This chakra alleviates the heavy metal and syphilitic miasms.

The first chakra is especially linked to the etheric body. When this chakra is awakened, one initiates spiritual practices.

"The color red opens this chakra, and the color green closes it. Chakras need to be properly stimulated and balanced. Too much energy in a chakra can be just as unhealthy and even dangerous as too little energy.[8]

"The second chakra is associated with the testicles and ovaries; when properly opened it eases all sexual diseases and problems of infertility. Arthritic diseases associated with protein imbalances, general stiffening of the skeletal structure, and diseases linked to stress from internalized anger can be eased by balancing this chakra. Detoxification, particularly in the urinary tract, is augmented, and the gonorrhea, syphilitic, and radiation miasms are alleviated. This chakra also balances the body after overexposure to the earth's natural radiation.

"When the second chakra is properly balanced, creativity and an ability to integrate the emotions increases. The second chakra and the mental body are linked together. Orange opens this chakra, and turquoise closes it.

"All crippling diseases, ulcers, intestinal problems, spleen imbalances, psychosomatic diseases, and emotional problems can be treated by balancing the third chakra. And the psora and radiation miasms are eased. The white corpuscles and all nutrients are notably stimulated, and the emotions are integrated, so sensitivity and intuition increase. The astral, emotional, and etheric bodies are linked to this chakra. Yellow and white open the third chakra and brown closes it.

"The quality of Divine Love manifests in a person when the fourth chakra is awakened. All miasms, all nutrients, and all heart and childhood diseases are affected when this chakra is awakened. When this chakra is properly stimulated, one attains mastery of the immune system and thymus, particularly in the first seven years of life. Complete tissue regeneration can also develop. The astral, emotional, and spiritual bodies are connected to this chakra. Emerald opens and orange closes the fourth chakra.

"When the fifth chakra is properly awakened, diseases in the immune system, neurological system, throat, and upper bronchials are relieved. And health in the entire endocrine system improves. Psychosomatic diseases and illnesses resulting from suppressing the self can be treated by stimulating this chakra. There is greater interest in spiritual affairs, and this interest is stimulated in others. Blue opens this chakra, while red, orange, and yellow close it.

"The sixth chakra stimulates the pituitary gland, the immune system, creative visualization, and visions. It is linked to the spiritual and soul bodies. Indigo opens and scarlet closes this chakra.

"When the seventh chakra is properly stimulated, there is alignment with the higher forces. Other activities concerning this chakra will be discussed in the future."

In this revised edition new information is presented on the five key chakras above the head. Thus, when there is reference to the eighth, ninth, tenth, eleventh, or twelfth chakras that is in reference to these five chakras. Further information on these chakras is presented in *Gem Elixirs and Vibrational Healing,* Vol I.

The nadis are petals inside the chakras. They distribute the life force and energy of each chakra into the physical and subtle bodies. Their energy sources are within the chakras, and these are magnified in patterns so that different resonances of each nadi provide energetic pathways into the physical and subtle bodies. They also exist at the boundaries between all the subtle bodies and the physical body. They are also particularly active in the interacting points between each chakra and the associated subtle body. There are approximately 72,000 nadis or ethereal channels of energy in the subtle anatomy, which are interwoven with the nervous system. The nadis are like an ethereal nervous system.[9] There are not too many flower essences that influence the nadis, but they are so important that it was felt best to include this subject when discussing each flower essence.

In considering the subtle bodies, there is the etheric body, emotional body, mental body, astral body, causal body, soul body, and integrated spiritual body. The integrated spiritual body represents a combination of these other subtle bodies and the physical body. These subtle bodies spread out from the physical body in the above order, respectively. There is also the aura, the ethereal fluidium, and the thermal body, which are connected to the subtle bodies.

The information in this text on the subtle bodies is among the most important in the book because of their great role in health, disease, and spiritual growth. One of the important new steps in modern medicine will be to understand the role of the subtle bodies in health and disease.[10] The subtle bodies have been discussed by many authors, but Steiner and Bailey in their many books provide real detail on the proper role of these bodies in our daily lives.

"In true health, the subtle bodies are perfectly aligned with each other. There is a thin wall encasing each subtle body, and they should exist in a certain area about the physical body. Flower essences often restore imbalances in these bodies. For instance, zinnia essence generates a good balance between the physical and emotional bodies, which creates a good sense of humor. A few flower essences such as lotus, pomegranate, and redwood temporarily align all the subtle bodies. When this happens, toxicity is released from the physical and subtle bodies, so vibrational remedies work better and positive personality changes result.

"Psychological problems and disease result when the subtle bodies are misaligned—they are too close or too far apart from each other or the properties of one subtle body spills over into another subtle body.[11] For instance, when the mental and emotional bodies are improperly linked with the etheric body, anxiety results. When the mental body spills over into the emotional body, mental lethargy and a loss of confidence ensues. Or when the mental and emotional bodies are too close, frustration, unknown fears, and an inability to divide emotional and mental issues transpires.

"Except for the etheric body, all the subtle bodies enter the physical body mainly through one area. The physical and etheric bodies are so intertwined that there is no one focal point. The emotional body is usually connected to the physical through the stomach, the astral body through the kidneys, the mental body through the left brain, the causal body through the medulla oblongata, the soul body through the pineal gland, and the spiritual body through the pituitary gland. The right brain balances all these associations.

"This subject can be confusing partly because esoteric groups in different cultures call the same subtle bodies by different names. For instance, the eastern atmic body is almost the same as the western astral body. The arrangement and even the actual existence of some subtle bodies varies in different cultures and amongst different people as individuals make spiritual progress.[12] The chakras and subtle bodies are quite alike in this regard.

"The ethereal fluidium is part of the etheric body that surrounds every cell in the physical body. It is the vehicle used to feed the life force into each cell. Such a vehicle is needed to transfer energy between the physical body and the ethereal dimensions. These higher energies are then organically bound and assimilated into the physical body. Nutrients are assimilated more easily and miasms, genetic diseases, and viral or bacterial attacks are averted when the ethereal fluidium functions normally.

"In health, the ethereal fluidium is evenly distributed throughout the physical body with a slight enhancement in red blood cells. Its crucial points of storage are the colon, lymphs, muscles, skin, stomach, and thermal body. Even a non-psychic person can see its activities under a microscope. Occasionally it is observed as orgone energy. It is orgone in a more stable state as it makes a transference to the physical body. The place to observe the ethereal fluidium is on the outer walls of cell tissue.

"The etheric body is the interface between the physical and subtle bodies. It maintains a proper balance between these two areas. When the etheric body is weakened, diseases and karmic problems residing in the aura and subtle bodies tend to move into the physical body.

"The thermal body is a force field about the physical body that consists of the outer extension of the etheric body and the physical body's heat. This heat, which comes from normal cell division and the body's electromagnetic energy, is regulated by metabolism and the thyroid. While the etheric body consists of just ethereal properties, the thermal body is the by-product of physical body activities.

"The emotional body provides a sense of emotional stability and psychological security. In contrast, the mental body enables people to think in a clear and rational manner.

"The astral body is the total accumulation of the personality. It acts as a screen to filter karmic patterns and information from past lives into one's consciousness.

"The causal body links the entire personality with the collective consciousness of the planet. It is a doorway to higher consciousness and a key to attunement with astrological influences. Past life information is coordinated here and then released by the astral body.

"The soul body holds the essence of the spirit that is as God.

"The aura is different from the subtle bodies. The aura's field is a general pattern of biomagnetic energy that surrounds and reflects the physiological and metabolic processes of the physical body. It creates a balanced polarity in the system. While subtle bodies also reflect the activities of the body's physiological and metabolic processes, they are specific fields of energy that incorporate magnetic, orgone, and electromagnetic energies. The various subtle bodies are specific bands of different types of energy at set distances from the physical body. The subtle bodies coordinate and regulate the soul's activity on the physical plane."

In this revised edition new information is presented with each flower essence regarding their affect on animals, plants, the twelve rays, and with various astrological configurations. Later, there will be more information presented on how flower essences can be used in these areas.

"Some information has been withheld or has been deliberately presented symbolically with individual flower essences to stimulate the reader's intuition. Otherwise, this would be but an intellectual exercise. The intellect must always have flexibility so that the mind may translate into spirit. The brief comments on the karmic background and signature of certain essences exemplify this pattern.

"There is little data presented on some flower essences because they are more enhancers that are best used in combination with other flower essences or other healing agents. As to slight differences in clinically using these flower essences when two or more of them have similar impacts on the same area, such as fear or depression, this, for the present, is left to discerning researchers.

"While some might be skeptical in believing that flower essences can create noticeable, positive changes in people, especially in physical diseases, there are now numerous cases in the medical literature in which advanced physical diseases have been cured mainly with meditation and creative visualization.[13] Western medicine is only now beginning to appreciate how much the mind can cause and cure disease."

1 *Medicines For the New Age* (Virginia Beach, VA: Heritage Publications, 1977), p. 27-28.

2 John Diamond, *Behavioral Kinesiology* (Los Angeles: Regent House, 1981).

3 Ann Ree Colton, *Kundalini West* (Glendale, CA: ARC Publishing Co., 1978), p. 38-39.

4 Alice A. Bailey, *Esoteric Healing* (New York: Lucis Publishing Co., 1980), p. 72-73, 465-466.

5 *Sri Chinmoy, Kundalini: The Mother-Power* (Jamaica, New York: Agni Press, 1974), p. 7.

David Tansley, D.C., *Subtle Body* (London: Thames & Hudson, 1977), p. 26.

Swami Vyas Dev Ji, *Science of Soul* (Rishikesh, India: Yoga Niketan Trust, 1972), p. 66-67.

6 C. W. Leadbeater, *The Chakras* (Wheaton, IL: The Theosophical Publishing House, 1977).

Ray Stanford, *The Spirit Unto the Churches* (Austin, TX: Association For the Understanding of Man, 1977).

7 David Tansley, D.C., *Subtle Body* (London: Thames & Hudson, 1977), p. 26.

8 Alice A. Bailey, *Esoteric Healing* (New York: Lucis Publishing Co., 1980), p. 37-38, 76-81, 207-209.

9 _____. *Ibid*, p. 195-197, 333.

10 _____. *Ibid*, p. 2-4, 197, 273.

11 _____. *Esoteric Psychology* II (New York: Lucis Publishing Co., 1975), p. 313.

12 _____. *Esoteric Healing*, (New York: Lucis Publishing Co., 1980), p. 343-344.

13 Francine Butler, *Biofeedback: A Survey of the Literature* (New York: Plenum Publishers, 1978).

Lois Wingerson, "Training to Heal the Mind," *Discovery*, Vol. 3, No. 5 (May, 1982), 80-85.

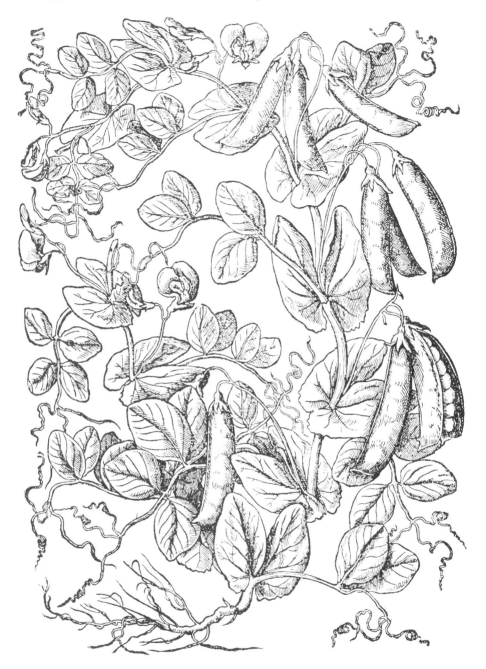

Garden Pea

Chapter II

Flower Essences Effecting Primarily the Physical Body

Almond
Aloe Vera
Amaranthus
Apricot
Avocado
Banana
Bells of Ireland
Blackberry
Bottlebrush
Camphor
Cedar
Celandine
Centuary Agave
Chamomile (German)
Coffee
Comfrey
Cotton
Dandelion

Date Palm
Fig
Forget Me Not
Four Leaf Clover
  (Shamrock)
Ginseng
Grapefruit
Hawthorne (English)
Hops
Jasmine
Khat
Koenign Van
  Daenmark
Lilac
Loquat
Luffa
Manzanita
Marigold (French)

Mugwort
Pansy
Paw Paw (American)
Redwood
Saguaro
Self Heal
Snapdragon
Spice Bush
Spiderwort
Spruce
  (Colorado or Blue)
Squash
Star Jasmine
Star Tulip
Sugar Beet
Watermelon
Wisteria (Chinese)
Yerba Mate

Flower Essences Effecting Primarily
Ethereal and Psychological States

Angelica
Bleeding Heart
Bloodroot
Blue Flag-Iris
Bo
Borage
California Poppy
Carob
 (St. John's Bread)
Chaparral
Clover (Red)
Corn (Sweet)
Cosmos
Daffodil
Daisy
Dill
Eucalyptus
Garlic
Green Rose
Harvest Brodiaea
Helleborus (Black)
Henna

Hyssop
Lavender(French)
Lemon
Live Forever
Loosestrife
Lotus
Macartney Rose
Madia
Mallow
Mango
Maple (Sugar)
Morning Glory
Mullein
Nasturtium
Nectarine
Onion
Orange
Papaya
Passion Flower
Peach
Pear
Pennyroyal

Petunia
Pimpernel
 (Scarlet or Red)
Pomegranate
Prickly Pear Cactus
Queen Anne's Lace
Rosa Webbiana
Rosemary
Sage
St. John's Wort
Shooting Star
Skullcap
Stinging Nettle
Sunflower
Sweet Flag
Sweet Pea
Thyme
Tuberose
Wood Betony
Yarrow
Yerba Santa
Zinnia

Description of Flower Essences Effecting Primarily the Physical Body

ALMOND
Prunus Amygdalus

This popular nut tree produces white flowers tinged with pink. Almond, and its oil, are used to treat kidney, bladder, and respiratory problems.

Q What is the karmic background of this tree?

"Karmically this particular plant form arose from dissension in the consciousness of the Atlantean people and from the development of personally applied will power. This essence eased karmic patterns that became internalized tensions and developed into stress-related diseases. Individuals bent their will unto the self in Atlantis and then internalized same so that cancerous accords sometimes developed. This particular plant form was developed in the time periods stretching between Lemuria and Atlantis when dissension developed as to the application and direction of society and its social framework. Cancer, in part, then began to develop more rapidly because of environmental stress and the use of radiation."

Elsewhere John has pointed out that nuclear power was extensively used in early Atlantis, but the dangers of this power were soon understood. As solar and quartz crystal technologies developed, nuclear power was completely abandoned. Much of this nuclear material was buried in the American West; this is one reason why uranium is now being discovered in this region. As early Atlantean society developed an interest in advanced technologies, many people, accustomed to the Lemurian attunement with nature, experienced tensions that caused diseases. Many Atlanteans misused will power. Almond was developed to solve these problems.

Q How is the tree now used as a flower essence?

"Almond fosters maturation by stimulating growth patterns for children undergoing any form of stunted growth such as dwarfism, and it helps one mature mentally. The key is its application to the pituitary and somewhat to the thymus and adrenals. These organs are important for the proper distribution of hormones throughout the body. But more than anything else, almond invigorates the entire endocrine system, which is the key to the maturing process. Cancer especially if caused by tension can also be treated with almond.

"On the cellular level, it stimulates the exchange between the DNA and RNA. As an interesting test, add this essence to a culture of bacteria, perhaps with cells from an older person. Cells treated with almond would divide and grow faster than the same untreated cells.

"Almond strengthens the etheric body, which augments its role as the gateway between the physical and subtle bodies. If you have trouble solving a problem such as constant fear, almond brings this fear into consciousness from the mental body so it can be confronted and resolved.

"The flowers appear a long time before the leaves in young almond trees and just before them on adult trees. This signature is a clue to the fact that the almond essence influences the aging process.

"The one psychological syndrome to look for here is a fear of aging. Almond can be used to treat the petrochemical miasm, it mildly influences the throat chakra, and it can be used externally. The second ray is enhanced. The test point is the joy-of-life point just above each elbow. Orgone energy is concentrated here, thus this point vitalizes the body.

"There is some enhancement of the parent-to-infant animal relationship. Thus, it is excellent to provide after an animal has given birth, especially in the early part of an animal's life until it is about six months old. This is particularly true with birds, dogs, cats, and other domesticated animals. It is also useful as the animal is beginning to reach adulthood, when there are signs of stress in dealing with the outside environment and influence of other animals outside those of the immediate family of the animal.

"There is a strengthening of plants in their final stages just before going to seed. For those who have difficulty bringing a plant to seed and getting sufficient quantities almond may increase seed production. Some negative aspects of the planet Saturn are alleviated."

ALOE VERA

This plant originated in Eastern and Southern Africa. It has been cultivated in the West Indies since the sixteenth century and is often called Barbados or Curacao Aloe. Yellow to purplish flowers evident much of the year grow in long racemes. Aloe vera contains a jelly-like pulp which has been used as a cosmetic and healing agent since ancient times. Aloe vera is mainly prescribed for burns, boils, cuts, psoriasis, insect bites, and internal and external ulcers.

Q What is the karmic background of this plant?

"This particular plant form was developed in Lemuria to bring forth balance and the ability of personal survival in harsh climates. That it is now native to desert-like climates is a perpetuation from those origins."

Q How is aloe vera now used as a flower essence?

"Some of the plant's herbal properties are transferred to the flower essence. It is excellent for treating most carcinogenic conditions, especially tumors, leukemia, and cancer in which there is a general breakdown or degeneration of tissue."

Q Would it be wise to combine the flower essence and aloe vera juice to treat cancer?

"Yes, it would often help to take aloe vera juice internally, and in certain skin cancers or tumors the juice can be massaged over the body.

"Aloe vera is effective for many skin conditions, especially burns and lacerations. It can be added to essential oils. Put a few drops of the essence on your hands and rub that over the person's body. Then apply the oil, or oils, that you use. This enhances the transference of energy from the oil into the person.

"Another function of aloe vera is to stimulate the nervous system. The circulatory flow is also increased, particularly when the essence is rubbed over the skin. If rubbed on the feet, it improves the effects of reflexology. In addition, upset stomachs and indigestion are relieved by aloe vera.

"Insights normally stored in the heart chakra are activated. The essence makes you more sensitive to other people. It augments the etheric body which allows the ethereal fluidium to flow freely between the cells, particularly for healing various skin conditions. Lacerations or holes in the physical and etheric bodies are alleviated. Prescribe aloe vera in some cases of obsession caused by holes in the aura. Such cases are often associated with past life emotional obstructions that seek to fuse with the aura in a disjointed manner.

"Aloe vera stimulates the astral body leading, in some cases, to mediumistic properties such as clairaudience or hearing inner voices or sounds perhaps from your spirit guides. This process can be enhanced by putting a few drops from the essence on the end of a cotton wick. Put that into your ear and remove the wax, but do not touch your ear in the process.

"Concerning its signature, the leaves are rather tough with little points along the edge. This symbolizes its ability to heal lacerations on the physical and etheric bodies, for if the plant were abused it could cause lacerations in a person. The test point is the palm side of each thumb on both hands.

"Significant trauma can manifest in behavioral difficulties when animals do not seem to follow patterns already set up for them by an owner or keeper. As these may relate to deep emotional states otherwise inaccessible to the animal's will, aloe vera brings this closer to consciousness allowing the human working with the animal to assist in rebuilding behavioral patterns. This essence is indicated when a deep traumatic stress is the clear cause of these behavioral difficulties.

"Two or more years after a fire, if there is continued difficulty in growing a plant in that area, particularly a plant that previously grew there with some success, use this essence. Aloe vera will close the etheric hole in the earth that is sometimes created by a fire. Normally, these etheric holes close in about 12 years. Place three drops in the center and one or two drops in the corners of the land. This should be sufficient even though it may cover a fairly large area. Some prayer and meditation along with the flower essence will also assist. Negative aspects from the conjunction of Neptune and Mars will be eased. The second and third rays are stimulated."

AMARANTHUS
Amaranthus Hypochondriacus

This tall annual is native to the tropics. Its flowers are deeply crimson-red or gold, densely packed on erect spikes. The bloom appears in August. It was prominently grown by the Aztecs as a food crop, but the invading Spaniards destroyed it. Today, in the United States, it is again becoming popular as a garden flower and food plant. To the ancient Greeks it symbolized immortality. It is an astringent and is taken internally for diarrhea or dysentery.

Q How is this plant used as a flower essence?
"This essence stimulates the thymus and pituitary glands, and it augments the immune system to repel viral and bacterial inflammations. It increases interferon in

cells to fight invading viruses. Prescribe amaranthus in a wide range of diseases in which the immune system is under strain."

Q Is amaranthus effective in treating mental illnesses?

"Yes, for disorientation or stress placed on the body from the body's chemical imbalances. A person subject to hallucinations, attention-span disorientation, too many radical dreams, or autism and schizophrenia can be treated with amaranthus.

"Amaranthus' gold flowers stimulate messages from the higher self and activate visionary capacities from the pituitary gland. One experiencing hallucinations could need an essence from the gold flowers. In contrast, amaranthus' red flowers tend to treat disruptive dreams coming from the biological levels, especially imbalances in the immune system.

"Amaranthus is good for treating AIDS. It also assists in bringing out negative thought forms around issues of courage and sexuality, especially intimacy with individuals who already have AIDS. Amaranthus and corn are soothing to the spine, but this is a rare occurrence. If you attune to other properties of these essences, this property may apply.

"Protein assimilation and enzyme activity are stimulated. Absorption of nutrients from the amino acids increases. Dysfunction in the physical body's biochemical patterns on the cellular level are corrected.

"The emotional, mental, and spiritual bodies are aligned. This generates clear thinking in hallucinations or disruptive dream states. The heart and pituitary chakras are activated by amaranthus. The test point is the medulla oblongata.

"A balancing of an animal's emotional state after the death of an animal close to it will be noted. This is because amaranthus increases the sense of courage within an animal.

"Plants not native to a particular area will sometimes be enhanced by using amaranth. They will grow more easily in areas that they had not previously been used to. This must be within the bounds and constraints of usual temperature and growth conditions, but within these boundaries there can still be occasional difficulties in growing plants not native to a region. Transits of the Moon through the natal sun will usually be eased, and the fourth and sixth rays are enhanced."

APRICOT
Prunus Armeniaca

This popular fruit tree produces flowers with white or pinkish obovate petals. An oil extracted from the seed is used in the manufacture of perfume and soap.

Q What is the karmic background of this plant?

"This particular plant was developed by a group of Lemurian horticulturists who wanted a supplement to the properties of papaya, but in part, through deliberate horticulture development, it has deviated from same developing its own peculiar properties."

Q How is this plant now used as a flower essence?

"Apricot has applications similar to laetrile. It alleviates cancerous tumors and relieves gall bladder stones and crystals, especially when they lodge in the muscles. Inflammations associated with these problems can also be treated with apricot.

Apricot also treats what are considered dormant parts of the body or secondary organs or glands. To illustrate, the appendix, when not in an acute stage, can be purified. If it is swelling and ready to burst, it might be thrown into remission with large doses of this essence, but it would be safer to also use other remedies.

"Apricot strengthens the pancreas. It changes one form of sugar into another, so sugar imbalances in the system can be adjusted. Glucose is distributed more evenly, blood sugar levels are regulated, and extreme behavioral patterns associated with high or low blood sugar levels are modified. The moodiness of hypoglycemia and diabetes ease. The assimilation of proteins, all minerals, and vitamin C and B are enhanced.

"Apricot develops women's breasts and the fatty tissues in the buttocks is strengthened. This is associated with the nature and shape of the fruit. Apricot controls weight because it has such an influence on blood sugars and fatty tissue.

"Mental agitation in the mental body is kept from moving into the etheric body. Such movement causes allergies in the physical body by causing blockages in the eliminative tissues and organs such as the kidneys. Stress placed on the kidneys produces many allergies and toxemia in the physical body. Apricot stimulates the mental body in a specific manner, so stress in the kidneys is relieved.

"Various concepts or ideas generally present in the mental body may be difficult for a person to live with. They may be difficult to understand, apply, or work with, yet they remain. They must in some way be denied in order for one not to be obsessed with them or to struggle with them. This will often cause some part of the other subtle anatomies to interfere. Usually, the emotional body will create an emotional block. The etheric body can also transfer subtle energies throughout the nervous system, particularly in the brain, where mental body energies may coordinate with physical presence. The physical cells, in capturing these various nerve impulses and working with them on a physical level, can be interfered with by the etheric body. The trouble with this is that the energies transferred to the etheric body must manifest in some form. Usually, it will begin as a mishap or difficult aspect with one's image of oneself. Thus, that part of the body begins to shift. This can relate to such difficulties as problems with the complexion, skin cancer, or other difficulties with the skin. This changes fairly rapidly.

"The chakra opened is at the very tip of the shortest finger on each hand. This chakra stabilizes various pulses throughout the body. The devas associated with apricot have a certain gaiety and lightness. This is again related to the plant's influence on moods. Apricot can also be applied externally, and it eases the petrochemical miasm.

"This is a general tonic and strengthener for animals. The canine kingdom will be particularly receptive to using this essence to release negative thought forms relating to the cancer miasm and other difficulties associated with cancer that are absorbed from humans. This may be especially prevelant if you have a dog and you or someone close to you is struggling with cancer. In about five or six years, this will also apply to cats. Leukemia is now moving through the feline kingdom, but the full permeation of the cancer miasm and negative thought forms associated with it have not yet been fully transmitted from humans to cats. However, this process is nearly complete with dogs. Squares between natal Mars and natal Pluto are eased. This is a lifelong tendency for most people. The fifth ray is stimulated, and the test point is the jaw."

AVOCADO
Persea Americana

While this tree is native to Central America, it is now found in many tropical regions. The small greenish flowers are followed by pear-shaped, green fruit, which have an unusually high protein content.

Q How is this tree now used as a flower essence?

"It works with the body's eliminative processes, specifically the liver, kidneys, and lymphs. Avocado is a blood cleanser, it rejuvenates the muscular tissue, and it eases ulcers. It isolates tumors and restores the appetite to people with advanced cancer, but this would only delay the progress of cancer. However, avocado could be used in combination with other remedies to reverse cancer in the system. And it removes inflammations in the mid-brain. This particular effect was more applicable in Lemuria when the mid-brain was the seat of consciousness.

"Avocado helps the body to more efficiently assimilate proteins and chlorophyll, particularly in the lower intestinal tract. It stabilizes radical emotional fluctuations because of its influence on the proteins. And it actualizes telepathic abilities, intuition, and the ability to see auras.

"A heightened sense of touch develops, so a person becomes more sensitive to being touched. It could even be considered an aphrodisiac. Client and massage therapists could take this internally or rub it on their hands, and it would assist each person in the process. It would, for instance, prevent the magnification of negative emotional states in either party.

"Some of the new touch therapies could be enhanced with this remedy. Emotional states become clarified and amplified, which puts the individual in closer touch with these feelings. The overly intellectual person develops increased understanding of suppressed feelings, and some cases of impotency and frigidity can be overcome.

"It is a common misunderstanding that touching each other is primarily associated with infantile needs. Touching people is also a mature expression and normal balancing of masculine and feminine qualities. Avocado partly creates these influences because it augments the emotional body dissolving emotional tensions, and it opens the third chakra, which is associated with emotional issues.

"The green color of the flower and fruit symbolizes its impact on chlorophyll in the system. Under a microscope the flowers look like neurons in the mid-brain. Central parts of the tree, under magnification, look remarkably like the muscular cellular tissue, which is strengthened by avocado. The test point is the solar plexus where many emotions and nerve endings are stored.

"Growth spurts are sustained in animals. Thus, when you change the diet and new minerals or new substances with growth potential are added to the animal's diet, better assimilation will result. Similar growth spurts through enhanced absorption will be seen with larger plants. This is an especially useful essence to provide in the spring with trees. The first and sixth rays are stimulated. "

BANANA
Musa Paradisiaca

This tropical plant, which grows to thirty feet, produces yellow flowers in clusters. There are many cultivated varieties of this popular fruit.

Q How is this plant now used as a flower essence?

"Banana is very physical in its effects. It treats the bone structure, including the subluxation of any bones, particularly in the sacrum and spine. It also strengthens the bone marrow, especially in its attachment to the teeth. Banana could be used in certain periodontal diseases in which there is a loss of support in the bone level at the gum line. The bone structure in the jaw is rejuvenated. It can be used in temperomandibular problems. It can be applied to the jaw as a salve, or it can be ingested as a mouth wash. Take three to seven drops in one or two ounces of pure water several times a day until the overt problem eases, or for several weeks.

"The assimilation of calcium, iron oxide, phosphorus, and zinc increase. If there is a tendency for poor absorption and low body weight, take banana essence with germanium. The body assimilates such sugars as fructose and glucose and transforms them from one form into another to properly utilize these substances as energy.

"Banana is a tonic, more than a cure, for blood sugar problems such as diabetes and hypoglycemia. It helps in weight problems when sugars get assimilated improperly into the system. Inflammations in the skin tissue, which are allergic reactions to the transference of one form of sugar into another, are eased with this essence. Some forms of acne and eczema result from too much sugar in the body and an attempt to eliminate this through the skin because the skin is an organ of elimination. Banana is more effective in treating the moodiness caused by these states.

"The sweetness of the fruit represents its association with yin qualities, which the essence accentuates, while in the interior of the fruit there is an astringent taste symbolizing the yang qualities, which the essence weakens. While the essence balances male and female sexuality and thus the yin and yang qualities, it is more applicable for the male. The shape of the fruit symbolizes its relation to male sexuality.

"This essence deals with the male and his relation to women in sexual issues and insecurities associated with male sexuality. Banana is applicable in Freudian psychotherapy to help men, and to a lesser extent women, establish a truer sense of identity with their feminine nature. This essence negates male sexual machismo. As part of its signature, notice that it grows in Latin countries, where this is often a problem."

Q Autistic children often love or hate bananas, but no one really understands why. Why does this attitude exist, and would banana essence be relevant to this condition?

"Autism, in part, is caused by mixed brain dominance or an imbalance in the left and right spheres of the brain. As stated above, banana—the fruit and the flower essence—eases an overly yang nature and accentuates the yin qualities in an individual. When an autistic child craves a banana, it is because he is too yang, and when that person abhors a banana, it is because he already has sufficient yin attributes. There is a mild opiate-like substance in the banana, mostly in its peel, which relieves some of the chemical imbalances associated with autism. A similar substance exists in the pineal and pituitary glands. It also maintains a proper balance between the left and right brain. It has been isolated by orthodox scientists, but its properties are not yet understood.

"Banana essence enables general mineral and sugar substances found in banana to be more assimilable through pathways in the physical body that are not usually accessible by other means. This also transfers to the banana essence in that these vibrations become more assimilable into the subtle bodies and other pathways than people have normally set out for themselves in their lives. In autism there is usually a powerful pathway of withdrawal that excludes much communication with others. Banana essence creates new bridges so that the person may more easily choose ways to better communicate with others.

"Banana balances the emotional and mental bodies, which helps resolve sexual conflicts. The ninth chakra is stimulated. It alleviates the syphilitic miasm, and the test point is the bladder or kidney meridian points on the outside of the ankle.

"Food patterns significantly affected by humans working with domesticated pets can be a problem. This occurs when an animal in eating scraps, leftovers, or other food provided by humans, seemingly becomes addicted to such foods. Banana will assist in releasing this addiction, as animals may then find it easier to reacclimate to food appropriate for them. This is particularly true with sugar substances or sweet foods in general. For nondomesticated animals there is also benefit. This is particularly true when the foods these animals are being fed are produced in unnatural ways, such as with chemical fertilizers and pesticides. Banana will not directly counterbalance some of these effects but it will help rebalance the animal's own ability to correctly absorb the proper nutrients from such foods.

"There is some ability to ease difficulties that most plants have with excessive salinity in ground water. This may be noted during a drought or when increased agricultural use of water has caused certain minerals to leech into the soil and through the soil into the water table. Salt will increase at the same time. The movement of water will sweep away most effects of salt within a few days, so banana essence can be directly applied to water used with such plants. There may be a well near the plants so that the ground water moving up through the well is the same source of water that is available to the plants through secondary absorption by the plants' roots through the soil. Add three drops of banana to the well water about once every three or four days to counteract the effects of excessive salinity.

"Positive aspects, particularly trines between Jupiter and Venus are enhanced. And the third and fourth rays are activated."

BELLS OF IRELAND
Malluccella Laevis

This annual originated in Asia Minor. Its green flowers bloom from late winter until early spring. When the flowers are picked a white sticky sap gushes from the stem.

Q What are the clinical effects of this flower essence?

"The main application of this flower essence lies in its signature, i.e., the plant's sticky sap. It works with portions of the physical and subtle anatomies that act almost like binding agents or glue. This notably includes the connective tissues and ethereal fluidium. It also increases male and female fertility and infertility, and it revitalizes the vaginal fluids. This is because male sperm is a binding agent between the male and female, and the ovaries and vaginal fluids are part of this process.

"While bells of Ireland has tissue regeneration capacities for the entire system, this effect is accentuated in the above described parts of the anatomy. It alleviates the radiation miasm, and connective tissue degenerative diseases. All degenerative diseases involve a misalignment of the ethereal fluidium surrounding the cellular walls.

"Bells of Ireland makes one more sensitive to receive light therapies such as color therapy. When the etheric body is stimulated light therapies become more effective because this is the connective point into the physical body by which light therapies are carried into the cellular structure vibrationally.

"Intense stress, anxiety, or nervous tension are eased with this remedy. All nutrients are more easily absorbed into the system, and the test point is the solar plexus. Psychic abilities, especially communication with nature spirits are stimulated by this essence. This usually occurs with green flowers.

"It is useful in the breeding season with animals and in old age when an animal is injured and regeneration appears impaired. This is similar to its properties for humans. There is some difference with the breeding season and certain issues of regeneration. Receptivity to new pictures about regeneration and correct breeding practices are made more available to the animal. Within about ten minutes of giving animals this essence, visualize or focus the new change within the animal. Receptivity to your thought picture will be enhanced within animals.

"Use this essence during cross-fertilization, particularly when intervening processes such as bees are involved. The properties of this essence will be strengthened when the Moon or Mars are in Scorpio. The effect of the fifth and eighth rays increases."

BLACKBERRY
Rubus Villosus

This perennial plant is commonly found in the Northeastern and Midwestern United States. The white, five-petaled flowers appear from June to September. It has traditionally been used for treating diarrhea, leucorrhea, bleeding gums, and appendicitis.

Q How is this plant now used as a flower essence?

"Blackberry is efficacious when an individual is in a lethargic or disassociated state that dissolves when the person sits down and rests for awhile to collect his or her thoughts. It is also appropriate for the fears of a dying person or for an unusual fear that someone is going to die. And it eases depression that sometimes results from the passing of a loved one. It would be perfectly ethical to give this to people to help them confront these feelings; however, this should often be done in combination with therapy.

"It stimulates the kidneys, liver, and various rhythmic processes throughout the body.[1] This includes, for instance, the heart and lungs. It helps the blood absorb food throughout the body. Through the capillary action, the blood penetrates deeper into the ductless glands receiving more of their hormonal properties. In this process, the entire endocrine system is purified.

"Fertility in barren women is stimulated. In addition, blackberry treats the tubercular miasm and certain forms of genetic diseases. Researchers can explore this. On the cellular level, it enhances mitosis. Excessive concern with death has a negative effect on the reproductive rate of cells. Cells divide a specific number of times; in fact, the rate is highest in youth and slowest in old age.

"Blackberry brings the causal and spiritual bodies closer to the physical body in an integrated fashion. This essence then becomes almost a liquid meditation. Put some blackberry essence into a bottle, then meditate and project a thought form of a specific problem into the bottle. You would often have a vision or dream revealing a solution to the problem. Dormant talents from past-life experiences might be released. It is also excellent to take before going to sleep as higher teachings may be revealed in dreams.

"The chakra point by the armpits is opened. This chakra helps the body to more consistently take in orgone energy, which creates a greater sense of vitality. Vitamin E and all the minerals, especially iron, are assimilated more easily into the system.

"The small cluster of flowers looks somewhat like the inner nucleus of the cell, particularly the red and white corpuscles. The plant is associated with certain Kachina devic orders. It is also attached to a devic order that is associated with the mound builders in the center of the United States centuries ago.

"There is an increased ability to work with unusual environmental situations causing the animal depression and with states similar to those described for this flower essence with humans. When the animal is by itself for a while it appears to recover. However, going deeper, this essence assists animals that are seeking to make changes in their own nature. They may be attempting to learn something new. Use blackberry, sometimes with other essences, when you are teaching an animal something that is entirely new but is something they also have enthusiasm for.

"Take it when Venus and Mercury are in conjunction. Added strength may be felt. The effect of the first and second rays increases."

1. Rudolf Steiner often spoke of the rhythmic processes in the body.
Rudolf Steiner, *Spiritual Science and Medicine* (London: Rudolf Steiner Press, 1975).

BOTTLEBRUSH
Callistemon Viminalis

This evergreen tree, which is native to Australia, is now common in Florida and California. The red flowers are densely packed in terminal, cylindrical spikes resembling a bottle brush in size and shape.

Q What is the karmic background of this tree?

"Originally, in early Lemuria, there was the development of conditions wherein that for all to be able to develop their faculties to the fullest accord the limited resources of the crystalline technologies in those days called for a strong need and ability of cooperation. This plant was specifically developed and given for levels of cooperation under high degrees of population during the time periods before the development of other mineral resources and crystalline beds. This was in early Lemuria before there was the ability of fully materializing the properties that they needed."

In early Lemuria, as the science of luminosity developed, quartz crystals were used in various meditative and spiritual practices. Gradually, it was discovered that many other minerals could be used in these practices. Bottlebrush was then created in the then developing science of luminosity. This cooperation was especially important because there was such a high population density.

Q How is bottlebrush flower essence now used?

"This essence can be used for treating the muscular tissue when there is physical exhaustion. It is good for athletes specifically because it eliminates lactic acid, which develops during strenuous exercise. It also strengthens the kidneys, and it is a good tonic for the nerves. Bottlebrush counteracts the syphilitic miasm, and it can be used when there is a deterioration of muscular tissue because toxemia is not being eliminated from the cellular tissue of the muscular structure. Bottlebrush augments the ethereal fluidium in the cellular walls to better eliminate waste products. In doing this, it also aids in the general assimilation of various nutrients into the system.

"If an individual experienced a general sense of anxiety, that would be a clue to using this essence. Sometimes anxiety might lead to tics or nervous body shaking. Many plants native to Australia will be important flower essences as this work develops in the coming years. Bottlebrush, with its strangely shaped flowers, exemplifies this trend.

"When separate groups of animals, such as birds or even schools of fish that have been previously separated are brought together, difficulties will sometimes arise. This is a good time to use bottlebrush. It can be added to the animals' food, but one drop should be sufficient for each animal. The instincts towards greater cooperation at the higher group mind level will become more conscious and available to the animals. Of course, in reuniting animals that have long been separated there will also be some beneficial effects, but it is primarily with larger groups, particularly more than 12 that the effects will be especially noted.

"When planting repeatedly creates overcrowded conditions, regardless of how the person doing such planting may adjust the seed patterns, consider using this essence. It is best placed in the soil about two weeks before planting to prevent such overcrowding. When there are no interfering conditions regarding the mineral and water content of the soil and thinning of an excessive nature is noted, this essence will correct this condition. The essence is self governing in correcting overcrowded or thinning conditions. Many negative aspects of Pluto are eased, and the first and fourth rays are stimulated."

CAMPHOR
Cinnamomum Camphora

This evergreen tree produces small whitish-yellow flowers, which grow in clusters. Medically it is used for calming the nerves, for inflammatory conditions, and for heart problems.

Q How is this tree now used as a flower essence?

"As a flower essence it temporarily aligns the subtle bodies, especially the etheric, mental, and astral bodies, almost reaching the spiritual body. When this alignment occurs, information from the higher self is more easily received, toxicity in the body is discharged, and vibrational remedies work better. Camphor and caffeine no longer impede the life force in the circulatory system, nervous system, and spinal column. Camphor essence raises the physical camphor in the body to a homeopathic frequency, which activates the meridians, nervous system, etheric body, and nadis."

Q How should one take camphor flower essence with homeopathic remedies?

"In some cases you can take the camphor essence along with the homeopathic remedy, while in other cases in which people have physical camphor in their system, first take the essence for two weeks and then start the homeopathic remedy. If you treat people with physical camphor in their system, usually first prescribe camphor essence homeopathically prepared to discharge the physical camphor. In such cases 10MM, or to a lesser extent, 6c would usually be the best neutral homeopathic potencies to use. This places the treatment closer to the homeopathic frequencies. If a person took a homeopathic remedy and then took some physical camphor or caffeine which interfered with the homeopathic remedy, taking the camphor essence would usually, to a degree, negate the effect of the physical camphor so the homeopathic remedy would then work better. But this essence does not negate the long term physical effects of camphor and caffeine in the body. It can discharge these substances from the physical body, but rarely does it permeate deeply into the physical body to adjust the physical problems they cause.

"The penetrating quality of camphor oil expresses the penetrating quality of this essence on the ethereal levels. It activates the meridians, it can be used externally, and it eases the psora miasm. But if someone wants to also take a homeopathic remedy, do not take this essence internally or as a salve with any camphor oil. That oil is close enough to the physical level so that it would interfere with the homeopathic treatment.

"A gentle cleansing effect develops when camphor flower essence is used with animals. This is a gentle thing, so it is best to use it about two or three weeks before using other essences for healing and change. If you know you are going to move, for instance, about a week before the move give your animal this essence. Then after the move you might treat any difficulty or stress developed by the animal with other flower essences. Camphor essence paves the way for correctly using other flower essences.

"This essence can be used when seeds have been contaminated by excess environmental difficulty of any nature including radiation, microwaves, or diseases. This could also include the excess use of heat, cold, water, or dryness. In cleansing the negative aspects of environmental difficulty associated with such stress, the ability of the seed to germinate is enhanced. Apply camphor again about two weeks or so before actually planting the seeds. The correct ratio would be three drops of camphor flower essence to a gallon of water. The gallon of water is sprayed very lightly on the seeds, and they are allowed to dry slowly at room temperature without direct sun.

"Some easing of negative aspects between Saturn and Venus occur, and the fourth ray is enhanced."

CEDAR
Thuja Occidentalis

This species of Cedar is native to the Eastern United States and Southeastern Canada. In April and May liver-colored flowers appear on the ends of the branchlets. The two sexes are separate and distinct from each other. While the American Indians have traditionally burned cedar for purification, its medical use was discovered by Hahnemann, the founder of homeopathy.[1] It is one of the main remedies in homeopathy and is used to treat many conditions, including skin disorders, gonorrhea, and urinary problems.

Q How is this plant now used as a flower essence?

"This essence cleanses the intestinal tract and restores fresh tissue to the colon. It is a mild laxative similar to psyllium seeds. Cedar induces autolysis in the intestines during fasting and is almost a liquid colonic. It facilitates the assimilation of germanium and of most foods, especially cholesterol and protein.

"In many cases, the relationship of the root chakra to the digestive tract will be aided by cedar. This is particularly true when individuals have a physical response in taking cedar that they feel in the root or crown chakra.

"Cedar stimulates and restores hair to its natural strength. This is because cedar affects the male hormone testosterone, the female hormone estrogen, and the cholesterol levels on the physical and cellular levels. It strengthens hair shafts, giving them a thicker quality, perhaps even a body. Cedar can be applied on the scalp and skin for most imbalances.

"It alleviates intestinal tract poisons or toxins, bubonic plague, and scalp disorders, especially hirsutism or excessive body hair. It eases stress caused by an over-analytical mind, over-aggressiveness, or hair loss.

"The signature of cedar is quite esoteric. It allows energy flows of a transformative nature between the tree and the dimensional shift points that exist between the eighth and ninth dimensions (and other dimensions as well) and the physical three-dimensional world that you are aware of. Many of these dimensional shifting patterns relate to energy that changes one's perception of time and the ability to understand one's self within this context of time. In addition to such interesting energy flows between these dimensional realities, the source energy from which all life on earth springs is also affected. This is what is planted in the eighth dimension and harvested in the ninth dimensional level.

"The etheric body is stimulated by the hair and nails, which are crystalline in shape and content. This evenly distributes the body's energies. Cedar is a good remedy for problems associated with an imbalance in the subtle bodies. Ulcers caused by a strong imbalance in the mental body exemplify this. This essence, with a remedy for the mental body, manifests a quicker healing of the total problem. The test point is the crown chakra.

"As with people, apply cedar to the exposed part and internally for animal with hair loss. There will be enhanced ability to regenerate where hair loss has been significant. It is good to mix with some massage oil. Most oils would be sufficient, but almond oil is excellent. Massaged this gently into the place directly on the animal's body, and a drop or two of cedar should be taken by the animal. Some strengthening will be noted in animals exposed to environmental contaminants. This toxicity is released so that an inner cleansing and strengthening will result.

"This is an excellent plant to burn in fields around plants when significant cleansing is required. The essence can be added during such a burning. A mixture of sage and cedar is beneficial. There is some vibrational impact of a cleansing nature when this is added to water, so if you know that your water has pesticide contaminants, adding these essences to the water will relieve some of this difficulty. The positive aspects of Jupiter are enhanced, and the fifth ray is activated."

1 J.H. Clarke, M.D., *Dictionary of Materia Medica,* Volume 3 (Saffron Walden, England: Health Science Press, 1977), p. 1418.

CELANDINE
Chelidonium Majus

This herbacious perennial yields bright-yellow flowers, which appear from April to September. It commonly grows in Europe and the Northeastern United States. Herbally and homeopathically this is a prominent remedy for liver disorders. As a poultice, it heals various skin conditions, including eczema, herpes, and ringworm.

Q How is this plant now used as a flower essence?
"Celandine manifests one characteristic, which is the ability to transfer information. It sharpens whatever sense is necessary to do this. It effects the throat chakra, the nadis in the throat chakra, and the thyroid; thus the essence also stimulates the metabolism distributing energy throughout the body. Because metabolism is activated the meridians are strengthened.

"This is an exceptional remedy for singers and lecturers for articulation and for receiving information. Student-teacher communication is stimulated, telepathic transference of information increases, and lucid dreams and instructions from one's spirit guides are activated. All forms of dialogue are enhanced.

"Any problems in the throat, particularly the vocal cords, can be treated with celandine. This is from the remedy's strong relationship to the throat, not from its being a specific for any diseases. The essence likewise heals the syphilitic miasm.

"Another function of celandine is to stimulate the tantric experience. Tantra is, in part, the exchange of male and female energy. Many believe the male loses energy and the female gains energy from the sexual act. This is a bad observation. Most observers agree the male is relaxed and the female is somewhat active after sexual activity. This is, to an important degree, because the intuitive faculty of the female has been transferred to the male. He has a heightened intuitive and meditative quality, while the female has received the male's analytical outlook. As a result, the female wants to explore these analytical and logical thoughts, while the male expresses increased sensitivity and emotions. Celandine stimulates these traits. Ingest the essence before any sexual communication begins.

"Celandine benefits people unable to receive information clearly. Autistic children, stubborn people, and individuals with short attention spans exemplify this.

"It mildly stimulates the mental body, and the etheric body is strongly activated, which generates a smoother flow of the odic force into the physical body. And the emotional and astral bodies are aligned. This and its effect on tantric experiences make celandine an important remedy for Reichian therapists.

"The white powdery substance of the plant expresses the pure spiritual information that can be received with the assistance of this essence. Another more subtle part of the signature is that during one stage in its bloom the flower resembles the larynx. The test point is the thyroid and the medulla oblongata.

"New life's lessons applied to animals will be better absorbed. This can relate to many areas including new owners, new interrelationships with other animals, or a new environment. When the animal struggles with these areas and shows behavioral difficulties or stress, the animal is not learning the new lesson. This information transfer is not at the conscious level but is still available to animals. Animals will be particularly receptive to humans around it when receiving this essence.

"Celandine can also be used to train wild animals, when there is already a bond between the owner and the animal and the animal is being shown something entirely new in which the animal's own conscious ability to integrate and work with what is being shown is part of the process.

"Some benefits will be noted in cross-breeding plants. The essence can be mixed with water and sprayed on the ground immediately before planting those plants that you wish to crossbreed, and then again immediately before planting the seeds that have resulted from this cross-breeding. The most positive aspects of Uranus are enhanced, and the second and third rays are made clearer."

CENTURY AGAVE
Agave Americana

This tree grows in Mexico and warm parts of the Southern United States. It takes some years for the greenish-yellow flowers to appear, after which the tree dies. Medically it is used for intestinal, liver, stomach, and respiratory problems.

Q How is this tree now used as a flower essence?

"This essence brings the emotional, mental, and soul bodies into alignment, which creates wisdom, maturity, and patience. People displaying immature behavior patterns such as anger, impatience, or sulking can benefit from century agave. Excessive stress from hearing or memory loss can be treated with this essence. Many individuals develop a deep strengthening of the ear canal.

"There will be added energy in the entire nervous system and brain cells, but this will probably not be very noticeable. You are not likely to have increased memory or perception as a result of this essence. There will be some cases of Alzheimer's or mental deterioration in old age that are helped by century agave, but this is primarily due to the individual's willingness to attune to new subject matter, new contextual understanding, and new forms of mental stimulation.

"The circulatory system, endocrine system, heart, and lungs are also strengthened. Century agave brings relief in senility, stroke, cardiovascular disease, hardening of the arteries, or deterioration of the brain cells.

"On the cellular level, tissue regeneration is stimulated to reverse the aging process. It is a general tonic enhancing longevity. Calcium, gold, iron, magnesium, RNA, phosphorus, silica, vitamin C, and E, and all the B vitamins are more easily assimilated into the system. Most of these nutrients are critical for the nervous system, circulatory system, and mental faculties.

"It strengthens the heart and emotional chakras. The longevity of the plant and the fact that it takes some years to bloom shows its relationship to patience and aging. The test point is the medulla oblongata.

"Longstanding difficulties with prana will be eased for most animals in old age. If an animal has shown a tendency towards bursitis or arthritis during its life, and then in old age this becomes a particularly difficult and irritating condition, this essence may be indicated. In easing the attitudes around this, the animal's healing energy will be made more available. It is useful about once a week, if you give this essence to an animal, to use hands-on healing to bring more energy into the animal.

"There is some benefit in using this essence mixed with water applied to areas of land where the same plant is being grown repeatedly. Rotation of crops is always beneficial, but sometimes repetitive growing will still be necessary for economic or environmental reasons. This essence will not increase the plant's absorption of minerals available in the soil, but it will reacclimate the plant to gain greater etheric energy from the earth during the growing season. Therefore, use this essence just before planting and at regular intervals of about ten days under such soil depletion conditions until the plant reaches maturity.

"The rare occurrence of a conjunction between Neptune and Pluto are excellent times to utilize this essence. The fifth and seventh rays are stimulated."

CHAMOMILE
Matricaria Chamomilla

German chamomile is a Southern European annual with small white-rayed flowers and yellow disks in the center. As an herb or homeopathic remedy chamomile is prominently used in a wide range of children's illnesses. It relieves inflammations, asthma, and neuralgia.

Q What is the karmic background of this plant?
"This was one of the first plants developed in early Lemuria. Meditative practices and then the Lemurian science of luminosity evolved with the aid of this essence. The gold and white flowers, the plant's physiological properties, and its geometric patterns stimulated meditative practices. Meditation was the cornerstone of early Lemurian society."

Q What are the clinical effects of this flower essence?
"Chamomile augments the entire nervous system, especially the autonomic nervous system. The entire ductless system, the respiratory system, and the kidneys are strengthened. It stimulates the pineal gland, which creates a sense of harmony and organization through creative passive states applicable to meditation. On the cellular level, it stimulates morphine-like properties scientists recently discovered in the brain.

"It aligns the mental body, even touching the soul body's outer extremities. Higher wisdom, philosophies, and factual academic and linear information are absorbed more easily. And people become more susceptible to hypnosis."

Q Would chamomile influence the emotional body to reduce emotional tension?

"In aligning the mental body, emotional tensions are released. When the emotional and mental bodies are integrated, emotions are examined with more objectivity. The increased emotional stability creates a calmness in the stomach.

"Chamomile relieves the syphilitic miasm, insomnia, and kidney diseases, particularly genetic diseases in the kidneys. It is universally applicable to alleviate stress in the nervous system.

"Chamomile regulates the flow of the meridians, and it awakens the pituitary associated chakra and the chakra at the upper point of the index finger. This minor chakra facilitates assimilating higher wisdom and specific linear and academic information.

"This plant is affiliated with devic orders originally associated with various Arabic and Egyptian dieties. Previous to that, it was connected to certain Lemurian devic orders in which it was prescribed for spiritual growth and healing. The minor signature is that the color and texture of the plant and flowers are related to the nervous system. The nadis are slightly stimulated. It promotes digestion of the B vitamins, and it can be applied externally. The test point is the shoulder blades.

"Greater contact with the overall uniting animal thought form or animal soul group will be intensified for most animals. This may bring greater instinctual energy to the animal; thus, use chamomile if a wild animal has been taken at a young age, raised under domesticated conditions, and then is released into the wild. For about two weeks before such a release, apply this essence every day both externally and to the animal's food. This will help the animal acclimate to instincts that are natural but may be suppressed due to living with humans.

"Absorption of all minerals, particularly calcium, manganese, boron, and molybdenum, is enhanced. Thus, adding this essence to water used for most plants will have a beneficial effect. An extremely dilute concentration is sufficient. As little as one drop of the essence to 100 gallons of water will provide sufficient vibrational effect to enhance a plant's absorption of these minerals.

"There is an easing of negative aspects between Mercury and Mars. The influence of the fourth and ninth rays increases."

COFFEE
Coffea Arabica

This small evergreen tree is native to parts of Africa. The white, scented flowers appear in clusters for only a few days in the spring. While it is a popular beverage, coffee is also used as a stimulant, for heart problems, and for cases of snake-bite.

Q What is the karmic background of this tree?
"It was used in early Atlantis to stimulate the then developing nervous system. As more complex nervous tissue developed, coffee was used to give dominance to the sympathetic nervous system, cutting off and atrophying some of the ability in the parasympathetic nervous system. This allowed an expansion of activities in the left-hand portion of the brain."

Q How is coffee now used as a flower essence?
"On the physical level, its major impact is on the sympathetic nervous system, with little or no influence on the parasympathetic nervous system. It also stimulates the motor nerves and the kidneys. A wide range of neurological diseases can

be treated with coffee. On the cellular level, it removes fatty tissue from the heart, pituitary, and thyroid. As to psychological impacts, it eases indecisiveness so that one can make quick decisions. This is particularly so for one who overanalyzes."

Q Why does coffee sometimes block homeopathic remedies from working, and can coffee flower essence ease this problem?

"Ingesting coffee that contains caffeine, which is what blocks vibrational remedies such as homeopathy or flower essences from working, imbalances all the meridians. This in turn causes a leakage effect on the etheric body, causing emotional instability in a person. Caffeine also causes an imbalance between the emotional and mental bodies. This is why caffeine upsets the stomach, which is the main seat of the emotions in the physical body. Caffeine acts as a depressant on the nervous system, the nervous system is influenced by the imbalanced mental body, and, to a lesser extent, drinking coffee weakens the circulatory system. Coffee flower essence raises caffeine in the body to a higher vibration so that it becomes equivalent to a homeopathic frequency in the system. It then stimulates the meridians, etheric body, nadis, nervous, and circulatory systems, so they are more receptive to vibrational medicine.

"If people have caffeine in their system, coffee flower essence can ease the problem. Take coffee essence at the neutral homeopathic potency of 10MM for a month once or twice a day in the morning, three or four hours separation with each dose. Or, it could be taken in the neutral potency of 6c or 12c once or twice a day for two weeks. This usually nullifies any physical caffeine in the body.

"The heart chakra is stimulated, which results in higher inspiration or mental acumen. The emotional and mental bodies are enhanced, and the etheric body is aligned with them. This allows for a smoother distribution of the ethereal fluidium. Coffee flower essence also aids in the assimilation of calcium, iodine, iron, zinc, vitamin A, and all the B vitamins. And it relieves the petrochemical miasm. That the blooms appear for only a few days relates to the fact that the essence enhances quick decision making. The test point is anywhere along the spinal column where there is a high concentration of neurological activity.

"The ability to make quick decisions for those training animals, utilizing them for behavioral experiments, or attempting to breed greater intelligence in animals, will develop. This essence also stimulates quickened thought and decision making in animals. For instance, use coffee with pigeons or rats running through mazes. There will be an improved response. These animals are now being focused on for such enhanced quickness of thought. These include dolphins, sea otters, elephants, and thoroughbred horses. The essence is utilized simply by putting it in water that animals are near, if it is not possible to put it directly into the mouth of the animal. This also improves the ability of these animals to relate to humans, particularly under domesticated conditions.

"When Mercury is stationary and will shortly go retrograde or direct, consider using coffee flower essence. One can prepare for such times by taking coffee essence internally and perhaps in a bath three days before and three days after the day Mercury goes retrograde or direct, that is, stationary. It is applicable for both moving in and out of the retrograde period. In addition, the fifth ray is activated."

COMFREY
Symphytum Officinale

This perennial herb is native to Europe, Asia, and the United States. The pale-purple or white flowers appear from May to August. Medically, this is one of the most popular herbs. It is used to treat sprains, respiratory problems, bruises, female illnesses, ulcers, and many digestive imbalances.

Q What is the karmic background of this plant?

"This plant was developed in early Lemuria when there was a need to develop the physical body to increase telepathic abilities. Its impact upon neurological tissues allowed for these tissues to act as a secondary form of telepathy. This reinforced telepathic training since the nervous system can often act as a grid or a screen for receiving information through the transmission of the physical body's biomagnetic field."

Q How can this plant now be used as a flower essence?

"This is a powerful tonic for the nervous system, particularly the autonomic nervous system. It increases neurological response, and it invigorates the activity of the synapses between nerve cells. Any diseases such as shingles associated with the nervous system can be treated with comfrey. If a person is trying to regain use of the nervous system after it has been in an atrophied state from, for instance, muscular degeneration or being in a wheelchair from an accident, this would be a powerful remedy to reeducate the body. Comfrey eases phantom limb pain because it heals nerve endings, allowing individuals greater strength and control over the healing process.

"Comfrey can be used when brain tissue has been damaged or destroyed. Alcoholism or a blow to the head often exemplify this. Comfrey does not rejuvenate brain tissue, but it allows dormant or atrophied portions of the brain to be used. Your scientists are increasingly realizing that there are many unused portions of the brain and people can regain lost abilities by tapping into this resource.

"Comfrey helps rechannel brain messages. As various energy patterns associated with the nerves are stimulated by comfrey, incomplete patterns in the brain will naturally be associated with nerves that are then unused or regenerate under the influence of comfrey. These nerves will begin to fill in some of the patterns that were missing in the hologram patterns of memory, understanding, and consciousness that might have previously been lost. This transfer into new patterns will gradually be established as comfrey is used by a person.

"Comfrey assists in the process by which higher levels of consciousness, spiritual understanding, and the purified vibration of the mental body allow penetration into other areas. This penetration can allow previously unconscious thought patterns and ideas from the subconscious mind to surface, and then they are much more easily released.

"In balancing the left and right brain, it increases physical coordination. It enables one to gain better control over the body processes such as heart regulation and glandular functions, and it also quickens reflex responses in the body. Thus, this essence increases biofeedback response, and it is excellent for athletes and practitioners of hatha yoga. This is a good tonic for the entire endocrine system, particularly the adrenals and spleen. Tension-caused ulcers and the syphilitic miasm can also be treated with this elixir.

"If you ever sprain yourself lifting something so that a vertebra gives out, take a few drops of comfrey, wait three to five minutes, and then do a few cat-like stretching exercises. Continue doing these exercises over the next few days, especially when you get up in the morning, and it will help the vertebra fall back into place. This is partly because there is a sympathetic bond between the nervous system and the muscular structure. This essence has many applications in massage work and with chiropractors and osteopaths. It can be used as a salve.

"A healthy nervous system is very important in many forms of meditation. It is then easier for a person to relax. Comfrey helps one release tensions stored in the nervous system and the subconscious mind. This is particularly the case when a person is coming to the end of a cycle. This essence also improves the memory. Students cramming for exams or people trying to find lost objects or to remember dreams upon awakening should consider using this essence.

"Comfrey integrates the mental body influences evenly throughout the nervous system. This allows the intellect to directly enter all levels of the body, so that the mind exerts greater control over the normal reflexive acts of the body. It activates the first, or sacral, chakra. This chakra acts as a tonic for the nervous system because it is a major reflex point to the nervous system.

"If studied under a microscope, it would be discovered that some of the plant's structure has similarities to the nervous system. The stickiness of the plant symbolizes the essence integrating the intellect and the physical body. Comfrey aids in assimilating all the B vitamins, and the test point is the medulla oblongata and sacrum.

"An accident to animals, particularly when there is structural or skeletal damage will be relieved, and regeneration will be significantly enhanced. This will not relate directly to the bones but rather to the nerves. The nerves must be dealt with rapidly or significant nerve dysfunction will result. Comfrey essence should be available as a first aid remedy for animals. Anytime within 12 hours of a significant injury is still within time to use this essence. Rebuilding nerve connections will deeply enhance regeneration and healing for the animal on multiple levels, because the animal often needs to feel what is happening in its body before it sees or gets pictures from humans. In taking this essence, as telepathy is enhanced, a picture of the animal's healed body will be more easily transmitted to the animal. A person and animal should take this essence together.

"There is some transmission of positive thought forms to plants. When growing plants for looks or for increased yield, and there is a clear picture of this in your mind with no hesitation or doubt, use this essence yourself and place a small amount of it in the plants' water to help transmit this image to them. Trines between Mercury and Jupiter are enhanced, and the influence of squares between Saturn and Mars are eased. The third and fourth rays are strengthened."

COTTON
Gossypium Arboreum or Gossypium Hirustum var. Punctatum

Gossypium arboreum or tree cotton is found throughout the tropics and subtropics of Asia. It produces a pale yellow to deep red-purple flower. Gossypium hirustum var. punctatum or upland cotton is native to Central America. Its flowers are whitish to yellow, fading pinkish-purple. Either bloom can be used.

Q How can these plants be used as flower essence?

"Cotton invigorates all the hair on the surface of the body with the protein content in hair being stimulated. Hair is the first immune system in the body. It protects sensitive skin tissue and areas subject to invasion from toxic microbes. This includes the nostrils, pubic area, arm pits, and surface of the head. The crystallized protein in hair is slightly toxic to invading microbes. During illness, unnecessary protein in the system is pushed out of the body. This process causes hair loss because hair is a channel of elimination.

"Another function of cotton is to allow more life force to permeate through hair. And there is an increase in the sense of touch as the nerves associated with the hair follicles are stimulated. While cotton is not used in skin diseases, it can be used to treat hair loss or excessive hair. It balances male and female hormones associated with hair growth. As one can imagine, it can be used externally.

"The spleen, thyroid, testicles, and abdomen, particularly the stomach's excretion of hydrochloric acid, are energized by cotton. This essence eases the Epstein-Barr virus and the tubercular miasm.

"There may be a sense of frustration with organized religion. Thus, there is often a need for further spiritual growth outside structured spiritual or philosophical systems of thought. Cotton helps one understand the inner spiritual essence of a spiritual path so that the experience is not an intellectual exercise in futility and frustration. Cotton translates philosophy into spiritual sensitivity. Another psychological clue to look for is a fear of association with a religious sect or cult. Cotton can be used to attune to future lives.

"Cotton invigorates the etheric body to more evenly integrate the energy of the etheric and physical bodies. A mild vortex or spiral of energy is created around each hair follicle. This is a good remedy for dowsers or people using the pendulum because it is the even distribution of the etheric body which enhances these talents.

"It strengthens the meridians, and any imbalances there are cleared up. Concerning the signature, there are many fine hairs on cotton. The flower has five petals, and the number five represents philosophy. The yellow, violet, and purple flowers represent the mental faculty extending down from the higher self to a single point of focus. The test point is the medulla oblongata or the center of the palm.

"Difficulty with animal fur, particularly with mange, is relieved. And enhancement of the animal's innate ability to absorb energy from water is increased. When animals do a lot of swimming in water in which they may be exposed to temperature extremes of hot and cold, utilize this essence.

"When attempting to again grow cotton on land that has been depleted, there will be some enhancement of cotton's ability to regrow if cotton essence is applied. But the cotton essence should be obtained from entirely nonpolluted sources. The seventh ray is enhanced."

DANDELION
Taraxacum Officinale

This perennial is widely distributed in nature. It bears single, yellow flowers in the spring and summer. The white puffball that succeeds the flower distributes the seeds. Medically, it relieves rheumatism, urinary problems, digestive illnesses, liver, gall bladder, and spleen diseases.

Q What is the karmic background of this plant?
"The ability of energy to be pulled from deep sources was an important part of the plant's natural mineral metabolism. This was recognized in Lemuria and was strengthened. This was to bring purer, more powerful energies from deep in the earth up into the plant. This developed some of its great strengthening and inner resolve properties which the Lemurians nurtured in the plant. The Atlanteans further strengthened these properties.

"This plant allows greater courage and strengthening within any species for the ultimate future. The exact species dandelion will move to has not yet been established, but it appears that its strong connection to the earth will require it to bridge to at least three more species after mankind has left this planet."

Q How is this plant now used as a flower essence?
"First, dandelion creates a tremendous relaxation throughout the muscular structure, especially if the essence is used as a linament. Then dandelion influences the mental body, and there is less stress. Mental stress often lodges in the muscles. The emotional body is influenced and the person may experience nervousness by confronting various emotional problems. At this point the individual may want to be alone to meditate. The life force dandelion essence represents settles back into the muscular structure, and tensions in the entire body are alleviated.

"Dandelion has an interesting signature because the clinical effect of the flower essence represents the natural cycle of the plant. This is a process of metamorphosis. First, the flowers bloom from denser levels associated with rich minerals in the leaves and roots. The mental body is represented by the yellow bloom, the emotional body is represented by the white puffball, and the seedlings falling to the earth represent the flower essence returning to the muscular structure to store calmer thought forms from the mental body.

"This essence is associated with the chakra at the base of the arch of the feet, which is connected to the small intestine. Activating this chakra stimulates absorption of various minerals to stabilize a person emotionally. This area is also the test point.

"Dandelion alleviates ulcers, fevers, leukemia, muscular degeneration, and the psora and gonorrhea miasms. When fasting to relieve various stages of cancer, this is an excellent essence to use. Its application externally relaxes the muscles. A high strung nervous person displaying poor posture should consider using this essence.

"The etheric, mental, and causal bodies are aligned. In addition, it strengthens the liver and its etheric pattern. Numerous devic orders are associated with this plant, but most of them are connected with ancient Greece.

"All difficult sleep states with animals are relieved. Dandelion provides deeper attunement to the earth for most animals, particularly to deep earth energies, and these are the energies animals often contend with in sleep difficulties.

"When there is particularly rocky or hard soil beneath the plant or a rock within a few feet of the surface where you grow a plant, consider using this essence. The ability of the plant to absorb deeper energies as symbolized by the deep tap root of dandelion and its ability to pull earth energy from deep sources will be enhanced with the plant grown under the influence of dandelion flower essence. This property will be strengthened if the essence is prepared at the homeopathic potency of 3x. Then this remedy would be added to water used with plants at a ratio of one drop to one gallon.

"In heliocentric astrology, any negative aspects to planet earth will be eased. The impact of the first and third rays increases."

DATE PALM
Phoenix Dactylifera

This fruit tree is native to North Africa and Western Asia. The white, fragrant flowers are male or female. Material from this tree has traditionally produced baskets, liquors, ropes, and oil.

Q How is this tree now used as a flower essence?

"It reverses the aging process by rejuvenating the entire cellular level and physical body, especially the skin. As research progresses in this area, there will be complete tissue regeneration, including complete organs and amputated limbs. It manifests these results because it rejuvenates the DNA, RNA, and parasympathetic nervous system. And it activates the etheric body and the ethereal fluidium, so they can better distribute the life force into all the cells.

"Date palm aligns all the subtle bodies in some individuals, but this is more likely to occur in people of North American descent, especially the Alaskan lineage. This is because they have not usually been exposed to certain energy and have not built bridges or barriers to it. Such individuals are generally separate and different from the growth energies effecting date palm.

"Its clinical effects are particularly pronounced for people who age too fast. A hypochondriac or anyone fearful of aging would also benefit from date palm.

"The signature is rather ethereal, but a psychic could see this. Its flowers look like prana as it passes in and out of a person occasionally forming small bell-shaped substances that tend to scatter or spark. The eighth and twelfth chakras are coordinated, and the Epstein-Barr virus eases with date palm. For centuries this desert fruit has supported life in various desert regions, which implies its life-sustaining properties. The test point is the center of the forehead.

"While some of date palm's regenerative properties apply to animals, its key use is to provide them with greater ease around stressful conditions when humans are involved in stressful situations and the animals do not comprehend their source. This, of course, involves all issues relating to civilization, such as money and job worries and things that animals do not understand. When humans undergo such stressful conditions sometimes the stress transfers to the animal, and relief of this will come by giving this essence to the animal.

"There is a similar use in agriculture. If you are undergoing great stress this essence can be utilized by both you and the plants. The plants will then better acclimate to your own energies and your ability to provide your own understanding, love, caring, and guidance to the plants. Trines between Venus and Uranus are strengthened, and the seventh and ninth rays are enhanced. Because date palm so rejuvenates the body, it is a good essence to use in combination with other flower essences."

FIG
Ficus Carica

While native to the Mediterranean region, this popular fruit tree is now culti-vated in many parts of the world. The flowers are clustered inside fruit-like struc-tures that become the fig. Twice in the Bible, in 2 Kings 20:7 and Isaiah 38:21, fig is mentioned as a poultice for skin conditions. It also has mild laxative properties.

Q What is the karmic pattern of fig?

"It is hoped that the full understanding of DNA code patterns will result as the complete understanding, at multiple levels, of the ability to regenerate any given body part is understood by humanity. This will naturally involve understanding the innate differentiation principles by which, only by arbitrary choice, does a being decide to be male or female. Then more male energy can be contributed to the fe-male and more female energy can be contributed to the male.

"It was used in Atlantis but more so in Egypt with good results, notably for fertility and infertility. The fig tree was very respected in ancient times. Jesus cursed the fig tree in the Bible, causing it to shrivel.[1] This symbolized peoples' higher abilities atrophying if they were not used, or not used in the proper fash-ion."

Q How is this tree now used as a flower essence?

"Fig is applicable on several levels. First, it is an exceptional psychological tool. It releases blockages and hidden fears stored in the subconscious mind. Insight into hidden or conscious fears or paranoias is attained so these problems can be overcome. In alleviating these fears, the individual experiences increased confi-dence. This increases acumen under emergency conditions, and peoples' telepathic abilities expand. Clairaudience and multidirectional clairvoyance develop. Fig can be applied in classical psychotherapy techniques, creative visualization, and biofeedback programming.

"This essence improves the memory. While it does not cause total recall, a few drops of this essence when you have forgotten something brings that memory to the surface. Fig expedites locating lost items.

"In conflicts, the essence produces solutions that please everyone. Even if there is not a basis for solving the issue, individuals can at least remain on good terms. In other words, it generates the wisdom of understanding that, even if the problem cannot be solved, communication should continue in a friendly fashion.

"Fig essence increases communication between the conscious mind, the sub-conscious mind, and the autonomic nervous system. This transpires because hidden fears are released; consequently, the autonomic nervous system is activated almost to the level of the sympathetic nervous system. To a certain degree, fig allows the mind to extend into the autonomic process. It enables the person to get in closer touch with his or her body."

Gradually there is an increased ability to handle the complexities of modern life in a calm, confident fashion. By projecting the mind's energies into the physical body, people can, for instance, exert increased direct control over the heart as certain yogis have demonstrated, to the confusion of western scientists. This is another lost natural ability that was common in ancient

Lemuria and Atlantis. This enhanced capacity is best expressed by fig's effect on the reproductive processes.

"Fig induces birth control, especially if ingested in combination with meditation and creative visualization. Take the essence and then meditate on the desire either to accomplish a drop in the level of fertility or to accomplish it on an anatomical level by temporarily closing off the fallopian tubes. Or acidity at the head of the cervix could increase. In the male, there could be a drop in the sperm count or infertility in the sperm could develop. To test the effectiveness of the essence with the male, meditate on reducing the sperm count and then test the results with a microscope."

Q Would there be any danger if someone later wanted to conceive?

"No, it is the thought process that triggers the entire mechanism, and these procedures can be reversed. Again, these processes work on levels of consciousness, which allow the individual to take responsibility. There must be a deliberate direction of the mental and spiritual capacities to create these results."

Q Could fig essence promote fertility?

"Yes, it works both ways. It likewise has the capacity to encourage celibacy or even spontaneous abortions."

Q How disciplined a mind is necessary to make this work? People may not have sufficient discipline to manifest the mental and emotional calmness and concentration to become fertile or infertile.

"The purpose of fig is to gradually generate these states. To an important degree, this is accomplished by the removal of fears from the conscious and subconscious minds. The reliability of the essence does indeed depend on the mental discipline of people. Once this mental clarity has been achieved, the desired state of birth control or fertility can usually be easily maintained.

"After developing this mental clarity, continue taking the essence and meditate briefly several times a day, including from two to four hours before sexual intercourse. If there is no sexual activity on certain days, ingest the essence in the morning because the life force is then strongest with the rising of the sun. Keep taking it several times a day until the physical body is adjusted. To achieve the desired state of birth control or fertility generally takes between fifteen to thirty days. After that, the essence could be taken once a day in the morning or two to four hours before intercourse on a continuing basis. While the unfamiliarity of the technique may initially create a lack of confidence, once the desired state becomes the norm there should be no complications.

"Use home instruments for measuring the thickness of the female's mucous. And there will probably soon be home-testing techniques for measuring the male's sperm count. These kits can be used daily to develop confidence in the process.

"When fig essence is used to develop birth control or fertility, the best results occur when it is utilized by cooperating couples. This is partly because of the shared responsibility between two individuals. In such instances, you would have practically a 100% fail-safe system of birth control. If just one individual took this essence and meditated in the fashion described, there would still be a very high degree of protection."

Q In other words, at the level of the physical body, fig essence assists the creative act of bringing children into the world, while at higher levels it gives birth to creative or visionary states. Would you agree with this?

"Absolutely, and this process of deduction is exactly the way you can expand your knowledge of how to apply the new essences clinically.

"The pineal gland is stimulated by low voltage electromagnetic activity within the brain. To illustrate, when you enter an alpha state, the longer brain-wave patterns exhibited by the brain stimulate the pineal gland. This is partly why certain psychedelics such as LSD often create extremely chaotic visionary states that are only occasionally instructive. The pineal gland is improperly stimulated by a foreign substance that is often a synthetic chemical. In contrast, fig essence stimulates the brain's electromagnetic currents and thus the pineal gland in a balanced and selective manner so that clear visions and increased mental clarity often result.

"The signature is several fold. Fig essence benefits the areas vital to fertility and infertility, and the tree's fertility is critically dependent on cooperation with a particular insect.[2] Before becoming an edible substance, the bloom is protected deep within the fruit. After the period of fertilization when everything has served its purpose, the fruit becomes a digestible element. The buzzing sound of the wasp, which fertilizes the fig tree, symbolizes the vibration of the electromagnetic current in the brain that stimulates the pineal gland.

"Iron, zinc, and B vitamins are more easily absorbed with this essence. It alleviates the psora miasm and some skin problems, and it can be applied externally.

"The throat chakra is activated and this in turn stimulates the abdominal chakra. The throat chakra is the vehicle for personal expression and release of many subconscious influences and fears that this particular essence stimulates. When the throat chakra is stimulated in this manner, this, not the flower essence, stimulates the abdominal chakra.

"The mental body and, to a minor degree, the emotional body are strengthened by this essence. The reason fig essence only slightly influences the emotional body when it influences fears so prominently is because such problems do not necessarily manifest in the emotions. They can be fragmented concepts in the mental body. Fig essence creates logical order from what may appear esoterically as cracks or disorganization of logical information in the mental body."

Q Would this remedy release improper thought patterns or conditions from childhood stored in the subconscious mind?

"Yes, there could be correct information that is merely out of context. For instance, if someone shouted at a child, 'You are going to die someday,' this is truth on the physical level, but the child may take it out of context and become extremely morbid. Fig essence augments the mental body creating a correct perspective. In this process of stimulating the mental body, the etheric body is likewise aligned.

"For most animals, fig is quite useful in the breeding season, particularly for females. Utilize it shortly before and after breeding. It will not only enhance fertility but the conception process is strengthened. Most animals are not fully aware of all things going on within their bodies during the process of conception and so there will be added absorption and enhancement of humans' thought forms around creation of a perfect growing body within the animal. This strengthening effect is one of imaging as well as direct physical effect, but fig is more beneficial with female animals.

"All negative or positive aspects between Venus and Mars will be eased or strengthened respectively. The second and fifth rays are augmented."

1 In the Bible, see Mark 11:13 and 21:19.
2 Pollination of the wild fig is carried out by the wasp, *blastrophaga psense*, which brings the pollen to fertilize the female flowers. This wasp enters the unripened fig to pollinate it.

FORGET ME NOT
Myosotis Sylvatica

This small, perennial plant produces clusters of pale pink, light blue, or white flowers in the spring.

Q How is this plant now used as a flower essence?

"This essence has its main impact on the physical body. It increases communication between the cells in the brain by influencing the synapses and by augmenting the brain's electrical activity. This increases memory capacity, clarity of thought improves, and negative thought patterns are released. With this increased mental perspicacity messages from the brain reach different parts of the body faster. One responds more quickly to emergencies.

"The pineal gland is assisted in its role of producing natural hallucinogens to stimulate the subconscious mind and the dream state. This gland restores or maintains emotional balance by releasing through dreams tensions stored in the subconscious mind. Disharmony in dreams can result in disturbed sleep, including constant nightmares, insomnia, somnambulism, or talking while asleep. General paranoia can be eased with forget me not, and this essence prevents anxieties that could lead to precancerous states from extending into the cellular level.

"Forget me not helps the pineal gland function more as it did in Lemuria. Then it acted as a primitive, reptilian skeletal brain. The rest of the brain now fulfills many of the functions that the pineal gland previously executed, and it is now atrophied to one-third its former size. The current shrivelled state of this gland is one reason why people are not so spiritually inclined as in ancient Lemuria. People were then able to better tap into the universal mind or the higher spiritual realms.

"This remedy aligns the mental and emotional bodies. The astral body is strengthened to close off what some call lower astral plane influences. It also integrates the activities of the crown chakra into the conscious mind, especially during meditation. It opens the crown chakra, so dreams and visions are stimulated.

"The flower clusters reveal a slight resemblance to the nerve structure of individual brain cells. The basic coloration of the flower is associated with the pineal gland. And the name of the plant expresses its association with memory. The test point is the crown chakra.

"Use this essence for first aid and accidents with animals as with people. Here, however, the effects will be felt for as long as one week, both before and after any accident. Therefore, as a preventative in taking on dangerous situations with an animal, there is some benefit in giving this to the animal as well. The information, thought forms, and ideas absorbed from the accident are made more available. There are really no accidents, and this also applies to animals. Indeed, the animals' guides arrange accidents so the animals may have something to learn from it. This learning is enhanced by forget me not.

"Animals' are better able to use nutrients including calcium, magnesium, potassium, and sodium in the correct balance. This effect is temporary and will generally last for about two weeks. It should not be repeated for about six to eight months. This is because the ability of animals to suddenly increase absorption of such minerals takes place on a deep cellular level. The rebound effect from this causes stress, particularly associated with the balance between these minerals and all other minerals in the body. Thus, absorption after taking the essence will be reduced.

"Enhanced mineral absorption will also take place with plants. This is an excellent essence to use when any of these minerals appear out of balance in plant analysis. This is particularly seen in plants that are poorly fertilized or fertilized with traditional chemical fertilizers with an excess or deficiency of potassium. The third ray is strengthened."

FOUR LEAF CLOVER (Shamrock)
Trifolium Dubium

While native to Southern Europe, this small plant is now naturalized in the United States. Its flowers are yellow.

Q How can this flower essence now be used?

"It activates the part of the left brain associated with mathematical abilities, co-ordination in the reflex responses is increased, and the neurological system is strengthened. The larynx and thyroid are strengthened, which enhances expressive abilities. This specifically helps one to speak better. The thyroid is a biochemical reflex system that augments the entire body.

"Four leaf clover makes one more intuitive, and the individual responds faster to intuitive insights. Increased reflexes to respond to emergency situations result. For instance, a falling brick may just miss you because you sensed it falling. Some would call a quick response to such emergencies good luck, but the essence also increases practical or logical thinking. People with poor intuition or individuals constantly complaining about their luck such as impulsive gamblers would like this essence.

"The emotional, mental, and astral bodies are aligned, causing increased clarity and a greater sense of self-identity and purpose in life, because this alignment releases knowledge of past lives. With this essence, this often involves information concerning present-day associates. And the heart and throat chakras are opened.

"It can be used in throat diseases, deterioration of the mental abilities in association with neurological diseases, and for the syphilitic miasm. It aids in the assimilation of vitamin E, all the B vitamins, and RNA. It can also be used externally. As to the signature, the flower looks like the neurological tissue in the brain. In addition, the number four relates to practicality, and this plant and green have traditionally been associated with luck. The test point is the heart.

"Mental acuity in animals is slightly increased, so there is some benefit in using this when teaching domesticated animals new tricks. However, hold the image or vision clearly in your mind before attempting to teach the animal. This will assist some animals.

"It is useful for plants that are exposed to sudden environment changes. For instance, plants not native to Hawaii may fall into such a category if they are being grown in Hawaii. The fourth and seventh rays are enhanced."

GINSENG (American)
Panax Quinquefolius

This plant is grown in the northern Midwest. It has long been used for mental and nervous exhaustion.

Q How is American ginseng used as a flower essence?

"This is a powerful essence for increasing humanness in the person. This is obvious in its signature, in that many shapes of the root remind one of the human form. This is very important because it creates for most people the strongest innermost awareness of what it means to be a human being. There is nothing innately male or female about the human form. Indeed, it is the proper blending of both sexes that gives rise to the capacities that one would consider highest and greatest in any given individual; that is what makes one a human being in the first place. Therefore, this beautiful blending of male and female takes place not simply for the purpose of physical androgyny; it actually takes place for the idea of spiritual oneness, in which the male and female halves of oneself are beautifully blended. It is not this way for other flower essences in which various male and female characteristics come out. Instead this is the sole purpose, as it relates to both male and female, that is so beautifully blended and strengthened by ginseng.

"Regeneration of the thymus, pancreas, pituitary, testicles, ovaries, and liver develop. There is a general strengthening of the endocrine system. Ginseng eases stress placed upon the immune system or ductless gland system. Cell mitosis increases, which aids the cells and promotes cell division for as much as two or three generations.

"Use this essence for any fevers, most genital diseases, and to balance hormones in the male and female when there is deficiency or overabundance. Ginseng also eases diabetes, diseases associated with the liver, skin diseases (especially inflammations), and inflammation of the neurological endings.

"Ginseng brings clarity to rational periods of thought, and the I.Q. increases. There will be help if one is slightly autistic or has trouble concentrating. A reduction of psychosis related to sexual anxieties develops. The creative capacity is released, and self-esteem improves.

"The etheric, mental, and astral bodies are aligned. The ninth, tenth, and eleventh rays are brought into coordination. A strengthened ability to communicate with people will be noted in most plants. Some cleansing effects may be noted with animals in taking this flower essence. Ginseng eases most negative influences of Neptune.

"The base and sexual chakras, as well as the heart, thyroid, and pituitary chakras, are activated. Ginseng brings energy from the five chakras above the head into the seventh chakra. This is a subtle effect that will usually take at least six months to develop, but this is an excellent benefit for most individuals on a spiritual path because they will then come to understand in a more direct fashion the purpose of the chakras above the head. In fact, ginseng is the only flower essence that can incorporate this principle. It makes these higher energies more human.

"It is useful to combine it with any essential oil, with any massage technique, or with anything that can be applied to the physical body, particularly when greater strength and stamina in the physical body are needed. The idea is to coordinate some of the spiritual side of the person with this physical property. This is usually brought on by nurturing and touching. Massage awakens in the individual, at an unconscious level, a capacity for self-nurturing.

"There is also benefit in applying ginseng flower essence to the spine. This can be done by placing it on a sponge and then touching the spine, or by placing a few drops directly over your spine. This is a generalized vibrational aspect that will gently bring a sense of inner energy and power to the spine. As this occurs, visualize currents of energy moving up the spine and then out the head, pouring around the body like a fountain and being absorbed through the feet. The test point is the medulla oblongata. All the meridians are energized, especially the kidney and bladder meridians.

"As to how often ginseng could be taken, this depends upon the individual. Some could take it quarterly. Take it for approximately two weeks daily, then do not take it for seven to ten days. Then take it for another two weeks. Throughout the course of the year this would stimulate the male or female. This essence could be used as a general overall tonic, particularly for westerners. In the east, ginseng could be taken as a daily tonic, almost as a nutritional supplement. But in western cultures, too much stimuli might trigger certain activities similar to a healing crisis if ginseng is taken in too great quantities. Westerners practicing vegetarianism for three years could take ginseng in a similar fashion as those with an eastern cultural background.

"We find some superiority in Korean and Chinese ginseng for the westerner, but this varies with each individual. Western vegetarians on a spiritual path should consider taking Chinese and Korean ginseng. Each ginseng has its own individual properties within a range. There is a certain similarity. Those people who are drawn to one particular variety over another should use that variety to the exclusion of the others."

GRAPEFRUIT
Citrus Paradisi

This tall fruit tree has been recognized as a distinct species since 1830. The large white or creamy white flowers appear alone or in clusters on the leaf axils.

Q What is the karmic purpose of grapefruit?

"In observing the growth of this fruit, it was seen that it had the potential for pulsations of sunlight energy as people might handle or be near it. This was developed in Lemuria. However, the direct action of this into the flower essence was not perfected until the Atlantean period, when this energy was seen to have many different properties. In particular, it strengthened the physical body and many aspects of regrowth that made it easier for sunlight energy to be transferred to people.

"This is ultimately to provide for mankind a greater sense of purpose and strength and a way by which the plant kingdom can share a certain inner peacefulness and resourcefulness with mankind."

Q How is this tree now used as a flower essence?
"It primarily adjusts and aligns the cranial plates, which relieves pressure from the atlas. It has a regenerative effect on the body manifesting in clearer thoughts and the release of tensions stored in the temples, head, and jaw bone. This is an excellent remedy for headaches. It acts as a mild tonic to the meridians, and the pineal gland is stimulated. It also stimulates a lustrous look in the hair because more blood is drawn into that region, which keeps the scalp in better condition. Adjusting the cranial plates releases tensions in the face that contribute to its aging, so you might call this essence a liquid face-lift. Manipulating the cranial plates usually balances the entire structure."

Q Before you said manzanita flower essence should also be used in cranial plate adjustments. Is there any clinical difference in using these two essences?
"Grapefruit is more effective than manzanita in adjusting the cranial plates. Grapefruit tends to bring the entire body into a correct posture or alignment, while manzanita does not.
"Although grapefruit releases stress in the skeletal and muscular systems, it is associated neither with specific aspects of stress in the system nor with specific emotional states. It merely affects the autonomic nervous system in the area relating to and controlling the jaw line.
"When someone massages your muscles, you might feel more relaxed, but this does not necessarily release stress from the body. Stress in the muscles often comes from the mental body and its association with the muscular system. An aggravated mental body often creates muscular tensions. On the other hand, tensions can be stored in the muscles that have absolutely nothing to do with mental tension. If you fought with someone there might be some fear, but the aches in your muscles would be from the direct physical contact. It is often wise to prescribe grapefruit essence with another remedy that will specifically relieve tensions stored in the mental body. Grapefruit has, at best, only a mild direct affect on the mental body. The mental body is aligned with the rest of the system. Healers treating the skeletal or muscular systems would find this a more effective remedy than would practitioners trying to eliminate psychological stress.
"There is a mild resemblance between some of the flower's structure and some of the cranial plates, but this resemblance was stronger in the past when the cranial plates were slightly different than today. Grapefruit eases the psora miasm, it can be used externally, and it helps absorb calcium and vitamin E. On the cellular level, protein assimilation is enhanced. The test point is either side of the temple.
"Injury from a fall will be assisted for most animals. This applies particularly to the neck and head region, as well as the heavier bones of the spine and pelvis. Better communication between dolphins and humans will also be noted if humans use this essence in communicating with dolphins. The vibrational rate of thought that creates a resonance between humans and dolphins is enhanced. Any negative aspects to Mercury are relieved, and the sixth ray is strengthened."

HAWTHORNE (English)
Crataegus Oxyacantha

English hawthorne is a shrub or tree native to Europe, North Africa, and Western Asia. The white, hermaphrodite flowers have round petals and grow in terminal corymbs. It blossoms in the spring in May and June. The flowers and berries are used in heart diseases and nervous conditions, particularly insomnia.

Q How is English hawthorne now used as a flower essence?
"This essence is very physical in its effects. It eases the spread of cancer, especially tumors. But it is not very effective against leukemia or bone cancer. English hawthorne alleviates the leeching effect of a tumor, and it can throw the tumor into remission. In cancerous tumors, it eases the thickening of the cellular structure and its spread throughout the physical organism. Its clinical effect is more on the cellular level. Research will also show that it can be effective against some forms of viruses. And it eases certain heart and nerve diseases.

"It dissolves organic compounds critical for the immune system. English hawthorne can be taken with a raw food diet, laetrile, and other organically bound substances used in cancer therapy. It helps the body's consciousness and intelligence decipher and synthesize the proper nutrient qualities. In addition, calcium, niacin, vitamin C, and vitamin E are absorbed more easily with this essence.

"Precancerous emotional states such as extreme stress or grief over the death of a loved companion can be treated with this remedy. It assuages emotional extremes that contribute to stresses that cause cancer. It augments visualization therapies now used to treat various stress-related diseases. Emotional affairs of the heart such as broken romances can also be treated with this remedy.

"The etheric body is strengthened to maintain a proper balance between the physical and subtle bodies. The test point is the hara, the forehead, and the center of the sole of the feet.

"It has been noted that many animals seek hawthorne as an herb in the wild. It is useful for many chronic conditions including added vitality and an inner cleansing. The flower essence enhances these effects, so if an animal naturally seeks out this herb, apply the essence as well. It can be rubbed into the animal's skin or fur or be taken internally to have some of these beneficial effects.

"Vitality with many plants also improves, particularly as a result of extended periods of cross-breeding or hybridization. It is as if some of the essential or beginning energy is again brought into the plant. This recreates some of its original DNA structure. The most positive aspects of Mars are enhanced, particularly when Mars is in the sign of Aries, Sagittarius, or Leo. The fourth and fifth rays are enhanced."

HOPS
Humulus Lupulus

This perennial vine is found in many parts of the world. The flowers are yellowish-green with the male flowers in hanging panicles and the female flowers in catkins. Medically this herb is often used to calm the nerves, ease insomnia, and solve restlessness.

Q What is the karmic background of this plant?

"This plant was developed in very early Lemuria when there was the need for increased size and physical capacity of the human form to develop from the lower primate state to adapt to the environment. Exposure to this particular plant essence enabled people to walk erect."

Q How is this plant now used as a flower essence?

"This essence stimulates physical and spiritual growth. It stimulates the pituitary gland, it eases dwarfism, and it increases the elasticity in the blood vessels. People yearning to amplify their spiritual growth should consider taking this essence. Moreover, it improves group interaction.

"The signature lies in the rapid rate in which it grows; moreover, in its growth there is an expanding and contracting phenomenon. This symbolizes the elasticity which it contributes to the blood vessels. Hops activates the etheric body and the ethereal fluidium. The sixth chakra is opened, the tubercular miasm is eased, and vitamins B, C, and D are assimilated more easily into the system with hops. The meridians are all strengthened because this essence augments the circulatory system.

"Playful instincts in animals are strengthened. However, there may be difficulty when playful instincts give way to greater bodily strength. In human growth this is equivalent to adolescence. This time period is governed in an easier and more conscious fashion by the animal and human when the animal takes hops essence. Some easing of obsessive or retarded growth spurts will be noted in plants. This is especially true when rainfall patterns that govern plant growth move out of typical patterns for that season. Negative influences of Uranus are eased, and the second and eighth rays are activated."

JASMINE
Jasmine Officinalis

STAR JASMINE
Trachelosperumum Jasminoides

Both plants are vines with jasmine being native to Persia and India, while star jasmine is native to Japan and China. They produce sweet-smelling white flowers that bloom from June to October.

Q What is the karmic background of these plants?

"These particular plant forms were developed because some Lemurians had overly developed meditative qualities, and these plants provided an ethereal stimulant to return to a more balanced principle. These plant forms allowed those individuals to harmonize more with society and yet maintain their individuality."

Q Here we have an unusual situation in that jasmine and star jasmine are two botanically different plants that can be used interchangeably as flower essences, with the same clinical results. Why is there this pattern?

"These are principles of healing based on cosmic energy. These relate to energies that affect individuals in their understanding the cosmos through astronomy and astrology and their ability to meditate in certain resonant principles with stars. This can also relate to understanding astrology and how one works with meditation and healing energies having to do with planets and stars."

Q How are these plants now used as flower essences?

"This essence regulates mucous in the system. It clears the nasal passages, the sinuses, the throat, and the lungs. It can also be utilized to improve the sense of smell; therefore, it increases the ability to quickly assimilate through the skin any nutrients or remedies used in aromatherapy. It is a good essence for massage practitioners, and it can be utilized as a salve for the skin or as a spray for the nasal passages. It increases the capillary action, and it is a general stimulant for the entire system. Do not take this remedy just before retiring, unless it is to clear the sinuses, because this essence might be too much of a stimulant.

"Another function of this essence is to ease diseases associated with mucous problems such as lung congestion, especially during pneumonia or the common cold. The essence dissolves and discharges viruses, eliminates excessive acidity, and removes stored toxins from the digestive tract, particularly the colon.

"Diseases associated with protein deficiency such as an inability to assimilate protein can be treated with this remedy. Hypoglycemia is one such disease. Protein gathers in congested areas to produce certain natural enzymes to attack bacterial and viral inflammations. Mucous is often a rejection of too much protein in the system. This essence is good for some vegetarians, especially if they eat only raw foods, as there can then, on occasion, be a problem of properly absorbing protein into the system. And it can also be used in treating the syphilitic miasm.

"A clue to prescribing this essence is low self-esteem or poor grades in school, especially in philosophy. The individual might also be an agnostic. It stimulates a sense of practicality and mental clarity. The person's philosophical skill is awakened so he or she gradually comprehends concepts of God. Otherwise, some might become emotionally unstable.

"Jasmine and star jasmine stimulate the God spark or permanent atom that resides in the heart chakra. This same permanent atom dwells in people from the soul's original creation through all incarnations.[1] To the psychic the God spark looks somewhat like jasmine or star jasmine. In addition, the mucous or liquid produced by these plants is biochemically related to the mucous in people, especially the mucous that exists around inflammations.

"On the cellular level, it slightly increases male fertility because by increasing the protein content in the system it also stimulates the production of male sperm cells. It acts as a bonding agent connecting the various subtle bodies to the ethereal fluidium in the etheric body. By doing this, it enhances the assimilation of other flower essences into the system. The test point is either the breast or the kidney meridian at the mid-point of the calf.

"With primates, an easing of mucus system problems will be noted. For most other animals this essence does not apply. Jasmine also helps animals channel the energy of repressed instincts and emotions associated with domestication into areas that are more beneficial and in greater harmony with those who might domesticate the animal. There is an easing of negative influences from Pluto, and the first and sixth rays are stimulated."

1 Alice A. Bailey, *A Treatise on Cosmic Fire* (New York: Lucis Publishing Co., 1977), p. 69, 71-73, 510-518, 527, 535, 694, 775.
_____. *The Consciousness of the Atom* (New York: Lucis Publishing Co., 1977).

Annie Besant, *A Study in Consciousness* (Madras, India: The Theosophical Publishing House, 1975), p. 66-88.

KHAT
Catha Edulis

This bush, which is native to Ethiopia, produces small bisexual flowers in axillary cymes and petals. Its leaves are chewed as a stimulant, and it is fairly popular in the Muslim countries of East Africa as a beverage.

Q What are the clinical effects of this flower essence?

"This essence stimulates the nerve ganglia about the throat region that connect to the autonomic and parasympathetic nervous systems. This gives one greater conscious control over the autonomic nervous system. This control is enhanced through creative visualization and chanting. All these spiritual practices, along with meditation, are strengthened by this remedy.

"Khat also improves cranial communication with the rest of the body. If you experienced pain in part of the body, khat would stimulate the immune systems, in conjunction with the autonomic nervous system, to resolve the problem. It activates the coccyx, medulla oblongata, muscular tissue, and the third chakra.

"While khat is not specific for any diseases, it acts as a general stimulant for the endocrine and immune system during illness. It retards the aging process and aids in the assimilation of vitamin E and all the B vitamins. It retards the aging process because it bring waves of vital force energy into the cells. On the cellular level, it stimulates regeneration of the neurological tissues. This is partly because khat strengthens the ethereal fluidium around the cells.

"This is a good essence for people who are anxious, lethargic, prone to a fear of aging, and lack vision in life. The small cluster of flowers, if observed correctly at the right angle, has a vague resemblance to the nerve ganglion spoken of above. The test point is the medulla oblongata.

"The nervous system is enhanced and some strengthening of thought processes in animals will be noted. This may be especially important in the mature years when an animal is being taught a new trick or something that might have otherwise been difficult to work with. There is some benefit for animals that have long been separated from their parents. When they are reunited, sometimes there are instinctual energies of a competitive nature. These are eased by khat. Squares between natal Venus and progressed Mars are eased, and the sixth ray is strengthened."

KOENIGN VAN DAENMARK

This double-alba rose is a hybrid introduced in 1826. The color of the flower is intense scarlet-pink.

Q How is this rose now used as a flower essence?

"This remedy regenerates the thymus, the pituitary, and the sympathetic nervous system. These areas revitalize communication between the conscious mental forces and the activities of the immune system, creating greater control by the conscious forces upon the immune system through the ability of mental calculus.

This essence enables the conscious mind to calculate, analyze, and deduce destructive elements within the body physical of the viral or bacterial accord. This can include cancer. This unfolds because the etheric, mental, and spiritual bodies are aligned. Bringing these influences into a trilogy activates the above described three major portions of the physical system.

"It also balances the mental activities in the right and left brain. A proper balance here stimulates the pituitary gland. It is the mild electromagnetic field, the low voltage of the brain, which bathes the pituitary gland and is critical to activating it into a state of balance to be the master gland that regulates the entire metabolism of the body physical.

"The heart and pituitary chakras are augmented. Visionary states increase so that the endocrine system can be consciously regulated. The endocrine system is the key to the major chakras within the physical body. It is the very seat of the soul in the physical body. Here the visionary capacity upon the physiological levels is produced.

"Complete regeneration of the endocrine system and glandular discharges takes place with this essence. And it strengthens the immune system. The test point is the thymus.

"There is little or no signature with this or any of the rose essences. Roses were fully formed by the angelic forces before the fall from spirit. They are a biological prophecy created in full perfection, so no further development of this species took place in Lemuria. Roses are as a process or system of medicine to help return to the realms of the spirit. In contrast, other plants and flowers, even with the extended development in Lemuria, are still achieving a state of full perfection. Even recently hybridized roses like koenign van daenmark manifest this state of perfection.

"This is helpful in strengthening animals exposed to diseases not normally found in the animal kingdom, particularly the newer viruses including: AIDS, Epstein-Barr, and some the new forms of cancer now appearing on the earth. Many forms of cancer previously restricted to humans are now spreading into the animal kingdom. Scientists are not yet fully aware of this trend. The impact of these diseases in an animal may not be directly physical. The animal may, however, experience emotional distress around people exposed to such difficulties. Such stress is eased with this essence.

"People who have these illnesses may find their plants growing better when exposed to this essence. This is helpful because many plants are helpful just by their life force energy to be around people who are suffering in such fashion. Trines between natal Venus and progressed Jupiter are enhanced. The impact of the fourth and ninth rays increases."

LILAC
Syringa Vulgaris

This popular garden plant originated in the mountains of Eastern Europe. The flowers appear in various shades of violet in the spring. It is used as a vermifuge and as a malaria treatment.

Q How is this plant now used as a flower essence?

"This essence mainly influences the spinal column. Lilac works immediately so it can be given by a chiropractor or osteopath just before doing a spinal adjustment. Lilac produces antibodies for spinal column inflammations, it cleanses and replaces spinal fluid if some has been withdrawn for medical tests, it eases paralysis associated with a pinched nerve in the spinal column, and it disperses solidification of the vertebrae that occurs in various diseases. Lilac also corrects the posture and brings flexibility to the spine.

"It brings mental clarity to chiropractic and osteopathic students studying or taking examinations in their field. It further activates the kundalini energy as it travels along the spine from the base to the crown chakra. In this process, lilac opens all the chakras. While it is specifically for chiropractors and osteopaths, lilac also relaxes the muscles so any body worker can use it.

"It aligns the etheric, mental, and spiritual bodies. The alignment between the etheric and spiritual bodies is one reason why lilac aids the spinal column. The alignment between the spiritual and mental bodies spiritualizes the intellect. Calcium, lecithin, and all the B vitamins are more easily assimilated with this essence. It can be used externally, and it is effective in treating the heavy metal miasm. Nature spirits use this plant to elevate their own consciousness. Various orders of fairies are associated with this plant.

"Healing abilities between animals are enhanced. When one animal appears to take on the role of parent or helper for another, some of these energies are transmitted. For those working with animals, such as veterinarians, especially if also involved in spinal manipulation, this essence helps the animal receive healing energy.

"There is some benefit in applying this essence to plants that repeatedly grow too tall or too short. This enhances some of the plants absorptive qualities for various minerals needed for correct growth. It is also useful if the person applying the essence supplies the correct mental picture of the plants' appropriate height and growth pattern. Negative aspects between Saturn and the sun are eased, and the seventh ray is stimulated."

LOQUAT
Eribotrya Japonica

This evergreen fruit tree is native to the Far East. It produces white flowers in the autumn with terminal panicles. The flower has a scent of bitter almond.

Q How is this tree now used as a flower essence?

"Its action is mostly on the stomach, especially the pylorus. It stimulates hydrochloric acid and some of the proteins that assist the digestive enzymes. Take this remedy with acidophilus culture. Loquat's most prominent use is as a first-aid remedy for nausea particularly from stomach problems.

"It balances the mental and emotional bodies, easing various fears and anxieties that can lead to agoraphobia, motion sickness, and nausea. Its signature lies in the bitter almond scent, which expresses the bitterness that can lead to nausea. The syphilitic and tubercular miasms are eased with this essence. The test point is the entire abdomen.

"For domesticated animals experiencing a dietary shift, particularly away from meat and animal origin foods toward vegetarian foods, this is a useful essence. It is quite helpful for the evolution of animals, and many people who are vegetarians may wish to attempt this with their animals. Animals will naturally require some of the proteins from meat, but part of the problem is also that their digestive system has acclimated to digestion of meat. This essence will often balance these digestive difficulties. However, it is not recommended to be utilized for extended periods of time. If it is used with the animal for more than about four or five months, there can be some difficulty with proper digestion reestablishing itself. Thus, it is best to wait about a month before attempting to use it again.

"When Mars is in Taurus, loquat will then be better absorbed. The fourth and seventh rays are augmented."

LUFFA
Luffa Aegyptiaca

This vegetable sponge, which is in the gourd family, is a tender vine native to the tropics. The male and female flowers are white or yellow. In the dried state, it is often used as a skin brush.

Q What is the karmic pattern of luffa?

"With luffa the point is to allow increased interchange through subtler dimensions so that people will understand the intertwining nature of cleansing and healing energies with those of inspirational energies. This will be shared throughout many species, including plants, animals, and mankind."

Q How is luffa now used as a flower essence?

"Luffa primarily rejuvenates the skin tissues' sensitivity, not only on the cellular level but also on the physical level. The skin better eliminates toxicity from the physical body. Luffa is a good remedy to use in any skin disorders, particularly eczema and skin ulceration. If an internal imbalance created a skin condition, luffa alleviates this disorder. This essence is used for the psora and syphilitic miasms. And skin is the test point for luffa.

"It affects the etheric body, which being closest to the physical body, closely interacts with the skin. By strengthening the etheric body, the life force is better able to penetrate the pores of the skin. This is another important function of the skin.

"Claustrophobic individuals and undisciplined or hyperactive people such as hyperkinetic children can benefit from this essence. Skin defines the space of the physical body; thus, people who are too introverted or extroverted can be helped by luffa. This is a rather esoteric part of luffa's signature. The interior of luffa in its dried state looks amazingly like inner skin tissue. Luffa aids in assimilating vitamin C, E, and all the B vitamins. This is an excellent remedy to use externally on the skin.

"Multiple difficulties of a karmic nature in the skin will be eased for the owner of an animal and the animal itself. These can relate to allergies, skin difficulties that are chronic and difficult for both the practitioner and the people working with this and for the animal itself. All these aspects of karma are released by luffa; therefore, it is also useful that a meditation be invoked or involved in this process so that some of the information received from the past life karma associated with these difficulties is felt. This will generally relate to a difficulty with animals in the past as well, so animals are excellent helpers in understanding this pattern. Luffa helps the animal to be your teacher of this karmic information.

"Diseases that affect the surface of the bark of trees, including different fungi, will be eased. Positive aspects of Neptune are enhanced, particularly when Neptune is in trine or conjunction with the Moon. The third ray is enhanced."

MANZANITA
Arctostaphylos Manzanita

This tree, which is native to Northern California, produces pink or white flowers from February to April.

Q How is this tree now used as a flower essence?

"It helps balance the cranial plates, especially alleviating pressure in the left brain, which causes stuttering. A leakage in the crown chakra can imbalance the cranial plates. It can also slightly raise the I.Q. The lungs are strengthened, and on the physical and genetic level, the substances that produce spinal fluid are activated. The spinal fluid is assisted in its critical role of nourishing and balancing various parts of the brain. Any deterioration of the spinal fluid, particularly when it becomes gelatinous as a natural process of aging, can be treated with manzanita. Manzanita can be used to treat sinus inflammation, lung congestion, deterioration of the diaphragm, and anemia, particularly when there is a disease associated with a breakdown of the red corpuscle walls. The signature dictates its applicability in the area of the chest cavity. The flowers imply this relationship.

"A person needing manzanita is often very timid or shy and in need of more attention and affection. There might be occasional outbursts of aggression expressing concern for other people with a sense of self-righteousness. This develops from an inability to express inner feelings. These people tend to go from one extreme of being too timid to the other of being overly aggressive. They need more emotional balance and identification with the physical body.

"It aids in the assimilation of all B vitamins, vitamin K, iron, and zinc, which strengthens the red corpuscles. The lung meridian is enhanced and the ethereal fluidium is strengthened and more evenly distributed throughout the cellular level. Manzanita can be used externally. The pinkish color of the bloom implies the action of the essence on the blood. The test point is the heart chakra.

"Animals are positively affected when this herb is used in a fashion similar to the way people are emotionally affected. This is especially true when animals appear to be suffering from domesticity or captivity in any fashion. Captivity may promote quietness, depression, or excessive sleep states until the animal is handled or removed from the cage. Under such a circumstance, the animal will lash out; there will be excessive anger. Then the anger stops and the animal again lapses into a period of seeming depression. The idea is to bring the animal out of this, but also allow the animal to channel such energy by giving it a place to play, an area to learn from, and something new to explore. As these things develop, the depressed states and aggressiveness ease.

"More rapid plant growth, particularly in a short growing season, will be noted for most plants. Most negative aspects of Uranus are eased, and the third and fifth rays are activated."

MARIGOLD (French)
Tagetes Patula

This popular decorative annual originated in Mexico. Its orange, red-brown, yellow, or striped flowers bloom from the summer until early fall.

Q How is this plant now used as a flower essence?

"French marigold eases inflammations in the inner ear and pancreas as well as inflammations or other problems in the muscular system where it is attached to the skeletal structure such as in the tendons. This extends to easing viral inflammations. And it eases genetic deterioration of the spinal column. It stimulates the pituitary gland and certain antibiotic properties in the thymus, particularly in the first seven years of life.

"This essence fuses the mental and causal bodies together. There is then an increased ability to hear what is spoken on clairvoyant levels, an increased ability to intuitively understand lay or academic information, and an increased insight into the mechanics of physics.

"French marigold helps one develop the psychic abilities. Or it can be used when one is not really in touch with what people are saying and when there is difficulty learning, perhaps because of trauma in childhood. This can include closing the self off from the world, as in states of schizophrenia such as autism.

"Devic forces associated with this plant desired to develop the predominance of the five senses, particularly hearing, as a supplement to the spiritual forces, so that the laws of physics could be observed and understood. Eventually, it was this branch of thought which evolved into thy allopathic system, which uses but the five senses and extensions of them in the study of the material.

"Greater attunement to inner purpose is felt by animals. This may assist them simply to have happier more productive lives, enabling them to live longer, if this essence is applied in early life from the time of birth until at least about halfway into the lifetime. Animals will also feel added strength as a result of this, so it is of great benefit to be provided from time to time during all periods of the animal's life.

"The chakra point in the center of the ear lobe is stimulated. This point opens and cleanses the nasal passages in the body physical. The test point is the forehead. Positive aspects of Jupiter are strengthened, and the second and sixth rays are stimulated."

MUGWORT
Artemisia Vulgaris

This perennial plant is commonly found in Europe and the Eastern United States. Small, greenish-yellow to red-brown flowers appear in the late summer. It has been used medically since ancient times in digestive problems, gout, and skin problems, such as poison oak.

Q How is this plant now used as a flower essence?

"Mugwort's most beneficial effect is its ability to reintegrate the synapses and enhance communication between the individual neurons in the brain. A person with damage to the left-brain from any cause could rechannel the energy from certain neurons, especially using creative visualization with this essence. Then the damaged portions of the brain could again be used. Brain damage involving the syphilitic miasm can also be treated with this essence. It increases one's I.Q., and it helps a person enter the alpha state.

"Using it opens certain psychic faculties such as telepathy. People taking this flower essence should be told that this might occur-it could be a shock to them. It is rare that we suggest such precaution because these remedies are self-adjusting. Of course, some will take this essence just to develop their telepathic abilities.

"It is a general tonic for all the subtle bodies, meridians, nadis, and chakras. Very frustrated people or individuals who feel life is structured against them would often benefit from taking mugwort.

"It stimulates fertility, especially in the male, so that twins or even quadruplets can be conceived. But again this could only happen if a couple were consciously striving for this using creative visualization techniques and other spiritual practices. It is not something that could happen as a side effect.

"Mugwort helps assimilate the B vitamins, and on the cellular level, it enhances the properties of RNA. The flowers in small clusters look somewhat like the clusters of neurons in the brain. The test point is the crown chakra.

"Nervous ticks or twitches are a good indication for mugwort. These may be eased at any time in the animal's life with mugwort, but this is particularly true in the later years.

"Stems or branches that grow in irregular patterns from what is normally expected with most plants are a good indicator for using mugwort. Straightening as if from the inside out, so that correction of such difficulties results, is likely after a few months of using mugwort essence. Most positive aspects of Mercury, particularly when Mercury is in the sign Gemini, will be strengthened using this herb. The influence of the first, third, and fifth rays increases."

PANSY
Viola Tricolor

This common garden annual flowers from March to October. The solitary, axillary flowers are blue, violet, yellow, or two-colored.

Q How is this plant now used as a flower essence?

"This is an exceptional remedy to prescribe against most forms of viruses from the common cold or AIDS to herpes or hepatitis. Since orthodox medicine has generally not overcome most viruses, you should have many volunteers for this essence without too much interference from chemical drugs, and the clinical results should be fairly easy to measure. Pansy is also effective against the radiation and psora miasms, but it is not put on the skin for any of these problems.

"Sometimes there is sudden tiredness or tiredness from meditation. Sudden tiredness may sometimes be the initial effect of interaction of viruses with the immune system. The person could extend the period of being awake for a short period with pansy, but do not take it as a stimulant. Do not depend upon pansy to keep you awake. Use pansy, but if possible, rest within half an hour.

"If tiredness develops after meditation, it is the immune system kicked into action from the meditative process. This focalizes powerful energy to destroy the virus, even if this means withdrawing energy from other energy centers, so some tiredness may occur.

"It stimulates the mental body by propagating and magnifying the essence of thought forms. It is effective in the right-hand portion of the brain, where the intuitive faculties reside. The signature is rather ethereal because pansy looks like the diaphragms or psychic membranes associated with the chakras. A psychic could see these patterns. Its devic origins are associated with latter Lemuria and some of the black races.

"No particular emotional states are associated with this essence because viruses are not influenced by intense emotional factors, except on occasion when there is lung congestion.

"A profound impact on viruses is going to take place with this essence for humans and animals over the next ten-year period. Therefore, as a preventative it is useful. When animals are exposed to viruses of any kind—which will cover just about all environments except those in strictly wild conditions as in Africa or South America—the essence of pansy, even at 3x homeopathic potency, will be of some benefit. When a virus appears deeply lodged, it can be taken at 30x and there will be some benefit also seen in most animals. This is because of the deeper acting effect at such a potency and the ability to dislodge negative thought forms associated with the virus. This may require a human working with the animal to understand its nature as it affects the animal. Homeopathic potencies of pansy are recommended because the virus thought form is not fully conscious, assimilable, or understandable to animals. Taking it homeopathically prepared intensifies mental body energy and strengthens the effect for animals.

"Pansy is quite useful in treating bovine leukemia and the new forms of AIDS characterized as HTLV II as well as HTLV I, which also affects bovine leukemia. This is a mutating form that will likely, in about three years' time, become a more common inflammation difficulty and experience for the cattle kingdom. As this is transferred increasingly to people, it will be seen that pansy essence will be useful in relieving some of the difficulties associated with AIDS in people. There are additional problems in dealing with the negative thought forms that are released, but if attention upon those is also taken, pansy will be seen to be more and more effective against AIDS with each passing year.

"New mutations of viruses may result from the overuse of herbicides, particularly those deriving from various chemical substances begun in the sixties as dioxin or Agent Orange and from many other substances that have derived from this. Some of these substances are causing viruses in the plant kingdom to mutate. The tobacco mosaic may be one that will shift in about two years time, and pansy is excellent to treat this.

"Squares between Saturn and Mars will be significantly eased for most people. The second ray is stimulated. The test point is anywhere on the face."

PAW PAW (American)
Asimina Triloba

This tall fruit tree is native to the Midwest. Its dull red flowers appear in late May. The American Indians use it as an emetic.

Q How is this plant now used as a flower essence?

"This is a catalyst for assimilating all nutrients into the system, so it is a good essence to take while fasting. It should be given to people suffering from anemia, anorexia nervosa, hardening of the arteries, obesity, and protein deficiency. Paw paw rebuilds the system after dehydration, over-exposure, and starvation. It is good autolysis and for people eating food in less palatable forms such as in a hospital.

"Look for psychological conditions associated with anorexia nervosa. This imbalance is primarily caused by ingrained low self-esteem created by conditions within society and lack of parental love. These people experience a fear of eating, an intense desire to be thin, and an inability to be outgoing.

"The ethereal fluidium is enhanced; this is one reason why paw paw aids in assimilating nutrients. The signature is that the high nutrient quality of the fruit extends to the flower essence. Its main value is for treating certain nutrient imbalances, especially if there is also an underlying psychological problem.

"An animal's inability to acclimate to new foods will be eased. And the shock of captivity will be lessened, but look for signs that the animal is having difficulty eating. It is not just absorption that is enhanced, but also the vibration of food as it is worked within the stomach. If an animal cannot accept human influence upon food, then it will not take this vibration in and will likely regurgitate the food. Squares between natal Mercury and progressed Mars are eased for most people. The second and third rays are made clearer."

REDWOOD
Sequoia Sempervirens

This tree, which is native to California and Oregon, is one of the tallest in the world. Tiny male and female flowers appear in the fall and open in the spring.

Q What is the karmic purpose of redwood?

"It is to understand all the natural kingdoms and to intertwine this with mankind's own purpose for increased patience. More patience will provide the essential energies of universal God expression within people and will become an important part of mankind's creative process."

Q How is this tree now used as a flower essence?

"Redwood strengthens the pituitary gland, skin, circulatory system, and red corpuscles. It increases longevity, tones the entire endocrine system, and increases the circulatory system's elasticity.

"On the cellular level, it regenerates cells, which increases longevity. Cell mitosis and red corpuscle production improves. Redwood stimulates red corpuscle consciousness to be more in tune with biofeedback techniques and the circulatory system. While this essence does not influence the pituitary gland on the cellular level, it does stimulate body processes augmented by pituitary gland secretions. Moreover, it can be utilized for tissue regeneration.

"It alleviates sickle cell anemia, toxemia, hemophilia, leukemia, varicose veins, hemorrhoids, psoriasis, leprosy, and acne if there is scarring. It also eases diseases affecting the red corpuscles. Imbalances from pituitary gland secretions such as dwarfism or obesity can also be treated with this flower essence.

"Digestion of calcium, gold, iron, oxygen, sulphur, and vitamin K improve with this essence. It properly balances and eliminates excessive aluminum from the body.

"All the subtle bodies are temporarily aligned, which discharges toxins from the system; thus, flower essences work better in the system. The emotional body is aligned more closely to the etheric body, which balances the emotions. Redwood increases the life force that enters the physical body, and it can be applied externally.

"It mildly influences the brow or pituitary chakra, and the alignment of this chakra to the pineal gland increases. This augments the impact of the pituitary chakra on the physical body. The test point is the brow chakra.

"Consider prescribing this essence with general stress, inflexibility, and difficulty in taking a firm stand on anything. This is the weak person who says yes to everyone. Its impact on the pituitary gland and chakra cause clearer insights into personal vision in life and greater spiritual awareness.

"The tree's shaggy bark relates to its impact on various skin conditions with scaling and flaking. The wood's red color implies its strong influence on the red corpuscles and entire circulatory system. That this tree is one of the oldest living organisms on the planet symbolizes the influence this essence has on longevity. It can be applied in many different ways such as mixed with water. Then the hands are dipped in the water and allowed to dry with the water simply evaporating.

"For the canine family in particular, many difficulties of old age are relieved. This can be utilized as a preventative as the animal reaches eight or nine years old. A tendency towards arthritic conditions, kidney stones, difficulty with blood, and urine will be eased. The root chakra for most animals is notably energized. Urinary or bladder difficulties, especially with the feline kingdom, are eased.

"A strengthening of most plants toward the end of their lifetime will be seen. Extending the period before a plant goes to seed will be the effect of this essence. This will depend on which variety it is utilized with, but plants that normally go to seed in the winter months toward the end of the growing season will be particularly assisted by this essence. The growing season will be extended, so the roots, leaves, and plant itself will have a chance to grow larger and stronger. This can be done in a balanced way, and the seeds that result will be slightly genetically changed to promote such growth in subsequent generations.

"Positive aspects between Pluto and Neptune are strengthened. The fifth and sixth rays are activated."

SAGUARO
Carnegiea Gigantea

This tall cactus is native to the Southwestern United States. Its large white flowers, which bloom in the spring, are five inches across. The male or female flowers can be prepared as a flower essence.

Q What is the karmic pattern of this plant?

"This plant was formed in Lemuria when there was a desire to create plant structures that reflected the selfless state and a balance within the self. The plant exists in a desert-like environment, so it can be used to develop more self-confidence. Lemurian souls who lived ascetic and monastic life styles used this essence.

"It provides cleansing with strength so that what is not needed anymore can be left behind. This is an important part of the educational process between mankind and plants, so it is hoped that the plant kingdom will also receive these energies."

Q How is this plant now used as a flower essence?

"Saguaro can be applied externally for many skin conditions, especially eczema. It assists the lymphatic system, particularly when there is swelling and tumors. It eases leukemia, cerebral palsy, and it strengthens the entire circulatory system's cellular walls. Saguaro can be especially useful for individuals with HIV positive but no AIDS symptoms, because it promotes continuous cleansing through the lymph system.

"It removes confusion from the emotional body, creating a clarity of thought. It balances difficulties associated with the father image, but it has little or no effect on the mother parental image. The essence may be used in treating the mental body for relieving senility, amnesia, and general tension that could lead to memory lapses.

"It strengthens the meridians and nadis, and the chakras on both heels are activated. This minor chakra generates more self-confidence and a sense of stability. Saguaro helps one absorb more vitamin A and C.

"The color of the flowers and the fine fibrous nature of the various patterns found within the inner plant structure are like the neurons of the flesh brain. The devic forces associated with Saguaro are the Kachinas, which are reflected in the Indian cultures of the Southwestern United States. The test point is the buttocks. In the future, many other cactuses will be used as flower essences.

"The lymphatic system is strengthened. Speeding up energy flows of the etheric body through the lymphatic system is enhanced. This is an excellent essence to utilize when building stamina or muscle in an animal, especially horses or animals that are trained for extreme muscular strength. Give the essence at the end of the training period and then once in the evening just before the animal goes to sleep. You may notice that the animal's stamina improves dramatically.

"This cleansing effect is transferred into the root system of plants. It enables them to release toxicity. If there has been an excessive use of pesticide or various chemicals, saguaro may help the plants relieve the resulting stress. Some strengthening of plants in the earliest stages just after the sprout stage will be seen. When you grow sprouts in water, put one drop of this essence into the water the day before you eat the sprouts. This will give an added strengthening effect beyond that of simply taking the essence.

"Some positive aspects between Chiron and Mars are strengthened. Stimulation of the seventh ray takes place."

SELF HEAL
Prunella Vulgaris

This perennial plant produces tiny purple flowers in dense, terminal spikes from May to October. Self heal is used to treat internal and external wounds, throat irritations, and diarrhea.

Q How is this plant now used as a flower essence?

"This essence aids primarily in fasting, particularly fasting for spiritual purposes. Put this essence in whatever form of mineral or distilled water you're drinking while fasting. It helps the body assimilate the mineral properties necessary to maintain a fairly good state of health during a fast. It helps the body become more self-contained. When properly attuned the body functions quite well on little more than certain mineral waters for some time. In other words, one could fast for sixty, or possibly even ninety days, on just the water and this essence. But it would take a number of years to develop that full capacity, so people should not just start out by fasting that long. If fasting for a few days, drink the water containing three to seven drops of self heal several times a day. For longer fasts drink this special liquid each day or in some cases just in the initial days of the fast.

"The actual influence of self heal on the body during a fast can be traced. What happens is that by living on waters rich in minerals, all the glandular forces in the body can recycle what already exists there. For instance, the nutrients stored in the body's fatty tissues can be released. Eventually, with this essence, the cells adapt to the minimal properties of minerals available and absorb these nutrients much more efficiently. Self heal helps absorb most nutrients. It has this effect even when one is not fasting.

"Surrounding the physical body is the thermal body,[1] which is a combination of the etheric body and the body's heat. Self heal strengthens this region, so you gain greater mastery over the skin's surface temperature. In the atmosphere there are tremendous quantities of various microbes that, being organic substances, could actually supply the body with its nutritional needs. The skin, which is the largest organ in the body, acts as a collecting agent, feeding the body intracutaneously through the pores of the skin. The thermal body acts as a proper breeding ground, which is hostile to unnecessary microbes and self-adjusting and positive toward needed microbes. The white corpuscles then become more enzyme-like in their properties to aid in this assimilation, while the spleen and colon become a concentration point for the re-assimilation of these nutrients. Thus, uric acids are cleansed from the system. This sounds quite esoteric, but it actually expresses the body's ability to live on prana. There are certainly factual records of people becoming breatharians.[2] The body always needs some form of tangible organic substance to survive and this is how it actually is accomplished. The only other nutrient the body needs to keep healthy is a source of pure water. The body gradually adjusts to what is really its natural and more evolved state.

"Self heal mildly enhances the meridians, and it can be used to ease self-doubts and confusions. It can be used to treat athlete's foot, and on occasion it can be used externally. It also has a minor influence on the cellular level of the system."

Q Because this essence has such a powerful influence on the etheric body would it be very good to use where people have a weakened etheric body from obsession or psychedelic drugs?
   "Yes."

Q Would this tend to be true with a number of flower essences especially effective in strengthening the etheric body?
   "This would often be the case.

"Originally in Lemuria the esophagus looked more like the present structure of this plant. Evolution has radically changed the appearance of the esophagus but there is still a rough resemblance.

"Self heal cleanses quartz. Many powerful flower essences do this, particularly if a drop or two are added to pure water and the quartz or other crystals are immersed in the water for ten minutes. Other essences that work in this way include cotton, date palm, saguaro, and lotus. After such utilization, those essences should be discarded.

"When people fast and are clear that this is for their benefit to experience greater awareness and purpose, sometimes it is useful that animals living with them should also fast. This is not usually possible unless the vibration of fasting is transmitted to the animal. Sit with the animal in meditation and visualization to pull energy as if from the ethers or from the sun into your own body.

"The animal may then also be able to have such a fasting state. Animals under such a condition will naturally seek food, but the influence of this essence may relieve some of this difficulty. Forcing your animals to fast is not a good thing, but when animals can take it on willingly, as they often will, this essence will speed up the process of cleansing and assist with bringing energy more clearly through the animal's body. Also, animals that have difficulty from overexposure to sunlight will heal much more quickly by application of this essence.

"Plants grown in nutrient-poor soil may experience added growth with this essence, particularly when there is strong sunlight. Use self heal when the sun is in Pisces. The eighth and tenth rays are activated."

1 Jerome Burne, "The Intimate Frontier," *Science Digest*, LXXXIX (March 1981), 82-85.
2 Hilton Hotema, *Man's Higher Consciousness* (Mokelumne Hill, CA: Health Research, 1952).
Wiley Brooks, *Breatharianism* (Breatharianism International: Arvada, CO, 1983).

SNAPDRAGON
Antirrhinum Majus

This plant, which is native to the Mediterranean, is now widely cultivated as a garden flower. It blooms from the spring into the fall with orange, pink, purple, red, white, or yellow-colored flowers.

Q What is the karmic background of this plant?

"It was developed in early Lemuria by the priesthood to aid in the development of speech and the larynx. Previously, the larynx was primarily associated with telepathy.[1] It was partly developed by the priesthood to exert control over the populace. This is one reason why its flowers are often purple. This plant was also, in part, developed with some humor behind it in the sense that certain people talked too much."

Q How is this plant today used as a flower essence?

"The name and shape of snapdragon's flowers show that it is predominantly associated with treating the vocal cords, lips, jaw, and facial tissues, and muscles. All the cranial plates are aligned. It treats tetanus, Bell's Palsy, lip cancer, some forms of arthritis, especially if associated with the jaw, TMJ (temporomandibular-joint) disorders, and imbalances in the throat region, including laryngitis and strep-tococcal infections. Inflammations in the esophagus and bronchial tubes can also be treated with Snapdragon. Another part of its signature is that the occasional spots on the bloom express the fact that the essence treats allergies that have a tendency to cause spots on the skin. Snapdragon should generally be used in the active stages of these diseases. It can be used externally to treat these problems, and it is effective against the radiation miasm."

Q Can snapdragon alleviate tic douloureux?

"While other remedies are more effective in treating this disorder, it along with meditation, kelp, and silver would partly ease this imbalance.

"Snapdragon reconstructs the larynx on the genetic level. If some larynx tissue still existed, in combination with hypnosis you could regrow its tissue. The concentration of energy in the throat can be very useful in many different processes. It is not just the tissue itself that is important but the person's ability to visualize the complete healing of that part of the body. The flower essence helps greatly in such visualization. On the cellular level it strengthens the enamel in the teeth, and the connective tissues and joint structures are also enhanced.

"It aligns the mental, emotional, and causal bodies to formulate the ability of speech. Damage to the brain's speech center could be treated with snapdragon. Any time there is mental irritation or an inability to speak or to express feelings, this essence should be considered. Stuttering is an excellent example. This can be associated with a problem with one's parents. While it is not associated with acts of violence, there can be a real release of suppressed emotions, which can include rage and screaming. This essence also improves logic.

"It opens the minor chakra on the palm over the area known as the mount of venus in palmistry. This stimulates the throat and kidneys. And it aids in the assimilation of magnesium, phosphorus, and silver. The test point is the crown chakra.

"Difficulties in the jawbone of animals and the muscles throughout the head, neck, and facial region are released and eased. A state of enhanced harmony and balance develops. This is also true for animals with any type of mouth, gum, and teeth difficulties, such as dentition or difficulty in chewing. In addition, flea infestation will be relieved especially when provided internally with garlic flower essence. The budding of fruit will be slightly enhanced by using this essence. The fruit will appear sooner and be stronger.

"Difficult conditions created between Saturn and Uranus will be eased by this essence. This can apply to both squares and trines when the energies released are not assimilated or utilized properly by the person. The fifth ray is strengthened."

1 Rudolf Steiner often pointed out that the human form including the senses only gradually developed in Lemuria.
Rudolf Steiner, *Cosmic Memory: Atlantis and Lemuria* (New York: Harper and Row, 1981), p. 100-109.

SPICE BUSH
Calycanthus Occidentallis

This is a wild flower native to California. It produces reddish-brown flowers three inches across.

Q How is this plant now used as a flower essence?
"It increases or decreases neurological activity in different parts of the body; for instance, place a few drops of this on the body where one is experiencing pain and the pain decreases. Or it might create a sense of pleasure in that part of the body, so this could be applied as an aphrodisiac. This increase or decrease in neurological activity occurs because the body intelligently understands its needs, and because spice bush strengthens the etheric body surrounding the neurological tissues.

"Spice bush is valuable in several forms of therapy. Optometrists using certain types of color therapy could use this flower essence. As the light permeates through the retina and the retinal nerves, it activates the nervous system, especially the parasympathetic nervous system's responsiveness to light as a stimulant to healing. This is a good essence for hypnotists because it increases contact with the parasympathetic nervous system, so that one is open to hypnotic suggestions. Acupuncturists stimulating the nervous system to promote health would also find this an excellent remedy. It can be used in creative visualization.

"The bloom looks like certain parts of the parasympathetic nervous system. It can be used in combination with other remedies for nervous system disorders. It has a slight effect on the cellular level stimulating the endorphines in the brain. Although it is not essential to make this essence into an external solution, several drops can be applied directly to an afflicted area or relevant acupuncture points. It stimulates various enzymes associated with the assimilation of food, and the test point is the medulla oblongata.

"Joyful states, a sense of playfulness, energy are enhanced in most animals. It can even temporarily create a feeling of youthfulness in old age. This inner joy within the animal is strengthened in relationship to people. Some of the playful aspects between animals and people are intensified by using this essence.

"Someone working with plants and growing them, particularly in the spring-time, will find the playful spirit, the energy of the devic order, intensified in themself. As they meditate with their plants, some of this energy will naturally be transferred. The essence assists the individual to be in greater contact with this inner joy, but it also assists the plants to absorb images of the person experiencing this greater joy. Positive aspects between the sun and Venus are enhanced. The second and fifth rays are augmented."

SPIDERWORT
Tradescantia Virginica

This herbaceous perennial originates in the Eastern United States. Its deep blue flowers bloom from late spring until the fall.

Q What are the clinical effects of this flower essence?
"This is a general psychological enhancer that releases psychological toxins from the system. Use this remedy anytime there is a need to reverse negative atti-

tudes. If a person is cynical, spiderwort makes him a healthier skeptic. If they are skeptical, it is almost the same mood, but the attitude has been adjusted. One attitude is constructive, the other destructive. Spiderwort produces these changes because it aligns the mental body, the ethereal fluidium, the etheric body, and the spiritual body, so people can experience their true identity. It merges the mind, body, and spirit. You might call it the holistic practitioner's dream essence."

Q Can you comment on the interesting fact that the blue cells in its stamen turn pink within thirteen days after the plant is exposed to radiation? These cells can even be counted under an ordinary microscope to determine the extent of radiation. Some have called this the flower of the anti-nuclear movement. It also detects auto exhaust, sulphur dioxide, and pesticides.[1]

"This is another reason why we call it a holistic plant. This is part of its signature. The three-petaled flowers represent mind, body, and spirit. It does not change conditions, but it offers the opportunity for creating an environment to make corrections.

"Each cell has its own consciousness. The resistance each cell experiences expresses its sense of mortality. When there is sufficient critical mass or resistance within each cell, it can translate physiologically into pain or discomfort throughout the neurological system alerting the body to its needs. This is amplified, for instance, in spiderwort because it has a dominant property of being able to visually communicate by changing its coloration.

"Spiderwort increases the body's ability to eliminate radiation, and there is heightened resistance to cancer cells caused by radiation. But as a flower essence, it is not too effective in treating radiation problems. As a homeopathic remedy, however, this is a powerful remedy for alleviating a wide variety of illnesses caused by radiation and other environmental pollutants.

"Research will show that the plant does, at times, change into white or various shades of purple depending on the degree of exposure to various pollutants. The exact meaning of these different colors is something researchers will resolve.

"Lecithin and RNA are absorbed more easily, which increases memory capacity. And this essence lowers cholesterol in the blood, which increases oxygenation to the brain. It mildly stimulates the chakras. The test point is the solar plexus and the bottom of the big toe on both feet.

"The radiation-releasing properties of spiderwort also affect plants and animals. This can be significant particularly under the influence of radon. Such radiation is usually difficult to detect. Animals may be particularly sensitive to this, even more so than humans. Aquatic plants growing near water released from nuclear power plants will be strengthened by this essence. There is a release of radiation toxicity and building of strength as resistance to radiation increases. When there is suspicion of radioactive contamination and sprouts are grown under such conditions, utilize this essence in the water used to germinate and nourish the seeds. Then also use it in the water that is used to wash these sprouts. This will communicate the energy and vibration of radioactive toxicity to the sprouts, thus eliminating some of the difficulty of transferring such radiation to people.

"Squares between natal Uranus and progressed Mars are eased. There is a strengthening of the fourth and tenth rays."

1 Karl Grossman, "Sacrificial Spiderwort," *Mother Jones*, IV (December 1979), 14.

SPRUCE (Colorado or Blue)
Picea Pungens

This tall evergreen tree is native to the Rocky Mountains. In early spring, the tree produces green or purple, ovate female cone-like flowers and male catkin-like flowers, yellow tinged with red. It is a popular Christmas tree, and its wood is used in carpentry.

Q What are the clinical effects of this essence?
"This essence bonds the etheric body closer to the physical body by enhancing the ethereal fluidium. This is important because a loose knitting between the etheric and physical bodies often leads to diseases such as cancer, even though the outer subtle bodies may be aligned. You might call this imbalance a precancerous state on the level of the subtle bodies. When there is a high level of toxicity present this is an excellent remedy which may prevent cancer from developing."

Such problems often develop in the female cervical region. When a person has symptoms here or in other areas of the body, but medical tests show no problem, this is often because the disease has not quite moved from the etheric body into the physical body. Current medical tests cannot yet determine imbalances in the etheric body.

"Spruce is good to use during a detoxification program; for instance, when people have been exposed to various pollutants such as asbestos. This is also an excellent remedy to take when undergoing chemotherapy or radiation therapy. It detoxifies the body to prevent side effects from developing. But once disease is manifest in the physical body, other essences should be used.

"Spruce should be considered when there is a general disorientation or a lack of direction in a person. This tends to happen when the etheric and physical bodies are not properly connected. Spruce stimulates tissue regeneration on the cellular level, and nutrients are better assimilated.

"With spruce, an animal is more comfortable when alone or when working in conditions of deprivation of light, sound, or food. An animal cut off from food or proper shelter for a period of time, though showing no overt illness, may experience difficulty at the mental level as if unable to eat properly or relate correctly to humans. Utilization of this essence under such conditions will increase the etheric fluidium flow between the human and the animal, and this will often restore a number of healing abilities in the animal and bring into alignment the animal's innate ability to heal and strengthen itself.

"After long periods of drought or conditions of a harsh nature, plants can be revived by this essence. Put one drop of spruce in a gallon of water and spray it upon the leaves, and put a small amount of such water into the earth. It is important that not too much be given at once. Let the plants revive in a slow fashion. The essence will help the plants revive so that their own natural flows get established more strongly. Then they will properly assimilate and work with whatever nutrients, food, and water are provided. Squares between natal Mars and progressed Neptune are eased, and the fifth ray is enhanced."

SQUASH (Zucchini)   SQUASH (Acorn)   SQUASH (Crookneck)
Cucurbita Pepo   Cucurbita Marima   Cucurbita Moschata

This edible fruit has male and female flowers yellow in color. There is slightly greater impact when men use the male flower's essence and women use the female's flower essence. Later, clinical distinctions in using these three different types of squash will be given.

Q What is the karmic background of squash?
"In the Lemurian epoch there were many different possibilities. The Lemurian use of simple thought processes was all that was needed to shape the development within only one or two generations of interesting shapes of this plant. This was true even with small groups such as three or more children. Its ability to respond easily to mankind's thought patterns allowed many capacities to go deep within the plant. The essential characteristics of male and female were imbued deep within the plant. This is more clarified in the flower essence than in the actual vegetables. Today several different varieties of squash exist in interesting symbolic shapes, including the round shapes that work with the female and the long pointed shapes that work with the male. In Lemuria, it was seen that if these thought patterns did not relate to something concrete and workable, the plant might be misused. And indeed, in certain genetic experiments in Atlantis this happened. However, the longevity of the plant and ability for such genetic mutations to persist was minimal, so such variations quickly died out.

"Squash provides this energy so that mankind can better understand and choose the ways of male or female to provide a greater sense of God's mirroring God within people. Then the balance of male and female, reproduction, and separateness points toward that of oneness."

Q How is squash used as a flower essence?
"The properties of squash are very physical. Hormonal imbalances are eased and fertility in both sexes is enhanced. It rejuvenates the organs of reproduction, the spleen, and the aging process is slowed.

"Especially concerning its physical properties, squash is slightly more effective for men. It eases an identity crisis concerning sexuality. It can be used in prison reform for the many sexual problems that develop there. Homosexuals experience a greater clarification as to their sexuality. Squash does not alter the sexual preference; it allows people to examine their priorities. This remedy increases sensitivity, especially in men.

"It releases frustration and anger, especially through meditation, by balancing the yin and yang qualities in both sexes. This is good for females who have suppressed their creativity and abilities because of personality difficulties or cultural conditions.

"Squash is an excellent remedy for sexual diseases, including the syphilitic miasm. There is a smoother flow of blood during menstruation, and it makes pregnancy easier. Toxemias such as kidney problems that develop during pregnancy are relieved. A weak spine is also treatable with squash. Or a drop in the male testosterone would be relieved with this essence. It is not so effective in treating these conditions if they are not brought on by pregnancy.

"Squash and other melons can be given in a gradual progression to treat many aspects of pregnancy and birthing. Initially you would give essences in which the fruit looked like the penis for cleansing the womb and then progress to the flower essences of fruit which is rounder and firmer in shape. More will be given on this strategy in the future.

"Squash aligns the eleventh chakra with the third and fourth chakras, particularly for women clearly devoted to a spiritual path. There is also an alignment with the chakras of the fetus. Chakras are not generally fully developed in the fetus until six months after birth, but there are many exceptions to this.

"Concerning its signature, the squash bloom looks like the male sex organ, and it has been associated with fertility. That the flower often opens close to the ground on this vine expresses the stabilizing nature of this essence. It has slight impact on the etheric body, germanium assimilation increases, and it awakens the lower two chakras specifically to activate the kundalini energy. The test point is just behind the kneecap. As will be seen in the future, many flower essences and gem elixirs can be used during pregnancy and birthing. Much of the information given for watermelon flower essence can also be applied with the squash essence.

"It is often useful to provide this essence to animals up to three months after birth. This rebalances many energies moving throughout female uterine system. It is also useful for balancing excessive sexual desires in animals, particularly relating to humans. This is commonly noted in domesticated animals when the energy they express is difficult to channel and thus naturally moves through sexual areas. Sexual attraction between animals and humans has a long history, and squash can bring much of this to consciousness so that it is released in the animal and the human master.

"Some beneficial effects in the springtime with most plants will be noted with increased attunement to earth energy and a greater ability to reproduce. There is a balancing of Mars' powerful influences, both positive and negative, especially when Mars passes through Scorpio. The second and third rays are made clearer for most people."

STAR TULIP
Calochortus Tolmei

This small wild flower is native to the West Coast from Southern Washington to Central California. The white, violet, or yellow flowers appear from April to July.

Q How is this plant now used as a flower essence?
"It initiates hair growth, but to complete this process other natural remedies such as nourishing oils and substances with a powerful vitamin content are needed. It has this impact because the hormone testosterone is stimulated. In women, cholesterol, a building block of testosterone (and with some women, minute quantities of testosterone) is released. Blocking these substances in both sexes stimulates hair loss, while their release stimulates hair growth. Star tulip also increases the skin's sensitivity, augments eyesight, and improves hearing. The inner ear, which is associated with balance, is strengthened.

"This plant was originally developed by a committee in Lemuria, so its effects are somewhat scattered and unspecific. It is a fine anesthetic, and it alleviates diseases in which the tongue is heavily coated. More specifically, this is an effective remedy in most bacterial inflammations, and it can be prescribed as a preventative measure. Hair, on the body, is one of the first lines of defense against bacterial infections. Finally, it eases the radiation miasm.

"Star tulip stimulates spiritual or psychic sensitivity, so, for instance, people can establish a more direct contact with their spirit guides. This may manifest as vivid dreams. This occurs more with the white or violet flowers, while the yellow star tulip flower essence mentally stimulates the individual.

"Star tulip mildly activates the third eye chakra. It also augments the ethereal fluidium, which when properly intensified, builds immunity on the subtle levels against bacterial problems. The hair on the plant expresses its influence on human hair. This is a fine essence to apply externally. A good test point is a sensitive area of the skin such as the wrists or palms of the hands.

"Difficult ultrasensitive states in animals will be eased by this essence. Such animals will be particularly sensitive to noise and touch, and will react with anger, frustration, or an unwillingness to be closer to other animals or people. Such sensitivity may extend to the physical level and cause hair loss. This is a good sign to use this essence. Positive effects, trines, and conjunctions of Pluto will be strengthened. The third and fourth rays are enhanced."

SUGAR BEET
Beta Vulgaris

This vegetable, which is native to Europe and Asia Minor, produces greenish clustered flowers. It has traditionally been used to treat skin disorders, to ease liver problems, and to purify the blood.

Q What is the karmic purpose of sugar beet?
"This provides a balanced flow within individuals to allow understanding of the great sweetness, strength, and gentleness of the earth as it helps sustain powerful physical energy in people. It is hoped that this will be extended by mankind, but this is humanity's choice."

Q How is this vegetable now used as a flower essence?
"This essence assists the pancreas in producing insulin. It works on the cellular level, stimulating the production of white corpuscles, especially in the spleen, which is strengthened. The etheric body is energized, and the ethereal fluidium increases the ability of white corpuscles to detect and discharge foreign objects in the body. Most invading bacteria or viruses are weakened by sugar beet. The white corpuscles are better able to expel diseased cells, but this also depends on the stage of the disease.

"Sugar beet treats radiation related diseases, leukemia, and blood sugar imbalances such as diabetes and hypoglycemia. Mood swings, especially depression, associated with blood sugar disorders are treatable with sugar beet. Furthermore, the assimilation of protein is greatly enhanced."

Q Does sugar beet balance the adrenals or liver in blood sugar disorders?
"No. The signature lies in the plant and its immediate effect on the physical body. Its very ingestion is a signature.

"This is an excellent remedy for many domesticated animals, particularly when addiction to food substances very high in sugar as provided by humans has taken place. Addiction to sugar can be difficult to break. The vibrational aspect made clearer for the animal may enable it to choose an entirely new food. Thus, it is wise to utilize this essence when providing new food choices for the animal, particularly when an animal is used to receiving table scraps or foods from humans that have a high sugar content.

"This essence can also be useful under certain circumstances when repeated use of sugar substances has weakened the immune function and viruses and other difficulties develop. But if changing the diet does not ease any of these problems, particularly resistance to infection and an improved energy level, this essence will probably not help. An enhanced assimilation of gold is noted, and in animals that need more love with people there will be enhancement of this function.

"Plants grown in very tough soil with a hard pan not far below the surface will function better. Plants can dig deeper and move through such substance and break it up more easily. This is temporary, so it is best to apply this essence during the new Moon after the plant has already taken full root.

"Some of the most beneficial effects of conjunctions and trines between Mercury and Venus are enhanced. The sixth and ninth rays are strengthened."

WATERMELON
Citrullus Vulgaris

This popular fruit is an annual and climber with many cultivars. It produces greenish-yellow male and female flowers. It is native to the Middle East and India.

Q What is the karmic purpose of watermelon?

"The ability of this plant to retain powerful energies, almost absorbing them like a sponge, was played with in Lemuria. Its small size then, similar to what is now called the Japanese watermelon, was seen by the Lemurians to be all that was necessary. The energies could be of many different capacities, but it was seen that those relating directly to the reproductive system, to root chakra energy, and to earth energies were best retained within the plant. This gradually gave the inner sections of watermelon their deeper color. This was eventually strengthened within the plant so that it could be utilized by all people.

"This is to provide an inner strength, not simply relating to more physical, root chakra, or reproductive system capacities. It is to allow its mutability to people so that they can use it as energy storage for many different healing and etheric energy capacities."

Q How is this plant now used as a flower essence?

"This is universally applicable in all aspects of the birthing process. It is best that the male take the male flower essence and the female take the female flower essence, but this feature is not essential. It stimulates fertility in the female and potency in the male. Even if a person has been taking birth control pills, watermelon overcomes the long-term effects of birth control pills to aid conception.

"It helps people develop a proper attitude before, during, and after conception. The emotional body is balanced, so there is less emotional stress during the pregnancy. The mother's emotional body is very important during pregnancy because it is vitally involved in creating the etheric body of the fetus. Furthermore, the initial emotional relationship between the mother and the infant is created in the womb. But while the emotions can be balanced, there can still be some mental tensions during pregnancy because watermelon has no impact on the mental body.

"On a psychological level, a deeper attunement and understanding is established between a couple desiring to have a child. Watermelon has a mild aphrodisiac effect, so sex appeal between the couple increases. But this is only in relation to birthing. An attempt to develop sexuality with watermelon outside the birthing process would not work. There is an easing of obsessive and depressed states, especially manic depression, and there is more understanding of psychic phenomena.

"One interesting effect from this essence is that during pregnancy the pain the woman experiences eases, and some of it can be transferred to her partner. This is part of the sympathetic bond that this essence establishes between the couple.

"Watermelon conditions and tones the male and female sex organs, so it eases imbalances in these parts of the body. This is particularly the case when someone is pregnant, but at other times, if someone is ill, watermelon should be considered as a remedy. For example, it eases the syphilitic miasm.

"In the female, you may see a slight weight loss especially in the stomach and waistline. And the hips and breasts may slightly expand. In the male, you may see an increase in muscular tone, the chest may expand, and there may be increased sensitivity in the area of the penis. Many of these things are accomplished by increased blood flow to specific parts of the body and by certain hormones being activated. While it is best that this essence be taken by a couple, if a single woman took watermelon it would still work, but the effects might be slightly less."

Q Does this effect on conception reside in the physical properties of watermelon at all?

"Yes, to a degree. Fasting on watermelon juice carries some of these properties for both sexes."

Q Would it be wise to fast on watermelon flower essence to become pregnant?

"Yes, fast on this essence for three to seven days every thirty days for three months prior to the desired period of conception. If the male also does this, then again it strengthens the bond between the couple, which enhances the process. Watermelon as a fruit or juice, not only as a flower essence, can also be taken during these periods to aid the process. But once the person became pregnant, physical watermelon would not have much impact on the person. Furthermore, do not fast once you become pregnant. These strategies can be repeated with squash essence and its physical fruit. In some cases, one may fast with squash and watermelon essences."

Q How should one take squash and watermelon essences once one becomes pregnant?

"Take three to seven drops once a day in eight fluid ounces of pure water in the morning. This should commence as soon as one realizes she is pregnant and preferably no later than the third month of pregnancy. In acute conditions, these essences can be taken more often each day. Again, it creates a greater sympathetic bond if the partner also takes the essence during this period. These essences should be taken by the male and female for three or four months after giving birth. This promotes the mother's milk. Taking one or both of these essences during the birthing process depends on the particulars of each individual case."

Q Elsewhere you said usually do not take any flower essences or homeopathic remedies in the final three months of pregnancy. Does this rule apply to squash and watermelon?

"Except in certain acute problems, this is a generally applied principle. Watermelon and squash are exceptions because they are specifically for pregnancy.

"As to the signature, watermelon looks somewhat like the penis. The many seeds relate to its capacity to create new life. The high liquid content of watermelon symbolizes the liquid in the womb during pregnancy. The inner red color so full of the water element symbolizes working with the emotions and root chakra.

"The assimilation of most minerals including germanium and most vitamins increases, which aids the birthing process. Melon is a perfect food. It activates the emotional, sexual, and heart chakras, and the meridians are all strengthened. The test point is the larynx.

"Watermelon is excellent for animals during pregnancy. It should be given to both parents during such a period, although in most animals you will not notice a great deal of interest from the father. However, the male is affected on a deep psychological level and is fully aware of this process. As suggested with people, the male watermelon is for male animals, and the female essence is for female animals. This is particularly applicable for the canine family because attunement to the developing puppy is extremely powerful at the current time in the development of this family of animals. There will be some benefit in using this herb after birth, but only for about one week. After that, with most animals, there will be less influence and squash is often indicated.

"There is some benefit to using this essence after germination has taken place and energy is forming within the plant to create seeds. For most plant this usually takes place in the fall. Watermelon utilized then will strengthen this process and probably increase the seed yield. When Mars is in Cancer or Virgo some of these beneficial properties will be felt by most people. The second and fifth rays are augmented."

WISTERIA (CHINESE)
Wisteria Sinensis

This Chinese native produces blue or violet flowers in long pendulous racemes in the early summer. There are white, dark-purple, and double flowered cultivars of this popular garden flower.

Q How is this plant now used as a flower essence?

"To begin, vitamin C and D, all the B vitamins, iron, lecithin, silica and protein, especially vegetable proteins, are absorbed more easily into the system. And it strengthens the DNA and RNA. The increased assimilation of these nutrients is augmented by a stimulation of the meridians. Generally when the meridians are weak it is because something on the physical level affects the channeling of their energy. Wisteria demonstrates that the reverse is also true. By strengthening the meridians through an interface with the etheric and mental bodies and their mild electromagnetic effects, these nutrients are stimulated in the system, generating improved vitality in the nervous and circulatory systems. In adjusting the etheric body wisteria bonds the nutrients closer to different portions of the subtle bodies."

As discussed in chapter V, the circulatory and nervous systems create a mild electromagnetic field that strengthens the meridians. The action of wisteria shows that this interaction manifests in both directions. The electromagnetic field in the meridians also invigorates the nervous and circulatory systems, and wisteria supports the etheric body in its role of feeding nutrients into portions of the subtle bodies.

"It assuages strong imbalances in the subtle bodies, particularly when the meridians are very affected. This essence is an excellent remedy for acupuncturists, acupressurists, and people using massage techniques. Although it is not recommended for specific diseases in the nervous or circulatory systems, it is a good general enhancer for such imbalances taken internally or as a salve. And it eases the tubercular miasm. The creeping flowers look like portions of the nervous system.

"Emotional difficulties with animals are eased. This may be useful particularly with animals when humans undergo great change as in a new job or new location. Animals moved to a new location or new environment may be unable to respond easily and appear depressed or withdrawn. Also, under certain circumstances of loss or separation, animals may experience some emotional difficulty. This balancing effect will influence an animal in many different ways. However, you may notice that with emotional imbalance, the animal experiences nutritional difficulty from poor absorption of food, perhaps with constipation, diarrhea, or unusual colors in the stool.

"The absorption of many nutrients improves and increased energy develops. This is excellent to give once or twice in most plants' lives, particularly in midlife. This is the point of greatest strength and the time when the most nutritional impact will be felt within the plant. Some negative aspects of Jupiter are eased. The fourth and eighth rays are augmented."

YERBA MATE
Ilex Paraguariensis

This small evergreen tree is native to Paraguay and Southern Brazil. The small white flowers grow in clusters at the leaf axils. It is the source of mate tea, a slightly psychotropic beverage popular in South America.

Q What are the clinical effects of this flower essence?

"Yerba mate increases tissue regeneration of brain cells, yet this is only the subtle aspect. It actually facilitates remapping cell patterns for unused portions of the brain: for instance, if there is damage to the left-hand portion of the brain, the right brain compensates for this. This essence increases memory, visualization, and development of the attention span.

"It is applicable in the full spectrum of mental diseases, particularly when psychochemical imbalances cause mental illnesses. It also affects the pituitary gland, which influences the personality far beyond that which western science now understands.[1] In addition, it alleviates the psora miasm.

"Yerba mate eases unwanted telepathic communication links with other people from present or past lives. Some of these communication links are made more conscious for individuals. But this is not an automatic thing. One needs to attune to this to ease the link.

"Yerba mate can be applied to a number of different points on the physical body. The minor chakras in the shoulders, hands, feet, knees, and elbows will be sensitive to receiving vibrations from this. In fact, the flower essence can also be mixed with an oil, usually not a powerful aromatic oil, and can be applied to these areas. A good oil to use would be almond. Greater absorption of some vibrations will be noted. It can also be added to an oil for use in massage.

"This essence influences the ethereal fluidium, enhancing its role of surrounding and nourishing the cells with the life force. Most psychotropic properties are transferred to the flower essence, which is part of the signature. The test point is either the medulla oblongata or the ear lobes.

"Animals belonging to owners who are struggling with drug addiction, who are in the process of quitting drug addiction, may have some enhanced ability to assist their owners through this essence. Animals with strong behavioral training, particularly seeing-eye dogs, will benefit by using this essence. This has much more to do with the transformation of light into thought for animals than direct stimulation of the brain. However, because some added nutrients are better absorbed in the brain it is wise, when giving yerba mate essence, to increase those brain-building substances such as methyline, lecithin, choline, inositol, and all the B vitamins, in particular B_6 and B_{12}. This will likely increase brain functioning and assist in these newly developing capacities.

"Some added attunement to people working with plants for the formation of new hybrids and entirely new species will be noted, as if their thought forms are more easily transmitted to the plants under the influence of this essence.

"The positive and negative aspects of Mercury become more available to most people. When Mercury is in retrograde, some emotional aspects become clearer and are better understood. When Mercury goes direct and is in positive aspect to other planets, this energy will be made more available in a positive fashion for people. The fifth and sixth rays are made clearer. This flower essence, in the future, will be part of a full system of psychotropic plants used to treat mental illness."

1 Alice A. Bailey, *A Compilation on Sex* (New York: Lucis Publishing Co., 1980), p. 63-64, 71, 74.

Description of Flower Essences Effecting Primarily Ethereal and Psychological States

ANGELICA
Angelica Archangelica

This plant is native to Europe and Asia. It is now a fairly common herb in many parts of the world. It produces greenish-white flowers from June to August. Medically the herb is used for many digestive ills, blood disorders, and skin problems.

Q What is the karmic background of this plant?
"It was developed by a small group of Lemurian botanists in the latter days of Lemuria. When the sensitive Lemurians visited the industrialized Atlantean society, some of them developed stress-related diseases. This is like the stress some people from rural countries today experience when they visit the United States or Europe. Angelica was developed to counteract these factors."

Q How is the plant now used as a flower essence?
"It is good for treating psychological imbalances such as disorientation, lack of confidence, sluggishness in response, and autism. Autism is often an inability to integrate information into the personality in conjunction with the reality of the world. Angelica is a bonding agent that ties together the many diverse aspects of the personality.

"When a person is schizophrenic, various aspects of the personality are so disintegrated that one's own thoughts, or those from another, can appear to be negative, attacking spirits. Although angelica can be used in cases of obsession, it is not the remedy of choice when a person is actually being attacked or influenced by negative spirits or when other people's energy is being directed at him.

"This essence actualizes clearer insight into the cause and nature of problems, but it does not create a solution. For instance, it helps an alcoholic understand the nature of his or her problem, but other remedies would usually be needed to ease the problem.

"This is an excellent remedy to use with meditation and many forms of psychotherapy. When pondering a problem, angelica provides intellectual or rational information to resolve the issue, but it does not actually solve the problem. This takes place because higher information manifests in the individual. This higher information manifests because angelica integrates and aligns all the chakras, nadis, meridians, and subtle bodies, but it does this without actually strengthening or changing these forces.

"Angelica augments the nervous system, particularly by connecting the sympathetic and autonomic nervous systems. Many neurological disturbances such as epilepsy can be treated with angelica. It enhances the effectiveness of the mind to extend and actually control all portions of the physical body. This is a fine essence to use in biofeedback, hypnosis, and hypnotherapy. It creates a sense of balance in a person, so it is a good essence for dancers. It eases various cardiovascular diseases such as arteriosclerosis or sickle cell anemia. And the absorption of germanium improves.

"Angelica rejuvenates torn tissue in the body. It relieves diseases such as skin ulceration or eczema when there is a loose knitting to the surface of the skin. The knitting-together effect of this essence extends to the cellular level. Angelica also reintegrates the biomolecular structure of the DNA to its normal pattern.

"The signature is one of the keys to using this essence. The plant consists of a vast complex of extensions, which become multifaceted. This expresses the effect the essence has on the nervous system, notably its ability to integrate diverse aspects of the nervous system. This also signifies the ability this essence has to integrate one closer to his or her higher self or to communicate with angelic forces. The name of the plant, angelica, correctly suggests an association with angelic forces. Information from these diverse levels can be integrated in an intellectual fashion, but to complete the process other remedies, therapies, or the will of the person must be activated.

"Praise increases one's connection to the angelic realms. Praise is sometimes seen in religious circles to mean shouting to the heavens, and this is not a bad analogy. It is the inner heart's voicing of this shouting; it is the great love bursting forth from the individual. Thus, take this flower essence and contemplate something about which one has a deep sense of praise. An excellent candidate for this is nature—look at the magnificent trees or a particular landscape. Let the sense of praise gather deeply within yourself. Then sit quietly. Allow the energies of the angels to be with you. Do not just imagine them there. They will be drawn to you when praise and the heart opening is accomplished. As the energies of these angels gather, allow their strength to be with you, as if acknowledging that they are standing to your left and right supporting your physical body. Then imagine viewing through the angel's eyes the nature that you have been contemplating. This exercise is enhanced by angelica, and feelings of praise may be more easily brought forth. And the angels loving energies may be more easily absorbed.

"Only in rare cases should this essence be used by animals, and this is under circumstances of extreme disorder, extreme behavior change, extreme difficulty in working with new owners, adapting to a new environment, or an inability to work with entirely new schemes of thought and understanding. For instance, when you teach the animal something entirely new there may be a severe reaction, as if the animal seeks not to even learn or care about the person trying to teach the lesson.

"This essence may have some applicability with the bird kingdom over the next five years because birds are now beginning to assimilate some human thought forms. When extreme variation of bird behavior is noted, this essence can be useful. For instance, sometimes it is noted that birds fight over territory and do so to the destruction of each others nests or young. People who have birds as pets may at times notice fighting or squabbling between certain of the birds that does not seem related to the size of the cage, feeding conditions, or the environment.

"When laboratory animals are suffering there will be a temporary alleviation of the suffering with angelica. As the animal attunes more clearly to what is happening, it will withdraw from the circumstances. Conjunctions of Mercury and Jupiter will be made more positive and helpful. The effect of the fifth, seventh, and tenth rays increases."

BLEEDING HEART
Dicentra Chrysantha

This small wild flower is native to California. Its bright, yellow, golden, and heart-shaped flowers bloom from May to September.

Q What is the karmic background of this plant?
"This plant originated during the height of Lemurian mental horticulture, when plants were created through creative visualization and meditation. It was developed to balance the heart chakra by coordinating the energies of the thymus gland and heart. The thymus was developed to approximate a crystalline structure, while the heart became the distributor of energies taken in."

Elsewhere John stated that in the original creation of life on this planet all creatures were to be created crystalline and quartz-like in structure, as in countless other worlds. But acts of free will caused life here to be carbon based. This was a radical shift away from the original Divine plan. The Lemurians understood that health and spiritual growth are easier to experience when life is quartz-like in composition. Thus they specifically developed the thymus gland and its etheric imprint to approximate and manifest these energies in the physical and subtle bodies. Even today there are numerous spiritual practices to transform the physical and subtle bodies into a crystalline structure. Wearing and possessing quartz crystals assists this process.

Q How is this plant today used as a flower essence?
"This is a fine remedy for stimulating the heart, the heart chakra, and the nadis in the heart. As a flower essence, and as an herb, this is a powerful stimulant for alleviating any heart disease. To a lesser extent, it regulates blood pressure, and circulatory diseases can be eased. It also is a tonic for muscle tissue. It harmonizes affairs of the heart, including extreme attachments to individuals. One generally experiences harmony and a sense of peace.

"The flower's shape symbolizes its relationship to the heart and heart chakra. If the flowers were opened and examined under a microscope, structures similar to musical instruments would be found. This essence helps people develop their musical talents.

"This essence aids in the absorption of vitamin E and most minerals. Bleeding heart can be applied externally, and it aligns the spiritual and mental bodies. Trines between Venus and the sun are enhanced, and the fourth and eleventh rays are activated. The test point is the heart.

"Animals' ability to respond to loving kindness from people will be enhanced. This is particularly helpful when past training of an animal has led to negative reactions around certain humans or certain behavior patterns that have allowed the animal to withdraw from human contact to the extent that a deep sense of love is prevented. Along with bleeding heart essence apply soothing music, particularly classical music, especially when it is close to the animal's heartbeat rate. This is generally a little faster than that for most humans. Also stroke the animal and create a greater sense of love.

"When new plants are created and worked with that they have not been around a person very much in the past and they are then transplanted, the loving energy of a human is sometimes required. This process is assisted with this essence."

BLOODROOT
Sanguinaria Canadensis

This small perennial plant is native to the Midwest and Eastern United States and Canada. It is one of the earliest and prettiest spring flowers. The plant bears white flowers with eight to twelve petals, several whorls, and golden stamens. Externally, it is used for sores, eczema, and fungoid growths.

Q What is the karmic background of this plant?
"Bloodroot was recognized for its properties in early Lemuria. This particular flower essence was, in part, developed when there was a radical shift beginning in the early phases of Lemuria. Then there was a need for properties that could aid in the development of the endocrine system. This early phase of Lemuria developed

soon after its separation from Atlon wherein there began the development of the first true humanoid forms as such even as androgenous in their state."

Atlon was an ancient civilization of ethereal fish-like creatures that ruled this planet for over one million years. When that culture collapsed, approximately 500,000 years ago, the Lemurian civilization gradually developed. Then the physical and ethereal humanoid form manifested. Flower essences were extensively used to develop the humanoid form.

Q How is this plant now used as a flower essence?

"Bloodroot enhances concentration, meditation, and creative visualization, especially in healing and for people who are too intellectual. The main psychological clue to look for is people who want to meditate. This essence is more a catalyst than a therapy.

"All the medical properties of the herb are transferred to the flower essence, but there is no danger from overdosing when it is used as a flower essence. However, when the essence is prepared homeopathically, there might, on rare occasion, be some nausea in the cleansing process. It is particularly valuable as a salve to ease blood clots, assimilation of Vitamin K improves, and it eases cancer.

"Bloodroot activates the heart chakra, strengthens the cellular level of the body, and eases the radiation and heavy metal miasms. The mental and spiritual bodies are brought into greater alignment to function more as a single unit. When this happens, the intellect is spiritualized. The single leaf that is initially wrapped about the area of the bloom gradually unfolds as the flower opens. This represents the single point of focus that gives meaning to life.

"The traditional herbal properties of bloodroot are transmitted in the flower essence to animals. In addition, bloodroot can sometimes be helpful when it is added to an animal's bath or sprayed upon the animal and then shortly thereafter a playful time is allowed between the human and the animal or between animals. This added playfulness is a natural enhancement of the animal's own ability to learn; they learn by play. From this essence, playfulness may be strengthened within animals.

"There is an added connection between iron and the soil and a plant's ability to absorb it. When iron deficiency is noted in plants, it may be appropriate to use this essence. There is some benefit to adding this essence to plants as well as to the soil. By adding soil high in iron along with this essence, absorption and utilization of iron within plants will be enhanced.

"There is some enhancement of trines between natal Venus and progressed Mars. A strengthening of the third, fourth, and ninth rays will be noted for most people."

BLUE FLAG   **SIERRA IRIS**
Iris Versicolor   Iris Hartwegii

This perennial herb is commonly found in the Eastern United States. From May to July, flowers bloom which are blue with yellow and white at the base. While rarely used as an herb, this is an important homeopathic remedy. It is used in digestive problems, pancreatic disorders, thyroid imbalances, and headaches.

Although Sierra Iris can be used, it is not as effective as Blue Flag. This small wild flower is native to Northern California in the Sierra Mountains. Its golden-yellow flowers appear from March to July.

Q How are these plants used as flower essences?

"They activate inspiration and creativity applicable to the arts. They magnify properties in the right brain, which is where much artistic inspiration originates. The right brain helps assimilate information arriving from the chakras, which is then released through the left brain. Some of the art forms influenced are dance, music, painting, and sculpture.

"They are applicable to all the moods associated with artists. This includes a sense of frustration from feeling alone, inadequate, or uninspired in one's work. Iris helps people crippled such as in a wheelchair to adjust to this condition and to release their artistic creativity.

"Iris opens the heart chakra, and blockages in the sexual chakra are released so that creative energy can be channeled to artistic endeavors. While iris does not cure sexual problems, some artists with sexual problems would find these problems eased with this remedy.

"Iris attunes your causal body to release hidden artistic talents from past lives. The causal body aligns with the mental and emotional bodies in a balanced fashion, activating artistic creativity. This also keeps an artist in tune with contemporary trends."

Q Does iris develop intuition?

"No, intuition is associated with several other chakras and the right brain. The pineal and pituitary glands and their chakras are associated with visions, not so much with intuition.

"The delicate gracefulness of the plant, with light tints of color, suggests its connection to artistic creativity. The yellow-golden flowers have a more cerebral influence extending to, for instance, ballet, while the bluish flowers are of a more spiritual influence, with inspirations toward tai chi as an example.

"Iris has little influence on the physical body, but it can be used to treat the syphilitic miasm. And it strengthens all the meridians.

"If a person is using this essence, it is wise to give it to their animals. That is its primary use with animals. Some beneficial effects upon trines between Uranus and Saturn will be felt, and the third and fourth rays are strengthened.

"In all aspects of decorative planting, planting for the effect of color—not just for the spiritual effect, but for the effect created visually by the plant—there will be enhancement. This is particularly useful with the bonzai tree, with herb gardens, and with sculpting of plants for mazes.

"The essence will assist in the joy of the creative experience of sculpturing, planting, and shaping for aesthetic purposes. As these things are felt together, this vibration will be transmitted to the plant so it will grow more in alignment and harmony with the creative vision of those governing and creating such gardens.

"New ideas may manifest for some individuals who become more attuned to their plants from such decorative features, along with meditation or visualization, these plants growing around you, and through using this essence. These ideas are stimulated by the plants' devic order and by the energy within the plant. These can be utilized as new forms of gardening and decoration. These are then created in co-ordination, cooperation, and harmony between the human and the plant."

BO
Ficus Religiosa

Native to India this sacred tree has long been associated with Buddhism. Buddha attained enlightenment under it.

Q What is the karmic background of this plant?

"It originated in the thought forms of children in Lemuria who saw that they wished a deeper enlightened state. The ease with which they achieved this began this plant, but no specific devic order was assigned to it for hundreds of thousands of years, until the specific entities associated with Buddhism came along.

"It was a very small plant in its original state and was used by the Lemurians to stimulate beauty and friendship. They knew that eventually it would be used more extensively and would be developed with the devic order associated with the process of enlightenment. In Lemuria, attaining enlightment was a difficulty only with little children, so the size of the plant was far less important. However, as beings came into existence in unenlightened states, as in Atlantis, more and more attention was placed upon this plant as a vehicle to assistant in attaining enlightenment. A soul volunteered to be that first Buddha, and this entity then came to assist the devic order. This is the Buddhistic devic order, the order that is associated with all forms of finding enlightenment. Although this devic order has been found more extensively in India and China, it is now spreading throughout the world.

"This devic order wants individuals to find enlightenment by choice. The karmic lesson is a way of choosing a path of enlightenment. The tree can be inspiring, and in learning about its association with Buddha, an individual may decide that it is a good way to begin looking at the process of enlightenment. For beings who freely choose this, it is wise to use the energy of the plant not only as an essence, but also to be in its physical presence, as in reading a book about meditation while sitting beneath it."

Q How is this tree used as a flower essence?

"This is a plant of significant importance for those seeking enlightenment. It stimulates the process that leads to enlightenment, but does not actually bring enlightenment. It must not be a path that is defined by an outward religion. Much of Buddhism is associated with self-discovery. A pattern is discovered in one's self, and that is what is explored and made deeper. Individuals may find that their consciousness changes in ways they did not expect. Thus, it is wise to have an open mind when using this essence. As psychic energy is transformed into spiritual energy, bo is of some benefit. Perhaps you had a period of a few years of deep spiritual searching, but recognized that it needed to be integrated in the world.

"Disharmony in a religious quest, not understanding some New Age ideas, or inner disharmony about one's purpose can be eased with bo. This essence will assist with schizophrenia because levels of hallucinogenic ideas, higher enlightenment, and states of fear are eased. This essence can promote states in which there is greater expansion, so one who may have never heard voices may go through a period in which they do hear voices. The essence should be continued during such states and the individual allowed deeper states of meditation to recognize that the voices are merely released energy from many levels. These are often past lives that they contact on the way to greater enlightenment.

"Because it is so etherically intertwined with the energy of Buddha, the signature is not so obvious. It is inspiring in its appearance, but it is the association with this tree that is important. In the many places that you will find this tree, someone may just come up and tell you about its past significance, alignment, and closeness with Buddha. It is now intertwined with this thought form and will likely remain so for at least a thousand more years.

"The physical body is nourished in an energetic sense. Those fatigued but on a spiritual path should consider using bo essence. Areas of the physical body especially affected relate to regulation processes. There is too much or too little energy expended. There may be exhaustion as a result of intense concentration or mental states. This may be the exhaustion that sometimes results in disappointment when someone seeks an inspired religious state and does not reach it as they expected. All nutrients that aid nerve growth and carbohydrate absorption, especially complex carbohydrates are enhanced.

"The sweat glands are sometimes unduly taxed. Sweat glands while releasing water are sometimes a part of the process of prana. That energy should be used appropriately. This pranic force is sometimes emitted in these higher states before enlightenment is achieved. And the sweat gland cells are regenerated. With deep breathing techniques, the cells in the lungs are stressed. Those using deep breathing techniques and seeking to give up smoking will be assisted by this essence.

"Many lung diseases are assisted including lung cancer, diseases associated with smoking of any kind like emphysema, and shortness of breath such as with runners. When a person is constantly fatigued, there may be a misalignment of earth energy. The person may contact colds easily. A paraplegic will benefit from bo essence if he is also interested in spiritual awakening. Other diseases assisted relate to nervous disorders associated with the spinal column. Multiple sclerosis will be eased, particularly when it affects the spinal column.

"This essence increases energy, particularly in the entire chakra system. It removes blockages in the chakras, in the sushumna, and in the way energy is brought from the earth into the feet, converted, and brought up through all the chakras. Those exploring kundalini energy will be able to use this if they have direct attunement with the feet to the earth. It affects the chakras on the feet in particular. This is not obvious, because it also works with the crown chakra. Use it when washing the hair because the crown chakra is stimulated more directly. It also focuses energy in the ninth and twelfth chakras.

"The causal, soul, and integrated spiritual bodies are directly assisted. Energy is added to them, but it must be filtered down into the physical body. This is not easy for many people, so if there is a heaviness from taking this essence, combine it with essences that align all the subtle bodies, like lotus and date palm. There will generally be a sense of guilt, as if they do not understand why they had an attraction to enlightenment. There will be no direct physical difficulty, but these individuals may be attracted to enlightenment but not be willing to look into it more deeply. Use creative visualization with bo essence to achieve spiritual goals.

"There are direct parallels in the symbology to Jupiter and Uranus, partly because of the surprising nature in which enlightenment is welcomed. An understanding of Uranus brings more clarity around this state, and Jupiter's expansiveness is assisted. In a chart, when there are positive aspects, particularly trines or grand trines between Jupiter and Uranus and other planets, there will be aid given with bo.

"Animals that have a particular affinity with the process of enlightenment, which includes many in the bird kingdom such as the eagle and falcon, would benefit from bo essence. Those involved in falconry will have some assistance in their visualizations and work with these birds. We suggest that it be applied for those working with free birds, not those kept in cages, but birds that prefer long areas of flight. Those working in intensive horticulture might take the essence as part of their inner meditative process while working with plants and trees. Perhaps apply it once a month or so.

"The gall bladder meridian is particularly energized, and the nadis in hands and feet have additional energy. The sixth, seventh, eighth, and ninth rays have increased energy. The test point is the sole of the foot."

BORAGE
Borago Officinalis

Borage is an annual that grows wild in the Mediterranean region. It is now a common garden herb in the United States and Europe. The bright blue and star-shaped flowers appear from June to August. It reduces fevers, decreases swelling in the skin, brings calm in nerve conditions, and stimulates milk in nursing mothers.

Q How is this plant now used as a flower essence?
"Most of the psychological effects of borage as an herb are transferred to the flower essence. Borage increases courage, drives away sorrow, and makes a person happier.[1] It opens the heart chakra, and any tensions in the emotional body are greatly eased.

"Stamina increases in the physical body, especially in the adrenals, circulatory system, skeletal structure, and thyroid. Calcium, iron, magnesium, zinc, and, to a lesser extent, iodine, are assimilated more easily into the system. This essence strengthens the heart meridian, which is also the test point. And the nadis are invigorated. Many feel its sky-blue and star-shaped flowers are among the prettiest in nature. Borage helps a few people assimilate air at higher altitudes, but this is mainly true with people who have direct astrological relationships to air signs.

"Greater bonding to one's animals will usually be noticed with this herb. This may be applied as an essence or given to the animal at times to eat as an herb. This bonding may extend to herds of animals, to farm animals, or to individual pets. However, because of the added life force generally created at the heart level in both the animal and the human, a more noticeable effect will be seen with herds or larger groups of animals. Indeed, at the solstice and equinox when the earth is affecting the animals more powerfully, borage utilized as an essence for the human and all the animals one is working with will increase yields and strengthen the animals' ability to survive disease, famine, and other difficulties that may not be foreseen at that time. This essence is an overall enhancer and thus has a subtle effect, but when utilized particularly at the solstice and equinox times, its effect will be especially noted.

"Some beneficial effect will be seen when one has a particular feeling of deep love for one particular plant. Thus, one may be seemingly attracted in an unusual fashion to just one particular plant or species. That is a good essence to utilize with that species and with yourself so that this bond may strengthen with time. Again, there will be some enhancement of this effect during the solstice and equinox.

"During conjunctions and oppositions of the sun and Moon, energies released will be better balanced. Greater clarity and strength will be noted within the third and eighth rays."

1. Claire Powell, *The Meaning of Flowers* (Boulder, CO: Shambhala Publications, 1979), p. 48-49.

CALIFORNIA POPPY
Eschscholzia California

This hardy annual is native to California and the Pacific Northwest. Solitary, saucer-shaped, and deep-orange flowers germinate. It is a mild narcotic, and the Indians apply it for toothaches.

Q What is the karmic background of this plant?
"This plant was created by Lemurian devas as a thought form to augment the body's evolution by cleansing the meridians. Evolution is the direct sculpturing of the life force along the meridians and the chakras into the physical body. The more intelligence that is projected into the body, the more rapid its evolution."

Q How is this plant now used as a flower essence?
"The need for psychic and spiritual balance is a major indication for prescribing this essence. A sense of inner balance is maintained during psychic awakening. Past life information and psychic information in general are released and properly integrated. Much of this information is released through dreams. Used over a six-month period, some people would start seeing auras and nature spirits. The recommended dosage is several times a day with up to five or seven drops of the essence being taken in pure water with each treatment.

"The essence creates these effects because it aligns the mental, causal, and spiritual bodies with the astral body to release past life and psychic information in a coordinated pattern. The integration point of this psychic information is the solar plexus region because past life information residing in the astral body enters the physical body through the solar plexus. The other three bodies assist in this process.

"California poppy energizes the heart, throat, and navel chakras, and it activates the minor chakra behind each knee. This minor chakra increases negotiating skills and physical flexibility. All the nadis are strengthened and cleansed.

"Most people could employ this essence because it is universally applicable in expediting emotional cleansing. But this essence is applicable neither to any specific emotional states nor to releasing emotional traumas that occurred in childhood. Artists' creativity is stimulated with this essence through the release of past life and psychic information.

"By the early 1990's many individuals will seek to stop their cocaine addiction. It is likely that injecting cocaine and other uses of cocaine that can be extremely addictive may be made clearer at mental levels for most individuals, thus easing some of these addictive properties. This is a new quality that is being transferred from the heroin family into the cocaine family through this flower essence. It will only take place at the essence level, and at the homeopathically prepared essence usually at 12x and 30x. This will relieve some aspects of cocaine addiction. But this essence will not be so effective in treating heroin addiction or other types of addiction.

"It moderately invigorates the pineal and pituitary glands, but this is more the etheric portions of these glands. On the cellular level, it oxygenates the circulatory system. Moreover, it facilitates the ingestion of vitamin A. Since the psychic qualities in the eyes are strengthened, telepathic and clairvoyant vision is stimulated. The eyes are the physical vehicle involved in clairvoyantly seeing auras and nature spirits.

"It is easier to assimilate gold with this essence. This is an important remedy in multiple sclerosis and other nerve diseases in which a lack of gold in the system helps produce the problem. In addition, this essence heals the syphilitic miasm and hearing problems. Middle ear problems affecting balance can be treated with California poppy. It is utilized as a spray, especially over the eyes and ears.

"The signature is the universal attractiveness of the "cup of gold" shape of the flower. This is a signal for everyone to ingest it as a flower essence. It is intriguing that this is the state flower of California where many people are involved in various spiritual practices and they can benefit from the special effects of this essence.

"Most animals become more connected to the earth. A greater understanding of purpose at a very subtle and emotional level results. This may give more calm and ease some behavioral difficulties. There is less difficulty experienced with the opposition of Saturn and the sun. The fifth and eleventh rays are enhanced."

CAROB (ST. JOHN'S BREAD)
Ceratonia Siliqua

This evergreen fruit tree is native to Syria and Asia Minor. Its small, green flowers appear in the spring in elongated clusters.

Q How can this tree now be used as a flower essence?

"It develops a collective consciousness in a group of people, which enhances group communication and interaction. People in a group telepathically join their minds together to receive higher inspirations to experience a single, clear, and unified focus. Groups involved in any spiritual practices would especially enjoy this essence.

"It extends the etheric body directly into the mental body to improve their elasticity. This increases empathy in a group and between healers and their clients. If you were in good health and had a clear understanding of your anatomy, take a few drops of carob, internally and externally, and you would develop more empathy for the pain your client was experiencing. Or if a group took carob, they could more effectively send their healing energies to a sick person."

Q Since the causal body is associated with the collective consciousness of the planet, would carob influence the causal body?

"No, it is limited to the collective consciousness of groups.

"The signature is the fact that it tends to bloom in the more mature sections of the tree. Carob helps people have empathy with their elders and even to assume some of their wisdom. In Lemuria, it was used in this capacity. The test point is the medulla oblongata. This is another tree mentioned in the Bible that has much value as a flower essence.

"Some of the group-coordinating effects of this essence will be noted in animals, especially when horses are taken from a herd in the wild. This is also true with fish that traveled in schools but are separated from the school and transported to an aquarium or other setting. This essence helps the animal reattune to the group mind of that animal species rather than just merely the herd or school that was formerly known. This essence may be useful for animals that are joining new herds or working together in new groups. Apply it not just to yourself but to the animal.

"It is frequently observed that when people are involved in group meditation or group visualization, animals who are the pets of such people may sit at your feet and seem to be asleep or even meditating. Indeed, they are attuning to the thought forms and are involved in them. Many times, it is necessary for people to lead them in such activity, but animals have their own way of gravitating toward such energy fields and working with them. And some animals in the woods where you may be meditating or doing such group work may also be affected by such thought forms even though they may not be pets or be directly known to any people on the premises.

"Plants, particularly of wildflowers that occur naturally around houses where people have a common focus, where group energy is occurring naturally and repeatedly, will be enhanced by using this essence. When natal planets that figure prominently in one's chart pass through the signs of Libra and Aquarius, this is an excellent time to use this essence. The fifth, sixth, and seventh rays are better coordinated for most people."

CHAPARRAL
Chaparro Amargosa

This desert plant is common in the Southwestern United States. The yellow flowers bloom in the spring and winter. It is prescribed for chronic illnesses such as cancer, arthritis, skin problems, respiratory conditions, and kidney diseases.

Q What are the origins and karmic pattern of chaparal?

"The development of this plant was specifically regarded with a great deal of religious and ritual energy. This provided many of its cleansing properties and its ability to unite various vibrational levels within individuals. This was noted as the Lemurians worked with the plant because a deep sense of silence often resulted. As a method of exchanging this silence for energy, rituals were developed. This enabled the plant to grow easily, and great strength was imbued into it.

"Chaparral is to provide more sensibility amongst groups, ultimately leading to the development of new communication between all levels of vibrational beings. This karmic pattern is to eventually relate to the lower kingdoms—the non-hive insects, the kingdom of the insects, and the kingdom of the air. As this develops, mankind's loving energy may be a part of this process."

Q How is chaparral now used as a flower essence?

"It activates the causal and astral bodies. Taking this essence generates the ability of astral projection to any selected level upon earth, to any selected level of mind upon the planet, and to any selected level of information on the planet. And this information is incorporated into the mental body in an organized fashion to create mental clarity in the conscious mind. Creative visualization and, with the aid of meditation, conscious astral projection develops with chaparral. Past life recall increases, especially when past life events interfere with the present incarnation.

"Use chaparral for individuals experiencing insomnia, restlessness, memory loss, inability to recall dreams, and frustration from unknown origins. The minor chakras about each elbow are augmented. These chakras focus the odic or pranic forces in the system to remove blockages or congestion in the major chakras.

"Chaparral cleanses and aligns all the meridians. The correct alignment of the meridians stimulates the spleen, the body's immune system, the entire ductless system, and the circulatory system. Toxicity in the blood is dispelled, and, on the cellular level, the circulatory system is stimulated. The syphilitic miasm, AIDS, and tumors are alleviated. With creative visualization this essence stimulates autolysis. It can be prescribed externally as a salve or spray.

"Hopi, Apache, and Zuni Indian devic orders are associated with this plant. Chaparral was often used in ancient Israel among the Essenes. It is one of the more important plants on the planet. There is a lessening of any difficult effects of squares or oppositions of Chiron. The tenth ray is strengthened.

"Difficult sleep states for animals will be eased. More importantly, animals often have the ability to utilize astral forms with much greater ease than humans. Many times the reason for a close association in the waking life between an animal and human is so that during sleep the trust the human feels for the animal can be utilized by the animal's higher self to help the person to enter the astral states with greater joy. When you are aware that this is occurring with your animal, you and the animal should use this essence. Then as you fall asleep, visualize the animal leading you, taking you on a journey visiting astral realms. Animals will do this with far greater ease than most humans.

"Under circumstances of extreme difficulty such as fire, pestilence, locust infestations, or when large tracts of land are destroyed by various pollutants or difficult environmental conditions including drought, there is some benefit in using this essence. Sometimes the people associated with these plants will have dream states that help them understand more of the lessons and necessity for these difficult periods. With such information more clearly within their grasp, they can begin again more easily to work with such plants. The essence is given after the difficulty, when plants are again being regrown."

CLOVER (Red)
Trifolium Pratense

This wild annual grows all over North America and Europe. The red to purple flowers grow in dense, terminal, ovoid, or globular heads. Medically it is used for blood, liver, constipation, or respiratory problems.

Q What is the karmic background of clover?

"In Lemuria, this plant was utilized partly in ritual and partly as a decoration. It has a very powerful etheric energy flow which spiritualizes the emotions of the plant. It is as if people's emotions, their ability to be absorbed, shifted, and then released back into the environment is a natural part of the etheric flow through the earth with this plant. In exploring this the Lemurians saw many ways this could be strengthened. The flower essence was utilized to capture many different properties and it was by the mid-Lemurian phase that red clover was completed."

Q How is this plant today used as a flower essence?

"It fuses the emotional and causal bodies together causing a universal form of emotionalism. Certain emotional individuals run around agonizing over catastrophies. Red clover is effective for them. It treats mass hysteria. It breaks the chain reaction that starts with one individual and sometimes leads to panic. The state of mind that it engenders is calmness and an understanding of what is behind a disaster. Thus one can better deal with catastrophes in which many have suffered.

"It strengthens the blood vessels, and on the cellular level, it enhances the red corpuscles. In doing this, it strengthens all the meridians because there is a relationship between the circulatory system and the meridians in the operation of flower essences in the body. It eases the tubercular miasm and can be used with leukemia. The essence can be applied externally.

"The fuzzy appearance of the plant suggests its ethereal properties. To a psychic the plant's aura looks somewhat like the finer properties or energies connected to the meridians. Some of the classical devic orders from Ireland are associated with this plant. The test point is either the pulse or the wrist.

"Consider using clover when animals are forced into a group setting such as in a laboratory, kennel, and what is commonly termed the pound. Such circumstances are difficult for most animals, and many times hysterical states, states of consciousness focusing on escape, change, or deep anxiety, will be eased by this essence.

"When companion planting is difficult for reasons that are not immediately obvious, these problems will generally relate to soil or environmental conditions or the mental state of those working with such plants. This essence may be indicated. This essence will assist in greater harmonious states for companion planting.

"When natal Jupiter passes through Aquarius, consider using this essence. The seventh and eleventh rays are made clearer for most."

CORN (Sweet)
Zea Mays

This is one of the three main cereal crops in the world. It produces male and female flowers in long, spike-like racemes. The wild species originated in tropical America. There are now many cultivated varieties. Corn has traditionally been used as a demulcent and a diuretic.

Q What is the karmic pattern of this plant?

"Its seeds display different colors, expressing the goal of seeking balance amongst many diverse races. Corn was developed in early Atlantis with this goal. Numerous races then existed in Atlantis. It also established harmonious relations between newly divided male and female members of society. Karmically this plant is still associated with many of the red-skinned leaders of Atlantis, the American Indians.

"In Atlantis, corn was utilized for many interesting experiments in genetic engineering because it has a fairly simple DNA structure. This allowed many different mutations to be attempted. Few of these were very successful except for those leading to various colors. Even today, though rare, many different colors of corn are available. This strengthened purpose in working with the genetic structure had an unconscious effect with the Atlanteans in which some of their thought forms were captured and utilized by corn. It is a very absorptive and powerful substance, and corn flower essence can ease some of the karmic instability left with those who might still experience some guilt around difficulties associated with genetic engineering from their previous Atlantean times. This is also true with those who were present during such times and even for those who simply knew of such experiments."

Q How is corn today used as a flower essence?

"Corn is suitable for people living in large cities and high density housing because it helps people handle living in cramped quarters. If you have trouble paying rent take this essence; it calms the person down to handle such problems in an intelligent fashion. It can also be used in refugee camps. This essence helps people establish a spiritual relationship with the earth. This is one reason why it is so germane to people living in crowded conditions. This is an important reason why corn has long been a staple food crop for many American Indians. A spiritual relation with Mother Earth is an integral part of the religious beliefs of many American Indians.

"Daydreamers, overly nervous individuals, or those who cannot focus on various issues would benefit from corn. A child doing poorly in group tests, particularly if that was connected to peer pressure, exemplifies this problem. Corn can be used in mild cases of obsession, schizophrenia, or conditions generating such difficulties. But corn would not generally be sufficient to cure such conditions, so it should usually be used in combination with other remedies. This is a wonderful elixir to take when doing long-range planning. This can include buying a house or entering an agreement that will take some years to bear results.

"Corn is often the remedy of choice in psychosomatic illnesses, including stress-related cancer. It can be used in biofeedback and creative visualization therapies for treating cancer. It helps the individual focus the body's immune system, including the blood flows of imbalanced areas, and become emotionally detached to deal with problems in an objective manner. Psychological problems causing cancerous tumors or leukemia can be faced with this essence. If a salve of corn was rubbed over a cancerous tumor, it eases the problem. Corn can also be used to rejuvenate the white corpuscles, and it is usually effective against most viruses.

"With regard to androgyny, the acceptance of both male and female halves within an individual is encouraged by corn essence. Individuals who experience food allergy are also often affected with candida. Many common allergies relate to food substances that are taken repeatedly over time. Corn is often one of these. When an allergy to corn is noted, stop eating corn and add corn flower essence to the diet. Amaranthus essence can also be quite useful to provide some energetic pathways to release corn from the body. There are certain nutritional similarities between amaranthus and corn. Amaranthus can also be eaten, but not at the same time as a person is taking amaranthus essence. Taking the flower essence of the particular food that one is allergic to should usually be done with food allergies. This speeds the allergic response of the physical body in the educational process, particularly the etheric body and immune system.

"The emotional body is cleansed, so a person becomes emotionally detached. This makes it easier for the individual to accept what they are going through, which also affects long-range decision making. This process does not make one impersonal, just detached and objective.

"Because corn is a tonic to the astral body, it aids one in long-range decision making. All decision making involves, in part, dipping into the future. Corn can further be used to treat nightmares, which a weakened astral body can cause.

"The astral body is a dimensional state in which the mind travels along specific time flows into the past or future to retrieve information that is mostly relevant and personal to the individual. The astral body stores past life experiences, keeping this information from being released in a manner that would disrupt the current incarnation. Occasionally you will meet a person who always seems to have an intuitive understanding of events and to be in the flow of life. This is often because they have a balanced astral body, so they can project into the future. These individuals frequently become very nervous when others offer them too much advice. This is because their information is no longer personalized to them, so it no longer is in tune with their astral body. This can be an important issue with psychics.

"Corn opens the abdominal chakra, which helps balance the emotions. Massaging this essence over the body, particularly the medulla oblongata, is quite relaxing. It is a mild tonic for the meridians. For most people the negative aspects of Neptune are eased, and the fifth ray is enhanced. The test point is on the wrist where perfumes are traditionally tested.

"When an animal is in overcrowded situation for an extended period of time, anxious states may develop that are difficult to relieve. Corn is indicated at all times during such overcrowding, but particularly when the animal is readjusting. He is coming back to a place of less overcrowding or difficulty and attempting to form new bonds with humans. Then the animal is trying to assimilate and integrate this experience, as if then the fellows that the animal shared close quarters with are in some way psychically present with the animal. Corn essence allows a gradual release from some of the thought forms associated with such overcrowding."

Q How is corn different from red clover in this regard?

"It is significantly different in that with corn the circumstances apply to longer periods of time, not to short ones; and not to hysterical states, but instead to states of gradual anxiety that are created over time.

"Today much of the corn grown in the United States and most of the world is hybridized and has been treated and changed quite a bit over the last 30 years. It is useful to utilize corn flower essence, particularly if it can be derived from nonhybridized or older varieties. Then this essence may impart some new properties to the corn being grown, adding strength to it, resistance to disease, and, most importantly, increased ability to procreate."

COSMOS
Cosmos Bipinnatus

Cosmos is a common garden flower native to Mexico. It grows three feet tall with rose, purple, or white flowers and yellow discs. Orange and yellow flowers have also been developed. The plant grows best in a warm climate, and the flowers bloom from early summer until mid-autumn.

Q How is this plant now used as a flower essence?

"Cosmos has the rare ability of combining the heart and throat chakras. It generates composure before speaking or initiating an artistic expression. It is invaluable for actors, writers, or people in leadership positions. And linguistic abilities increase. It does not create a sympathetic link between individuals like some essences such as yarrow; it is strictly an individual thing. Two individuals, for instance, may debate articulately and not necessarily reach an agreement. They would just respect and listen more intently to the other person's position, for this essence does not necessarily resolve the conflict.

"This essence is more for certain types of people rather than for specific psychological dynamics. Introverted, shy, or procrastinating individuals would find this an excellent remedy. Such people could express more clearly their philosophies on given topics. The reason cosmos has this effect is because it brings the etheric, mental, and spiritual bodies into alignment. This, combined with its effect on the throat and heart chakras, enables people to better express themselves. It allows people to release emotional tensions stored in the heart.

"Circulation improves, metabolism is strengthened, sympathetic and parasympathetic nervous system sensitivity increases, and heart and thyroid activity are invigorated. Relief in heart diseases, sore throats, throat cancer, and bronchial conditions occurs, but in each case, the essence should be taken in combination with other remedies. It assists in the assimilation of iodine, silica, and vitamin E. Positive aspects of Venus will be enhanced slightly. The fourth and fifth rays are strengthened.

"This is a powerful essence for communication, including communication with one's animals. This is something that is developing gradually. There will, therefore, be added assistance with animals of great intelligence such as primates—gorillas in particular—and dolphins, sea otters, and other animals that have a greater tendency to communicate when given correct circumstances, greater love, assistance, and kindness from humans. In this way, both humans and animals are assisted. However, this essence may even assist animals of much lower intelligence as long as the human is willing to communicate at the level at which the animal may receive. This is often enhanced by voice communication. Speak quietly and clearly to the animal, and the animal is likely to understand this better by using cosmos.

"For those who perceive the ability of sound to work with various seeds to increase germination and to help young plants grow, consider using this essence. The use of sound around plants—by sharing songs, chants, and pure sounds, not just speaking to them, as has often been noted by many who grow plants—is all made better and more available to most plants when humans use this essence. It can also be added to the plant's water, but one should do this only when one is willing to speak or sing to the plants. Otherwise, various external sounds such as street noise or noise from machinery will also be more easily absorbed and assimilated by the plants. This can have a difficult effect when such noises interfere with a plant's growth patterns, particularly with machinery noises."

DAFFODIL
Narcissus Ajax

This popular garden plant produces golden and yellow flowers in the spring. The plant originated in Europe and West Asia.

Q What is the karmic background of this plant?

"This plant form was developed in Lemuria when there was the desire to develop certain systems of flowers in relationship to the separation of the subconscious and superconscious mind. In early Lemuria, there were suspicions and distinctions as to the three levels of consciousness. It was then desired to bring forth knowledge of the superconscious and subconscious mind independent from the conscious mind and to understand that unique distinction. The ethereal properties of this particular plant form were developed to comprehend this distinction. Greater spiritual progression was obtained when the separation of the subconscious and superconscious mind's influence from the conscious mind was understood."

Q How is this plant now used as a flower essence?

"Daffodil extends the conscious mind's activity through the mental body, which it helps organize, to certain levels of the higher self. This is desirable because the higher self is actually a fine attunement of all the subtle bodies, and it is never out of harmony. The higher self is always attempting to align the subtle bodies into their proper frequencies.

"This essence is applicable to transcendental forms of meditation and to hearing voices from one's guides or higher self. The conical shape of energy that can be observed appearing from the crown chakra feeding into the individual expresses this influence. The crown chakra organizes the conscious mind to receive information from the higher self. This is a splendid essence to deepen daily meditative practices."

Q When you refer to the higher self are you referring to the integrated spiritual body?

"No, I refer only to the higher self. To illustrate, if each of the subtle bodies were little rings and you were playing a game, attempting to toss them on a stake in a specific order, the higher self would be the stake. You would be attempting to place the rings on the stake in a specific order, but sometimes this does not quite happen. At times the subtle bodies are almost perfectly aligned, but still there are some imbalances. This is why perfectly healthy individuals function normally without the subtle bodies being totally aligned. If the degree of misalignment becomes too extreme physical and psychological problems can appear. It is a matter of degree."

Q Can you define what you mean by the higher self and how it differs from the integrated spiritual body, the superconscious, and the soul?

"The superconscious is the totality of the higher principles. It is synonymous with the higher self. The forces of the integrated spiritual body are activities that attempt to merge only the spiritual aspects. These are not necessarily, for instance, higher mental or intellectual attributes. The integrated spiritual body consists of all the integrated spiritual principles that an individual may work with. None of these forces represent the capacities of the soul. The soul is the all encompassing portion of the self that is united with God. The soul is that which is omnipresent in all quadrants of time and space."

Q Because this essence helps people attune to their higher self, would it be a good remedy to take before dowsing or doing any intuitive work?
"Yes, it makes the individual more sensitive.
"Daffodil vitalizes the body. This does not mean physically rejuvenating the body; it is more a vitality that manifests from a clarity of thought. It strengthens the thymus, eases stress, reduces high blood pressure, alleviates ulcerous conditions, and lessens the heavy metal miasm.
"It is excellent for treating manic-depression, psycho-spiritual imbalances, extreme frustration, low intellectual capacities, and constant self-condemnation. The conical shape of the bloom represents its ability to harmonize people with their higher self. It can be used externally, and the test point is the thymus.
"Some easing of behavioral difficulties where animals are very resistant to learning new patterns will be noted. This can be especially helpful when one is in greater attunement with one's guides and the guides of the animal. Together you visualize or create coordinated energies to show the animal new pathways, new ways of expression, or new ways to channel the energy the animal is dealing with.
"The ability to grow plants under difficult conditions and all types of crop rotation will be enhanced by this essence. Some positive aspects of trines between Jupiter and natal Neptune will be strengthened. The third and ninth rays are made clearer for most people."

DAISY (English)   **DAISY** (Shasta)
Bellis Perennis   Chrysanthemum Maximum

Either of these two plants can be used. Shasta daisy is a robust perennial. The large flowers on solitary heads are white with a golden center. While shasta daisy flowers only in the summer, English daisy flowers from early in the spring until the fall. English daisy is a low-growing perennial with small, white flowers, which are often pink on the outer surface. It is found all through Europe. English daisy is used for jaundice, liver disorders, and skin problems such as boils.

Q How is this plant now used as a flower essence?
"Daisy spiritualizes the intellect. Scattered information is brought into a crystal clear focus. If one had a collection of spiritual books on many different topics and you were trying to show how there was a consistent pattern in specific areas, this essence allows you to bring a semblance of order to this work. But this is not an intellectual achievement. Daisy facilitates intuitively understanding the process and unity behind what you are studying.
"It aligns the mental, causal, emotional, and spiritual bodies. This generates a clarity in someone to really understand what his or her feelings are in diverse areas,

particularly in spiritual topics. If you cannot decipher exactly what your philosophy is, or if you feel somewhat distant from how a process works, this essence should be considered. It stabilizes people who are constantly running from one spiritual or growth group to another without really finding what they are seeking.

"The chakra point stimulated is where the breast bones meet below the throat. This spiritualizes the emotions and increases humility.

"Daisy does not too deeply influence the physical body, but it relieves hiccups and shallow breathing. It also eases asthma, although other essences are often better in treating this problem. Daisy is a liquid tracheotomy, and it is used externally. Trines between the sun and Mercury will have greater beneficial impact. The sixth and seventh rays are activated.

"Daisy may be of benefit in the early phase of animal learning when new patterns are getting established. This is particularly true between parent and offspring in the way the elder one will move the younger animal, touch it, and then back away from it. Such animals may occasionally exhibit psychological disturbances as if they are unwilling to play, learn, or grow. These are indicators for this essence.

"Visualization of new plant types, new hybridization, new ways of working with plants will be enhanced when the person uses the essence and it is made available to the plant. This essence will increase understanding of plants under familiar circumstances that one wishes to change slightly as in correct companion planting or working with plants for new purposes as in using herbs for their spiritual effects. When two botanically different plants are sufficiently related vibrationally as these are, either is sufficient."

DILL
Anethum Graveolens

Dill is a hardy aromatic annual native to Southern Russia and the Mediterranean region. Numerous yellow flowers bloom in mid-summer. Dill resolves a wide variety of digestive ills, and it promotes the flow of mother's milk.

Q What is the karmic background of dill?

"The plant was directly seen by the Lemurians as providing interesting emotional interchange, particularly between animals and the other kingdoms. While working with this energy, some of the unconscious nature of those observing and feeling the energies of the plant began to come forth. It was hoped that such an energy might be strengthened for people to use. This has not been done to nearly the extent that was hoped for, particularly because the Atlanteans did not involve themselves in this process as was hoped. Thus, this is still one of the karmic possibilities for this plant."

Q How is this plant now used as a flower essence?

"This essence reestablishes a proper balance between the emotional and etheric bodies. When these two bodies become too bound together, this exposes the body to various forms of inflammation, particularly when the individual undergoes stress. People who cannot express themselves clearly may develop an ulcer, or a rigid unbending person may develop heart disease.

"People obsessed with aging or dying, morose people, manic-depressives, and overly self-critical individuals can benefit from dill. It uplifts a person to a lighter, more expanded form of consciousness to help him or her get beyond the basic difficulties to examine them in an objective light. This is definitely a healthier perspective. For instance, if there is an emotional problem, dill affords the person the intellectual opportunity to objectively examine the situation. This is not necessarily the solution to the problem, but it definitely is a less oppressive consciousness.

"Dill assists in the digestion and proper assimilation of most food. It also opens some of the synapses between various neurons in the brain. Tonsilitis and diseases involving degeneration of the brain tissue such as cerebral palsy can be treated with dill.

"The dome-like shape of the flowers symbolizes the extension of the primitive reptilian part of the brain known as the pineal gland toward the higher evolved portions of the cranium. The brain has grown from just being a primitive, biochemical regulator to having an expanded intellectual capacity. It has a mild impact on the pituitary and abdominal chakras. In astrology there is a strengthening of positive effects of Pluto and Uranus. The sixth ray is augmented. The test point is the kidney meridian at the mid-point of the thigh. This point mildly increases astral projection abilities.

"Arthritis, bone spurs, kidney stones, and stiffness in an animal's body will be eased by dill. And animals may find a greater ability to manifest love and patience.

"The period immediately following creation of seeds within the plant is an important time. Then plants are utilizing the lessons and understanding that have been accumulated during the lifetime. At this point, nearly all biological processes—germination, mid-growth, fertilization, and creating seeds—have been completed. This is an excellent time to provide dill so that the overall thought form of the particular species is strengthened. A direct effect will not be seen, but over several generations vitality and strength will be enhanced. Of course, this only applies to plants that create seeds and not to those that do not replicate by the use of seeds."

EUCALYPTUS
Eucalyptus Globulus

While native to Australia, this tree is now found in many parts of the world. Known as the blue gum tree, it reaches heights of almost 400 feet making it one of the tallest trees in the world. The flowers are solitary, axillary, and white with no petals. Eucalyptus essential oil is a powerful antiseptic, especially in various skin conditions, and it is recommended in many respiratory imbalances.

Q What is the karmic background of this tree?

"During the development of the ego in Lemuria, there was a need to bring forth balance within the emotional states. Eucalyptus, in part, evolved the ethereal properties of the lungs as an esoteric portion of the anatomy for the elimination of extreme emotional states in the Lemurians. It advanced the intaking and internalizing of the life force to stimulate physiologically and ethereally the entire subtle anatomies. This created the totality of balance within the entire system of the individual."

The current human form took shape in early Lemuria 500,000 years ago. Various flower essences and mental projection were then used to evolve the human physical and subtle anatomy. Eucalyptus essence contributed to the formation of our respiratory system and emotional body. There is a direct link between our lungs and emotional body, which creates emotional equilibrium. Rudolf Steiner discussed this connection; for example a sudden emotional shock usually causes people to take in a deep breath.[1] The formation of the lungs made it easier to breathe in the life force to shape people in mind, body, and spirit.

Q How is this tree now used as a flower essence?

"Many of the herbal properties of eucalyptus are transferred to the flower essence. It eases inflammations in the kidneys, liver, lungs, and nasal passages. It is quite effective in treating asthma, jaundice, malaria, and kidney deterioration.

"Iron and hemoglobin, which carry radiation in the system, are strengthened and cleansed, so parts of the body lacking oxygen are replenished. The entire circulatory system is activated to better carry nutrients and oxygen to various parts of the body, particularly the pancreas. These impacts take place more on the cellular level, especially in the skin tissue and the capillary action. Niacin is also absorbed easier with this essence.

"People who do not breathe well from any cause, individuals who almost drown, and people who suffer from smoke inhalation in a fire can all benefit from this remedy. Eucalyptus oxygenates the system and improves the lungs of people who have smoked for a long time. Partly because of its pronounced effect on the eliminative organs, it can be prescribed in any form of radiation sickness, particularly plutonium poisoning. And the psora and tubercular miasms are alleviated.

"The balancing capacities of the heart chakra are activated. This stimulates the thymus because it is associated with the heart chakra. In the first seven years of life, the thymus gland produces some hemoglobin. Disagreements in marriages or partnerships, and even sharp hostilities between people can be resolved with eucalyptus because it helps you understand the other person's position.

"People experiencing grief, especially over the demise of a loved one, can benefit from this essence. Sometimes in these situations kidney problems exist. Expansion of energy in the physical body can sometimes be necessary in moving through the grieving process. It also assists individuals to clarify their ability to understand what the other person is saying. In attuning to anothers energy, it sometimes appears necessary to shield your understanding, your sensibilities, and most importantly your emotional response. Eucalyptus relaxes this process.

"The ethereal fluidium, the etheric body, and the meridians are strengthened by this essence. This allows vibrational remedies to integrate closer to the cellular level. The pungent quality of eucalyptus oil is part of its signature because this expresses the penetrating quality of the essence. Eucalyptus can be used externally, and the test point is the tip of the index finger and any lung meridian points.

"Distress over loss of a loved one is also eased in animals. Here blame is often felt towards those involved who are human. This may run very deep for animals and may not emerge clearly until the animal again feels stress. For an animal to achieve its own degree of forgiveness, eucalyptus is recommended. This can be applied shortly after loss, and then repeated at intervals of about one week for two months. Then, for most animals, there will be added assimilation of many nutrients with eucalyptus, so it is useful to give this essence to most animals at least twice a year, particularly for difficulty in growth patterns in the period closest to adolescence. Then assimilation of various nutrients, especially iron, usually moves through several dramatic shifts. Such nutrients are then made more easily assimilable.

"Plants that require various support structures to hold them up, including beans and tomatoes, will be given added strength of a fibrous nature within their own physical bodies. These includes the root structure, stems, and points where the leaves meet the stems. There will be some strengthening when the plant is coming to the end of the support structure, when it nearly covers the structure, and it is then important that the plant's growth slow down. The plant may need new growth at its lower parts, and this will be enhanced by using this essence. Plants that appear to be growing too fast for the season and the growing conditions will also find such growth more easily self-governed by eucalyptus.

"Negative aspects, squares in particular, between Venus and Jupiter are eased. The third and fifth rays are made clearer for most."

1 Rudolf Steiner, *Spiritual Science and Medicine* (London: Rudolf Steiner Press, 1975).
_____. *What Can the Art of Healing Gain Through Spiritual Science* (Spring Valley, NY: Mercury Press, n.d.), p. 17.
Victor Bott, M.D., *Anthroposophical Medicine* (London: Rudolf Steiner Press, 1978), p.37, 85, 98, 121.

GARLIC
Allium Sativum

While native to Siberia, this herb is now a common food crop world-wide, especially in many Latin countries. It produces white, starry, and strongly scented flowers. It is a digestive aid, it eases insect stings, and it eases many blood and lung disorders.

Q What is the karmic background of garlic?
"It was observed that a pulsation was often seen in the flower as it worked with positive growing factors as earth energy moved through it. This was particularly observed at night. Insects and other creatures that came near the plant were noticeably changed. Part of this is due to the fairly high mineral content in garlic and its interesting chemical constituents. In observing this, the Atlanteans saw the obvious bridge to strengthen positive thought forms, to destroy negative thought forms, and to bring such energy particularly from the flower essence into people. It took a long period of development to bring this into action because the existence of negative thought forms was not fully understood in Lemuria. The Atlanteans continued this work. It was also utilized in many other areas by the Atlanteans. Garlic essence was an important component of many devices, and many ways of changing the plant by using mental energy developed in Atlantis. The karmic purpose of all this is to create for all mankind a full understanding of the necessity of negative thought forms, so the way of working with their essential energies can be understood and the necessity for negative thought forms may be ended."

Q How can this plant now be used as a flower essence?

"Garlic gets rid of any fear or paranoia because it crystallizes objectivity in the mental and emotional bodies, and the liver chakra is opened. This is partly associated with its legendary ability to banish superstitious creatures. Garlic also eases anger. It can be used for stage fright or to relax a person facing a difficult therapy such as surgery. Even if someone were afraid to release hidden fear or anger, these insecurities could be gradually released and faced with garlic. Classical Freudian psychotherapy is particularly enhanced with garlic.

"Interestingly, this essence can be used as an insect spray. Or you could ingest it, and it would revitalize the nervous system in a specific manner to create an irritating magnetic field in the aura antagonistic to insects.

"Many of its herbal properties are transferred to the flower essence. It cleanses the system of parasites, particularly those imbedded in the skin and muscular tissue, general inflammations are eased, and the liver is strengthened. The blood, especially the red corpuscles on the cellular level, is purified and invigorated. Interferon is also stimulated. Garlic eases the radiation, petrochemical, and psora miasms."

Q In traditional Chinese medicine fear is associated with the kidneys. Does garlic have any effect on cleansing the kidneys?

"No."

Q Would garlic be used differently from mimulus essence, which also eases fears?

"Garlic can be applied for all fears, while mimulus is applicable mostly to mental fears.

"The devic orders associated with garlic are from Lemuria, India, and Greece. Concerning its signature, a garlic clove looks somewhat like the liver. Garlic helps the odic force flow smoothly through the meridians, and the test point is the tongue.

"Use it with animals as an insect spray, but animals can also take garlic internally—not just for deworming and increasing digestion, but also to repel insects. Generally, it will take about three weeks before the essence will penetrate to such levels within the animal that the repellent effect will be noted. This is valuable. The negative thought forms associated with insects may be a part of the picture for some animals, particularly animals that have repeated problems with insects on only one side of the body. This applies more to ticks and fleas than to other insects, but as these are the primary difficulties with most animals, this essence is of benefit.

"In the newly formed diseases associated with ticks—particularly Lyme disease—there will be an easing and repelling of the negative thought forms associated with this disease. Such ticks will not penetrate or work with the animals as deeply. In the next twenty years there will be various new diseases originating from ticks. These diseases will affect people and animals.

"Lyme disease has its roots in many other diseases from the past. It is primarily a powerful mutation and combination of diseases relating to syphilis and rheumatoid arthritis at a very deep level. This new combination relates to the ways children approach the world. Adults, in viewing the world through the eyes of the child or in knowing the child within themselves, can have flexibility, and an ability to work with others. At the same time, they will not fear their own negative thought forms. One must recognize that even the smallest voice within is valuable and needs to be looked at, whether it is positive or negative.

"It is possible that variants of syphilis, AIDS, cancer, and several other contagious diseases will be seen in the next two decades. The most important of these may be related to a direct variant of bovine leukemia. This virus may be seen to be transmitted by ticks, mostly to other animals, but may eventually also shift in its ability to be absorbed by people. This is particularly dangerous because such variants may be difficult to note. The reason this information is given now is so that individuals may be on the lookout for it. It took several years after the first outbreaks of Lyme disease before the tick was recognized as the cause or carrier.

"Garlic essence should be sprayed in the air and given to animals. Garlic can also be incorporated in the water used to irrigate plants in such areas. By changing the vibration within plants, some of these problems will be eased. Thus garlic will repel; it will not kill. It will bring these negative thought forms into greater clarity so that plants and animals can dispel them.

"There is some assistance with the absorption of many nutrients, and plants are able to move such nutrients through the excretory system more quickly. Therefore, it is useful particularly when soils are mineral rich or when there are significant mineral imbalances within the soil. Squares and oppositions between the sun and Mars are good times to use garlic essence. The fourth and eighth rays are activated."

GREEN ROSE
Rosa Chinensis Viridiflora

This Chinese wild rose produces green flowers. This rose, a naturally occurring mutation, appeared in China in 1743 or 1855.

Q How is this plant now used as a flower essence?
"The green flowers appeared when there was a heightened interest in psychic development. When sports or mutations suddenly appear in nature, they usually represent some shift of consciousness in humanity. It first appeared in 1743 corresponding with the activities of Immanuel Swedenbourg. This was the start of a century of psychic development in the West. It was totally anchored on this plane in the 1850's with the activities of many individuals, including Andrew Jackson Davis and Daniel Douglas Home."

Q Most of the psychic work that you are speaking of took place in Europe and the United States, so why did green rose instead appear in China?
"China was a more sympathetic environment. It was as the polarity between the East and West. This symbolized the blooming of Eastern systems of thought within the West and the drawing of Western systems of thought into the Eastern sphere.
"This essence develops and enhances psychic abilities, particularly as examined within Western systems of thought. It specifically assists one to become a conscious or trance channel and to develop multidirectional clairvoyance. It is especially helpful to distinguish between soul and delusional messages. And it enhances spiritual healing such as laying on the hands.

"Green flowers, such as this rose, usually augment psychic abilities because the color green is an isolated spectrum and wavelength of energy similar to the frequency upon which telepathic energy travels. It is the wavelength of communication between the mental forces, so this essence amplifies telepathy within an individual.

"Green rose is a good essence for psychics who are emotionally unstable and for treating diseases caused by a perception of or a repression of psychic abilities. These imbalances include: allergies, asthma, colon spasms, epilepsy, Meniere's disease, migraine headaches, mucous colitis, night terrors in children, environmental problems, obsessional neuroses, manic depression, allergies that relate to past life memories, and solar plexus imbalances such as duodenal ulcers.[1] This essence can treat cases of schizophrenia caused by psychic trauma. Many of these problems are psychological imbalances, places in which individuals have come close to strong psychic awakening and have no models or groundwork to understand and work with such energies.

"Green rose also eases the tubercular miasm. In attuning to powerful psychic energies, the lungs are often put to great tests. This is often a powerful karmic pattern that people take from lifetime to lifetime.

"Green rose is quite potent because holding a spiral pattern as it does, enables it to duplicate the spiral energy of the pituitary gland, which is one of the critical, sensitive tissues for telepathy. Not only does it augment the pituitary gland, but it also increases the psychic faculties of the pineal gland.

"The spiritual and etheric bodies are aligned, the meridians are enhanced, the nadis are strengthened, and it can be used externally. The test point is the medulla oblongata and the center of the forehead near the third eye.

"Those opening psychic abilities may note that the sleep, or traditional or established behavior patterns of animals around them, are stressed. The animals have difficulty as you develop psychically. Under certain circumstances, allergic reactions to environmental pollutants or new foods may intensify. Green rose is often indicated for the animals as well as the person.

"Endangered species of plants, plants difficult to grow under ordinary environmental conditions, and plants being cultivated where they had only grown wild before will benefit by green rose essence. Use a very small quantity, as little as one drop to ten gallons of water. The individual working with such plants should meditate and visualize the plant growing in its own natural environment as much as possible. Even though this may not be supported in physical fact, the imagination and visualization will be enhanced if this individual also uses green rose. Under such circumstances, plants may reacclimate, but this will generally take at least three generations before the plant is able to work without the additional energy of the flower essence. This is a way of acclimating at very high vibrational levels assisting the oversoul of the plant to acclimate to these new growing conditions. Love is of great importance. After the third generation, one might stop using green rose essence so that the plant would then be acclimated on its own.

"Most of the positive aspects between Uranus and Jupiter are activated. There is a strengthening of the fifth and eighth rays."

1 Arthur Guirdham, M.D., *The Psyche in Medicine* (Sudbury, Suffolk, England: Neville Spearman Ltd., 1978), p. 206-254.

HARVEST BRODIAEA
Brodiaea Elegans

This perennial wild flower is native to California and Oregon. Its violet or deep-purple flowers appear from April to July.

Q How is this plant now used as a flower essence?

"This essence mostly affects the ethereal levels; however, it does influence the physical body. Harvest brodiaea helps spiritualize the mental body, which as a by-product in the physical level increases spiritual insight and acuteness of the senses. It also spiritualizes the intellect of more materialistic people. Such an individual may exhibit hostility toward religious concepts or be an agnostic. It alleviates certain forms of bitterness that can result from a materialistic life-style. This attitude can manifest as feeling isolated from society, self-centeredness, selfish behavior, or an intellectual form of hostility. Eccentric geniuses often fit into this category. More self-esteem, increased clarity of thought, and a less self-condemning nature are by-products of this remedy.

"It is a prominent essence for strengthening the eyes and can be used to treat eye problems including nearsightedness, farsightedness, cataracts, and glaucoma. At times certain eye problems result from an inability to release toxins from the system. It can be added to an eyedropper for the eyes, especially with such things as eyebright. In Atlantis, harvest brodiaea essence with a comfrey poultice was used. Comfrey is finely ground and the flower essence added to it. This can be applied to the eye.

"Harvest brodiaea has only a temporary influence on the other senses. It activates the pineal gland and crown chakra, increasing the dream state. The test point is the corner of the eye by the gall bladder meridian. The bulb-like shape of the plant is a clue concerning its effect on the eyes and spiritual insight. The spiritual value of this essence is suggested by the violet color of the bloom.

"Greater attunement to new patterns of behavior in humans will be felt by most animals. An ability to apply such information and understanding without becoming oversensitized is likely to result. Animals that have experienced much mental and emotional stress from an entirely new environment or difficulty in acclimating to circumstances beyond their control will respond well to this essence. However, the key is that the animal has always shown remarkable intelligence and instinctual ability to utilize such intelligence and to learn fairly rapidly and apply what is learned. After these difficult circumstances, this ability to apply and utilize what has been learned falls away. That is an indicator for using this essence.

"There is an enhancement of positive energies of trine and conjunction of the sun, Mercury, and Jupiter. There is a strengthened expression of the sixth and seventh rays."

HELLEBORUS (Black)
Helleborus Niger

This perennial plant is native to the mountains of Central and Southern Europe and Asia Minor. Its pure-white blossoms appear in mid-winter, so it is called the Christmas Rose. It has been used since ancient times with Pliny and Gerard referring to it. It alleviates amenorrhea, depression, dropsy, and hysteria.

Q How is this plant now used as a flower essence?

"This essence involves understanding the aging process, to gain a grasp of the purpose and spiritual impact of aging. This makes time an ally, not an enemy. This is not so much for the fear of aging, although it does cover that spectrum. One better understands why the body ages. It also affects the heart chakra; thus, it is good for people to overcome a broken romance. It is excellent for depression from aging or from a broken romance. This essence helps people understand and accept the conditions of life, particularly circumstances that cannot be changed.

"It mildly rejuvenates the skin tissues and the entire physical body and cellular level. It can be applied as a salve for some skin conditions. But this physical effect is more a by-product of a positive state of mind. Old people who have a healthy glow exemplify how a positive mental attitude can benefit health.

"It also aligns the spiritual and mental bodies. This brings more spiritual influence into one's mental processes. The signature is that it blooms at the end of the year. Older people will find this a useful remedy.

"Many of its properties with people are transferred to animals. It is useful for diseases associated with old age in animals even if occurring at a younger age. It is also indicated for difficulty urinating, kidney or bladder problems, arthritis, or cancer. All these largely degenerative diseases are symbolic of difficulty in the animal's assimilation of new ideas and new lessons. Therefore, after giving this essence look at the life's lesson associated with this difficulty regardless of the age. As you think of it and imagine it, the animal will receive some of the thought forms about this. This essence will assist in the absorption and understanding at the animal's own level of such thought forms.

"There is benefit in using this essence when animals have been closely associated and through death or other circumstances now must be permanently separated. Do not use this essence if such animals are likely to be reunited in the future, for this essence is best for establishing a permanent bond at subtle levels rather than at a temporary level. This permanent bond allows animals greater ease as if asleep and in circumstances where the animal is not fully within its body. It will have communion and understanding with the animal that it has grown used to.

"Use this essence just before a plant goes to seed. Then the plant's thought form is most receptive to understanding the cycles of life and death. Seed yield will not directly increase, but the essence will likely repel negative thought forms associated with this process. Therefore, there will be less difficulty with insect infestation as a result of using this essence at such times.

"Positive aspects of Uranus, Neptune, and Pluto are enhanced. Direct interaction of Pluto and Jupiter in trine, square, and conjunction as well as opposition are more intensified. The tenth and eleventh rays are made clearer for most people."

HENNA
Lawsonia Inerinis

This small shrub is native to the Middle East and India. The small, white and yellow, sweet-smelling flowers grow in large panicles. Medically it is utilized in jaundice, smallpox, headaches, and skin problems.

Q What is the karmic background of this plant?

"This particular substance was used in those days when it was desired to affect balance and conditioning to the portals through which the life force and many of the body's energies flowed, by allowing for the adjustment of the hair follicles upon the body physical. Even though the Lemurians were of very smooth skin and had little body hair, there was still the need to create a balance in the ethereal substances of the hair follicles and their activities. Pigmentation within the hair is a means to regulate specific ethereal functions. Henna was developed, in part, by a small body of Lemurian botanists who desired to work with such principles."

Q How is this plant now used as a flower essence?

"Henna is associated with the tempering of wisdom. Anyone seeking knowledge and spiritual wisdom such as people with an academic or philosophical background should consider this essence. It is also good in a transitional period when the individual is displaying unusual stress in either accepting or rejecting religious faith, spiritual wisdom, or philosophical wisdom. Usually the critical age periods for this are: one to six, twelve to sixteen, twenty to twenty-five, twenty-eight to thirty-two, and forty-nine to fifty-two. As the life span increases, and this will soon happen, the above noted time cycles will change.

"Although henna can be used when a person is experiencing an identity crisis, it is more effective when one is learning to accept philosophically the changes that come in life. During menopause, many women would benefit from this remedy.

"Henna releases past-life information from the genetic code in the DNA and RNA. The capacity for liberating the proper amount of past-life information contributes to decisiveness on the conscious mind level. An inability to intelligently translate this information from the cellular level to the conscious mind creates anxiety, headaches, and stress in the body's muscular tissue. This happens because part of the cellular memory and emotional factors are normally stored in muscular tissues. The type of tension created in the muscles blocks circulation to the brain causing a muscular tension headache.

"The signature is found in the physical substance of hair. Hair symbolizes wisdom, and henna penetrates, cleanses, and thickens the hair shafts. Henna is also a good tonic for that particular form of protein. The test point is the crown chakra and the hair in that part of the head. But the crown chakra is not influenced by henna. Sometimes the crown chakra is just a good point for assimilating light properties. And a perfect balance between the right and left brain can duplicate many properties of the crown chakra.

"Although henna essence does not have too much direct influence on the physical body, all the medical properties of the henna herb and homeopathic preparation are transferred to the flower essence. Diseases treated with henna as an herb or homeopathic preparation also can be treated, to a lesser extent, with henna flower essence. Researchers can expand on these principles. To varying degrees when an herb is prepared as a flower essence, certain of its properties are transferred to the flower essence preparation.

"There will be a slight overall strengthening in some animals. Positive aspects of Chiron are strengthened, and the fourth and fifth rays are enhanced.

"With certain plants there can occasionally be a profound effect when the plant is very separated from its original root stock by hybridization or continued inbreeding. Some of the essential characteristics of the overall thought form of the plant, the generalized soul, may come more powerfully into the plant. Using henna may strengthen this process to such a degree that new vitality will develop.

"Use henna during three stages in the plant's growth. When the seeds are in storage, apply a slight mist near the plant so that the seeds receive a small amount. Also use henna just as the seeds germinate in the soil and just when the plants begin to come out of the soil. At these three difficult times, the absorption and utilization of the energies associated with the essential life essence of the plant will have a profound effect upon the plant for the rest of its life, intensifying and restructuring the DNA so that some of that which is lost through hybridization and inbreeding may be regained in a gradual manner. The overall effects of this will probably not be noticed for many generations in terms of strengthened yield and the direct ability to see this through microscopes, but the enhanced vitality of the plant will probably be noticed at the very first generation."

HYSSOP
Hyssopus Officinalis

Hyssop is an evergreen herb native to Southern Europe. The rose colored to bluish-purple, pink, or white flowers grow in successive axillary whorls from June to October. It is used in many digestive and respiratory illnesses and as a poultice for skin problems.

Q What are the effects of this flower essence on people?

"Hyssop is primarily used to alleviate guilt. It is even mentioned in the Bible in association with guilt in Psalms 51:7, 'Purge me with hyssop, and I shall be clean: wash me, and I shall be whiter than snow.' The alleviation of guilt is not its suppression but is an honest confrontation with the basic cause of one's thoughts and actions. By acknowledging and releasing guilt feeling from within the self, more constructive tendencies within the personality can develop.

"As a by-product of alleviating guilt, hyssop becomes a veritable wonder. For instance, this is an excellent remedy to use with children and in prison reform. It can also be used in past-life therapies in which certain past-life actions have caused strong feelings of guilt that disrupt the present incarnation.

"Hyssop has a complex signature connecting the nervous system to guilt. This plant intertwines various etheric energies and encounter blocks within the atmosphere. As it intertwines these energies with earth energies, it overcomes many of the blocks. It is similar in many of its patterns to the way guilt is sometimes overcome, but not easily dissolved. As the plant grows older, the many flowers that appear on it will intertwine more clearly and powerfully, gradually dissolving each of these small blockages. These patterns can exist as set zones of energy from the ethers or as problems around the plant. This is why hyssop is often used in companion planting to provide nourishment to other plants.

"It alleviates tension throughout the system, especially the muscular structure and the nervous system. This is a good essence for massage practitioners. In alleviating guilt it takes the strain off DNA in the cells. Such tension contributes to many stress related diseases. Any disease caused by feelings of guilt such as cancer can be eased with hyssop.

"It helps the body to better assimilate gold. A lack of physical gold as a trace mineral is associated with an inability to assuage guilt."

Q Elsewhere you stated that low gold in the system helps cause most nerve diseases. Would hyssop be a good essence to use in chronic nerve disorders?

"While it could be used for such problems, this is not its prime function.

"It also affects the emotional or third chakra and the emotional body. In relieving tensions in the body, especially in the nervous system, this remedy is a good tonic for the meridians. It is a good remedy to enhance meditation, it can be used externally to ease tensions in the system, it is effective in treating the heavy metal miasm. Squares between Saturn and Mars are eased. The eighth and ninth rays are strengthened, and the test point is the lungs.

"Animals also have difficulty over making mistakes. When you are teaching an animal and mistakes must be punished due to the teaching methods, this essence is useful so that the animal may create self-forgiveness. Guilt and forgiveness are modeled within animal behavior similar to human thought forms. Thus, this essence will make the animal particularly sensitive to the person who is applying it to the animal. It is also useful for an animal to understand new patterns when humans feel they are doing something more "by the book" than that which they feel fully confident of within themselves. This is an interesting opportunity for many animals to be able to teach humans. An opening towards such teaching is enhanced by hyssop."

LAVENDER (French)
Lavendula Officinalis

This aromatic perennial is native to the Mediterranean region. The flowers, which appear in July and August, are small, blue, and strong smelling, in terminal spikes. Medically, it eases sprains, headaches, depression, and rheumatism.

Q How is this plant now used as a flower essence?

"Lavender activates the crown chakra and the chakra point about 1.5 inches above the medulla oblongata. This minor chakra creates keen awareness and alertness. When the crown chakra is activated, aspects of the higher self integrate into the personality. It cleanses the meridians, stimulates visionary states, and connects people to their higher self to remove karmic blockages that prevent spiritual progress.

"While lavender is not associated with specific emotional states, it can be universally applied to establish emotional balance. At the same time, it specifically removes old karmic patterns between two individuals. If two individuals are in sharp conflict and the cause of the conflict has been isolated to a specific past life, they could enter past-life therapy. With this essence the conflict could be resolved a lot more easily."

Q Why was it said not to use lavender flower essence externally when its oil is so powerful?

"The oil itself is sufficient for most uses. The exception to this would be individuals who have acclimated well to lavendar oil and have used it for many years. They might add lavender flower essence to the oil.

"Lavender's signature relates to the eighth and ninth dimensions. There is a blending of the source energies with those of people on earth, animal life forms, and other forms of intelligence. These change the energies, gradually allowing a blending with the third and fourth dimensions. Source energies are utilized to create the universe. They can be utilized to create such specifics as a planetary system, or a species such as mankind or a certain animal. Source energy relates primarily to the purpose of that which is to be created and thus transcends all dimensions."

Q Steiner recommended using lavender in a bath to rebalance the coordination between the physical and etheric bodies to the astral body. Does lavender essence have a similar or other beneficial effect if used in a bath?

"Lavender essence when utilized in a bath has similar effects to what Steiner suggested. The astral body is the portal from which past lives enter to influence people.

"From Lemuria there is a collective consciousness of many devic orders around this plant. It was a particular favorite in Lemuria. Lavender is quite valuable for people involved in spiritual practices, especially if they also have certain emotional conflicts blocking spiritual growth. Trines between Saturn and Venus are strengthened. The sixth and tenth rays are activated.

"This is a powerful essence to use with animals when there is a strong bond—an animal you care for deeply, one that you have felt closely connected to. As this bond becomes more spiritual, an awakening in the animal's consciousness may result. In many cases, the powerful attraction between a human and an animal goes far beyond this life. It extends into past life connections or connections to an energy very similar to the animal that you are now working with. Because of the mutable nature of the entire animal soul stream or all-inclusive connected thought form, the energies associated with that past life animal may present themselves clearly and powerfully in the present animal you are working with, even though it is not directly related to that previous animal. Under such circumstances, lavender increases the bond at the crown chakra level at a purely spiritual vibration. This goes beyond levels of understanding. It strengthens the bond in such a way that the animal is able to commune and communicate with the higher self of the person. This may sometimes involve pathways of communication not fully under one's conscious control. The ability to accept and allow this to occur in its own gentle way is enhanced by hyssop as well as lavender. The animal and the human should each take these essences.

"There is an increased understanding of the overall thought form associated with the animal you feel attracted to. This means that you begin to understand more about the entire kingdom of animals associated with this particular animal. This sometimes may bring great sadness, and therefore, it is also an essence that is useful for animal activists or those seeking to create new modes of working with animals in laboratory conditions, to take better care of animals that may be harmed. Animals also feel the need to understand and to release."

LEMON
Citrus Limon

This short fruit tree, while native to India, is now widely grown throughout the world. The white, deep pink, and highly perfumed flowers bloom in the spring. Its high vitamin C content makes this a valuable fruit in preventing scurvy. The fruit is also used for throat problems, heart palpitation, and jaundice.

Q What are the karmic origins of lemon?

"This plant was originally quite small and was primarily used for decorative purposes. The powerful energies observed moving through people when smelling the flower had a very nourishing, cleansing effect. Its scent was a very important component of many Lemurian rituals, and its similarity to other scents such as lemon balm was known. This was utilized for developing this plant, as if each energy factor released while under the influence of the scent, was to be added to the plant. This naturally imbued the plant with many of the Lemurian characteristics, including that of androgyny with an equal balance of male and female energy in much of their religious and earth-related rituals. This allowed much of this energy to pour naturally into the plant.

"Lemon is often seen for its holistic properties; it works on multiple levels at once, particularly as a flower essence. It rekindles much of Lemurian times for people today. In Atlantis, this was taken further and a refinement of some of these energies in the flower essence resulted. This also allowed the fruit to grow larger and brought increased regenerative properties to the flower. Thus, the regeneration capabilities are imbued from the Atlantean time, while the androgyny characteristics are imbued from the Lemurian time."

Q How is this fruit tree now used as a flower essence?

"Lemon has a strong impact on the mental body, creating clarity of thought in the individual. People needing this essence usually have mental blocks, a lack of humor, or extreme emotional states. Although often displaying a high I.Q., they cannot make decisions. There is an inability to link up issues or think clearly.

"The left-hand portion of the brain is stimulated so that mathematical or computer skills and the ability to learn languages are activated. Skills based on mathematical principles such as architecture can be learned with greater ease. Students studying for exams would like this essence. Lemon does not increase eloquence, but improves vocal capacity by enhancing your pronunciation. For example, it alleviates stuttering.

"Lemon is a valuable remedy to use in conjunction with color therapy. This is partly because it activates the mental body. For the mental body to be an active participant in color therapy, certain vibrational states must be achieved. Color therapy usually works with the etheric fluidium, the etheric body, and sometimes the emotional body in the way colors resonate deeply with emotions stored in the chakras. Lemon has the tendency to create resonances in the mental body which attune it to specific colors that are then representative of those particular resonances in the person's life. Thus, when one is dealing with important issues around survival, there will be many aspects of the emotions dealing with the color red, and the physical body may deal with orange vibrations. Certain other colors, perhaps silver, gold, or light blue, might also influence the mental body creating clear new pictures of how survival might be recreated in the physical world. Lemon allows a deeper resonance between the mental body and the emotions, thus allowing color therapy to proceed with other colors to stimulate the mental body.

"It aids many parts of the physical body because there is a general release of stress. The muscles are relaxed, the lymphatic system is cleansed, and the skin tissue is invigorated because of increased blood flow to that area. It is a good mouthwash because, in a manner more natural than fluoride, it removes plaque and strengthens the enamel on the teeth. Put three to seven drops of the essence in one or two ounces of pure water and drink that amount each day until the problem is solved. Lemon can be applied to teeth that decay from the inside. But the person's ability to transfer lemon's tooth enamel characteristics to the inner depths of the tooth through creative visualization will be very important to make it effective for this purpose.

"Lemon dissolves scar tissue in the body. This can be quite crucial in some areas of the body such as the fallopian tubes. Lemon is good to rub over the arm after an injection. Some of the effects of the injection will be reduced and healing will happen more quickly. Other essences that can be utilized here include lotus and saguaro.

"Lemon aids in the production of certain enzymes, and it assists in the assimilation of protein, calcium, zinc, and all vitamins, especially vitamin C. It could be used as a supplement in mega-vitamin therapy or when specific vitamins are needed such as vitamin A in certain eye diseases or vitamin E for the skin. In some cases lemon can be applied externally. Lemon reduces cholesterol in the system. These influences enable lemon to prevent hair loss and to regenerate hair.

"The yellow color of the fruit symbolizes the strong invigorating effect it has as an essence on the meridians and on the mental body. Yellow stimulates these areas. It has only minor impact on the cellular level, slightly stimulating that part of the body. It can also be used to treat the psora miasm. The test point is the navel. Lemon is another common fruit tree that is quite valuable as a flower essence.

"Lemon's primary use with animals is not in the flower essence form. As an herb and juice it is excellent for cleansing. It has some benefit in the essence form, primarily in the ability of the animal to understand mental pictures, ideas, and goals that the human working with the animal may wish to create. These are more easily transmitted to the animal.

"The strengthening ability of lemon is more important for plants. And people may create thought forms and images as to how plants should grow and how they should work with humans. Positive aspects with natal Uranus, progressed Mercury, and progressed Jupiter are enhanced. The fifth ray is strengthened."

LIVE FOREVER
Dudleya Farinosa

This wild flower is found along the West Coast from Central California to Southern Oregon. Its lemon-yellow flowers bloom in the summer.

Q How is this plant now used as a flower essence?

"This essence coordinates spirit guides and teachers into a single unit, so more evolved information from them can be received in an organized fashion. Information from spirit guides filters through the higher self into your subconscious mind and then into the conscious mind. This process takes place because dudleya activates the crown chakra, which temporarily cleanses the subconscious mind, and all the subtle bodies are brought into a temporary state of alignment. The astral, causal, mental, and spiritual bodies are especially affected by this process. Such higher information always comes through the subconscious mind because this creates a greater responsibility and involvement of the individual. Then his or her unique personality is included in the process. Any emotional confusion or subjective beliefs are temporarily set aside so that one can objectively receive this higher information without interfering with the process.

"This is an excellent remedy for trance or conscious channeling. Meditation, intuition, and the higher aspects of the psychic faculties increase. Dudleya gives the individual a greater awareness of one's self as a soul, and it increases the basic sensitivity and consciousness of the conscious mind to receive this sort of information.

"People experiencing a severe disruption in communicating with their spirit guides can use this essence. Some states of schizophrenia exemplify this. It also helps people in a quandary over their spiritual beliefs, so it can be used by theologians. This entire process helps unify the mind, body, and spirit.

"All nutrients are assimilated more easily, it generally strengthens the entire physical body, and it can be applied externally. It also can be used to treat the tubercular miasm and diseases in which people experience a rapid aging, especially with the young.[1] The test points are the medulla oblongata and crown chakra.

"The triangular leaf represents the mind, body, and spirit being unified. The conical-shaped flowers represent higher information penetrating down into the physical level, while the clusters of flowers represent this higher information being received as a single unit in an organized fashion. The coordination of all these things produces longevity. The name of the plant suggests this relationship."

What many consider intuition or inspiration is often information from spirit guides. When it is stated above that information from spirit guides is coordinated, this also applies to ideas or inspirations that may be received.

"Increased communication with the devic orders develops for most animals. The ability to commune with nature spirits is an important part of animal behavior, but this is not easily taught or recognized. This essence helps animals assimilate what occurs. Animals are able to perceive, sense, and feel the presence of nature spirits in many ways far better than humans. They also understand the essential energies and often feel the fears and difficulties that nature spirits experience.

"This is a particularly good essence for wild animals, or animals that have difficulty adapting to the conditions of living in a city and in the wild. Consider this essence when taking animals with you on vacation or to places that are far away from civilization. "There is a deeper bond between wild plants and humans who work with such plants. The essence should be given to the plant and the person working with these plants. It may enhance the ability to perceive the nature spirits; however, this occurs primarily with plants that grow under wild conditions. When returning to civilization, the ability to communicate with and understand nature spirits is very diminished.

"All the most positive aspects between Venus and Neptune, the trine and conjunction, are enhanced. The progression of Neptune into any positive aspect concerning the natal chart will also be enhanced. The fifth and sixth rays are activated."

1 Progeria or Hutchinson-Gilford disease is an example of this process. In this syndrome a relatively young person ages very rapidly, even having some characteristics of senility.

LOOSESTRIFE
Lythrum Salicaria

This perennial herb is native to Europe, but it is now common in the Eastern United States. Red-purple, pink, or white flowers grow in whorls, forming terminal spikes from early summer to early autumn. Medically it is used for a wide range of digestive illnesses, liver diseases, and internal bleeding.

Q Exactly how is this flower essence used clinically?

"This is a superior essence for New Agers. It is an enhancer for individuals who want to bring the three lower chakras into proper alignment so that they can apply spiritually inspired information, which is often received through the crown chakra. It brings the lower chakras temporarily into alignment, so one can achieve goal orientations and stability in life. In accomplishing this, the essence also mildly affects the other chakras, and it temporarily aligns the etheric, mental, and spiritual bodies.

"The heart chakra is frequently open with these people because they generally have a giving nature. And usually this essence works best with people whose crown chakra is already active, so they can receive higher inspiration. But this essence does not activate the crown chakra. Just because the crown chakra is somewhat open, these people are not necessarily saints. In these days, many people have the higher centers partly open. The test is if someone can at the same time remain steadfastly functioning reasonably well in life. This is where many New Agers have problems. When the heart, throat, and crown chakras are open, everything is usually fine, but when the throat and base chakras are closed you generally have an individual who is rather unstable.

"People who are blitzed out from spiritual or religious experiences, daydreamers, individuals who meditate as a form of escapism, and some schizophrenics would benefit from loosestrife. The signature is that purple flowers usually affect the higher chakras. The test point is the forehead or the medulla oblongata.

"Playfulness created between animals and humans when people are struggling with important issues may be enhanced and deepened. Sometimes the animal will give signals of a communicative nature, as if to say this is the time to stop playing, this is a time to be still. The human may better absorb and receive such a message when it is occurring. This is an essence primarily utilized only under temporary circumstances, when new information and ideas a person is assimilating begin to interfere in the relationship with the animal. Such times of playfulness with an animal one may be close to are useful and help individuals better understand and integrate the issues they are grappling with.

"When Mercury is in transition from retrograde to direct and back again or Mercury is stationary, consider using this essence. The second and ninth rays are enhanced."

LOTUS
Nelumbo Nucifera

Lotus is native to Egypt, Florida and several tropical regions of Asia. The white flower native to India is the best species and location to use as a flower essence. It produces a large flower on the top of water. The pink, purple, red, or white fragrant flowers appear in the summer.

Q What is the karmic pattern of lotus?

"Lotus in its normal state resonates easily with the crown chakra. There is a great similarity in the etheric patterns of the crown chakra and the physical makeup of lotus. This is obvious in many scriptures. The crown chakra developed along with the lotus flower. In Lemuria, the development of increased energy, in terms of movement between the physical and subtler levels, often required tremendous interaction at energetic levels of the crown chakra. This by itself tends to align all the other chakras to bring a state of harmony and energy in the other chakras. This is a similar energy to what was often provided to lotus. The lotus flower was often part of important healing rituals in Lemuria. Lotus was the prime flower of Lemuria. Thus, it grew more powerful. Even today those who meditate near a living lotus flower will notice that the flower usually takes on many characteristics of those around it by growing larger and its roots reach deeper.

"It acts as a bridge on many levels between the air and water kingdoms, between the energies of the sky and earth. In this way, it acts as an important symbol of bridging between multiple levels of energy. As a result of this ability, it was hoped by the Lemurians that a similarity between the etheric appearance of the crown chakra and the physical appearance of lotus would act as a constant and important reminder in other civilizations of this powerful energy. The crown chakra symbolizes this great and important shift point.

"The Atlanteans utilized this energy in many other ways. The flower essence was used not only in combination with other flower essences, homeopathic, herbal, and gem elixirs but also was used with important devices for constructing pure vibrational states. These vibrational states strengthened resonant principles between the physical and astral, etheric, and mental levels. In some cases it was used for out of body journeys. All this created a generalized unfocused lotus energy, and those who understood this often worked with this energy to focus it again into the plant. This allowed it to grow larger and to create a powerful odor that others could sense. Some of this is lost today. Its ultimate karmic purpose is to allow this uniting through the crown chakra of all of the chakras within the physical body, not just of people but of the earth herself."

Q How is lotus used as a flower essence?

"This is the equivalent of a philosopher's stone in healing with flower essences. It is a profoundly powerful flower essence. The philosopher's stone is an alchemical term traditionally signifying a powerful elixir or substance of which a small quantity will transmute a much larger quantity of base metal into gold or silver. All aspects of an individual can be treated with lotus. This remedy enables the entire body to assimilate any form of healing. If it were given in combination with other flower essences or vibrational remedies, lotus always acts like a booster to other remedies in the combination. This influence also exists on the herbal level. Lotus could be included in various herbal combinations and these remedies would be much more effective.

"All emotional problems are eased. It brings all the chakras, meridians, nadis, and subtle bodies into a temporary state of alignment. This rids the body of toxicities that block vibrational remedies from working. It aids in the assimilation of all nutrients, and it gradually rids the system of all miasms.

"Lotus has a major impact on the crown chakra and the pineal gland, which is part of its signature. Its name, the thousand-petal lotus, symbolizes the 1000 nadis in the crown chakra.[1] For thousands of years, especially in India and Egypt, this flower has symbolized spiritual enlightenment. This capacity is magnified when lotus is used as a flower essence. It is an excellent remedy to use in combination with meditation and creative visualization. Lotus temporarily coordinates the eighth and twelfth chakras. In some individuals all twelve chakras are aligned.

"Lotus, as represented in the crown chakra, is a point at which energy transfer takes place through an interference pattern that links multiple dimensional levels. These levels allow energy transfer into the physical form. The nadis act as receptors for such energy at the third dimensional level and transfer such energy back into multiple dimensional levels. Because of the appearance of nadis throughout these dimensional levels and their natural ability to align into beautiful patterns, they tend to swirl. This swirling motion moves at an extremely rapid rate when the nadis are fully energized, and this motion will, at multiple dimensional levels, give the appearance of many petals of a flower. They look as if they have about one thousand or so petals. The correct number as seen by the human eye will vary somewhat, but this idea of many energy pathways relating through different dimensions—all related to this beautiful interference pattern creating energy shifts between the crown chakra relating to physical form and crown chakra relating to higher subtle bodies and multiple dimensional levels—is the beautiful signature of lotus.

"Lotus helps attune to future lives, but this depends on the individual's psychic abilities. Many individuals have the ability to tune into the direction and force of certain energies from the past. This naturally leads to extrapolation about the future. Some individuals have the direct ability to understand the future, but there is sometimes fear around this. This is often an important keynote in using lotus for such a purpose. In easing such fears, which usually relate to their future lives, they will have a deeper understanding about the future in general.

"This essence energizes the heart, liver, and spleen. It brings any disease, including AIDS, to the surface, so these forces can be expelled from the system. Lotus as well as pomegranate, centuary agave, and mallow ease Alzheimer's. Lotus is particularly useful if taken in combination with these other essences. For many individuals, using any of these flower essences combined with homeopathically prepared alumina, usually at 30c, will be useful.

"It can be used extensively in all forms of tissue regeneration. Past life information stored in the genetic code is released and longevity increases. Obsessive states can be treated with lotus, and it helps one develop telepathy and other psychic powers. Lotus also helps distinguish between soul and delusional messages, and it can be used externally as a salve or spray.

"Certain children respond well to lotus because it encourages deeper meditation in children. But give it at the appropriate time. Do not give lotus to a child just before physical activity.

"Lotus can be taken once or twice a day for a month as a preventative and general cleanser to the entire system. In following this strategy, lotus should be taken as a flower essence in the stock bottle level or in one of the neutral homeopathic potencies, which include 6c, 6x, 12c, 12x, 200c, 200x, and 10MM."

Q Would any side effects develop, especially if one took lotus for a month?
"No, its effects are extremely benevolent. What you may call an overdose could produce a mild euphoria and peaceful feeling that would pass after twenty-four hours. Most flower essences can be taken in these doses and potencies.

"Lotus acts as a booster for most other flower essences, gem elixirs, and homeopathic remedies that can benefit animals. Lotus also temporary aligns all the chakras. In many animals there will be a deeper connection to the earth and through the astral body to one's owner. Thus, lotus is useful in creating such an alignment, holding it longer than might otherwise be the case, and allowing the animal to assimilate the messages associated with this. This may occasionally result in blissful states for animals, a state of greater peace and happiness.

"Lotus is also recommended during periods of stress when relaxation seems necessary. It is wise not to use lotus too often with animals. It can be useful to give as often as once a month or so when continued stress is observed, but to give it much more often than this can create imbalances in animals, as it is a powerful remedy. When a person takes lotus and is involved in a spiritual quest and is able to continuously assimilate information, it is usually all right to also give this essence to the animal, and indeed, it will have a positive and beneficial effect.

"Many powerful abilities of plants to reattune to their inner vibrations will be noted. Lotus also increases the effect of other flower essences and gem elixirs with plants. And the assimilation and release of water in plants is assisted. In times of drought, plants will need less water when lotus is added to the water that is used or sprayed near the plant.

"During most conjunctions, especially of the sun and Moon and of Jupiter and Uranus, positive energy is made more available. Lotus balances nearly any negative astrological influence. There may be some difficulty when individuals use lotus when progressed Chiron is in square to natal Chiron. Beyond this, however, from an astrological perspective lotus is a general strengthener. A strengthened effect will be noted for the eighth, ninth, tenth, eleventh, and twelfth rays."

Except for a few species of roses, lotus may well be the most evolved flower essence and plant on the planet. Having used it for several years, I can report that some experience immediate positive effects on their health and meditation, while for others the effects are more subtle. But then, flower essences in general work in this manner.

1 Ajit Mookerjee, *Kundalini: The Arousal of the Inner Energy* (New York: Destiny Books, 1982).

MACARTNEY ROSE
Rosa Macrantha

Macartney rose is native to Central and Western China. It is a species of wild rose. This vigorous shrub produces small pink petals.

Q How is this plant now used as a flower essence?
"This essence increases telepathic abilities. It balances the right and left brain, in part, by increasing the sensitivity of the neurons. This increased telepathic ability also creates a greater sense of self in comprehending one's total being. Macart-

ney rose eases epilepsy, alleviates various forms of schizophrenia such as autism, and balances motor neurological tissues.

"On the cellular level, macartney rose increases distribution of the RNA and stimulates tissue regeneration of the neurological tissues, particularly in the brain. It increases the ability of the cellular structure to hold an electrical charge. This has implications in tissue regeneration because electrical charges within cells activate cellular memory.

"The astral and mental bodies are brought into greater alignment, which also increases telepathy. An introverted person or someone who feels separated from their community would benefit from this essence. It can be used externally, and the test point is the crown chakra.

"Animals develop an improved memory with this essence. The ability to receive new teachings and new patterns of behavior will also be strengthened. With some, an ability to understand one's animals through telepathy will be slightly enhanced. For those communicating with animals and working to learn an animals' native instinctual language, there will be some enhancement of this procedure if the animal and human take this essence.

"Use this essence with animals that develop AIDS and Epstein-Barr virus. This virus has now mutated so much that it would be more accurate to call it chronic fatigue syndrome.

"Positive thought forms will be strengthened with plants given this essence. This assists in many areas when the plant life force essence is multiplied; for instance, in repelling insects or helping plants heal after difficulties with pesticide or excessive mineral content in the soil. All these things are more easily released. The thought forms held in the person working with this essence around plants will be more easily communicated.

"The trines between Uranus and Neptune will be slightly strengthened. The seventh and ninth rays are activated. This, and many other rose flower essences, will be crucial in tissue regeneration concepts to be discussed in the future."

MADIA
Madia Elegans

This wild flower is native to the West Coast of the United States. Its rayed, yellow flowers have brown or red spots at the base. It usually flowers from June to August.

Q How is this plant now used as a flower essence?

"This is a good remedy for people with great drive and stamina but who have an inability to complete something or to handle details. Such people over-burden themselves by doing too much work. Madia helps them develop concentration and a sense of perspective, so they can share their work in a balanced fashion with others.

"Madia heals a thinning of the walls in the mental body, which causes a leakage of some of its properties into the emotional body. This creates a lack of confidence, mental lethargy, and an inability to complete projects. This essence opens the spleen and sexual chakras, which activates the creative power of an individual. Madia helps to distinguish between soul and delusional messages.

"The flowers close each day with the afternoon heat. The opening and closing of the bloom and stickiness of the plant suggests the influence of the essence in sticking to details and a project until completed. The tiny red dots on the bloom symbolizes creative detail.

"Madia aids in the assimilation of vitamin E, all B vitamins, and the assimilation and processing of glucose. These nutrients are all associated with vitality. The test point is the thymus gland and hara, which is in the area of the navel.

"Some animals play until they wear themselves out, until they are "dog tired." They are so tired that they have a great deal of difficulty continuing to communicate or understand. Madia should be applied before the playfulness begins with animals that have this tendency. Then they will probably stop such playing before they are completely tired.

"There is significant easing of any difficulty associated with Saturn, especially Saturn returns that take place approximately every seven years. And progressed Saturn will be less likely to interfere with various natal planets. Many of these aspects are eased in a way the information revealed by the experience is more assimilable to a person, as this is ultimately Saturn's final purpose. The fourth and sixth rays are strengthened."

MALLOW
Malva Rotundifolia   Malva Sylvestris

Both these species of Mallow can be used. Malva rotundifolia grows throughout North America, except in the extreme north. Malva sylvestris grows in Europe, Mexico, and North America. Both plants produce pink or purple flowers, which appear from the late spring until the fall. Mallow has traditionally been used for many bronchial problems.

Q How are these plants now used as flower essences?
"Mallow mainly helps people overcome fear of aging. A sense of dignity in people experiencing the mid-life crisis is created, and it makes the menopause years in both sexes much easier. Stress or tensions that contribute to the aging process can be treated with this essence. Look for people who experience tensions that duplicate the symptoms of senility such as loss of hearing, loss of attention, and inability to focus and collect thoughts. It helps people psychologically and emotionally handle puberty, and it helps individuals overcome insecurity about their physical appearance. It helps a person reach hidden resources to attain real mental and psychological health.

"This essence is a good tonic for the entire endocrine system. The effect here is similar to the Edgar Cayce remedy atomidine. The pituitary gland is augmented, the skin tissue is invigorated, and the circulatory system is strengthened, particularly the veins associated with the brain.

"On the cellular level, mallow reinforces tissue regeneration, especially of the skin tissue. It helps the DNA to be reduplicated; it eliminates toxemia in the body that may interfere with this process.

"Mallow also increases cell memory, so that past-life information can be released to be applied in daily life. First gently massage the feet and hands. Pay particular attention to the palms of the hands and soles of the feet. Press them with small, point-like motions using the fingernails or fingertips. Then, mix mallow with an oil, use generous stroking motions around the hands and feet. These motions should move from the center of the body outward. Thus, you are always moving toward the fingertips and toes. This begins the process.

"Then begin a past life regression technique, such as remembering a time and place in the past that you already have some knowledge about, or look into a past life where you had left off previously, or discover deeper states within yourself. Then open your eyes and image yourself in that environment.

"While you are doing this, it is sometimes wise to visualize the flower and rub some of this flower essence mixed with an oil on the wrists as an anchor. This stimulates cellular memory. Many of these memories relate to past lives that relate to family relationships. These family relationships may be about ancestors, and sometimes the cellular memories will simply relate to past patterns very similar in physical conditions, or physical nature to their current physical bodies. This technique brings out physical difficulties currently found in one's life to relive them and experience their inner purpose. After completing the past life regression a deeper understanding results. Take the mallow essence under the tongue for three days, especially in the morning when first awakening. Do not then rush about; instead meditate on one's dreams, focus on the past life experience, and begin to integrate the information. This assists the cells to release more data, which often happens in the sleep state.

"Most diseases associated with the aging process can be treated with mallow. This includes varicose veins, senility caused by hardening of the arteries, and certain forms of heart disease, particularly deterioration of the cellular structure of the heart. Virility in the male and female can be restored. It eases hemorrhoids, restores the skin in most skin diseases, and treats the syphilitic and tubercular miasms. The ninth and eleventh chakras are activated.

"The signature is expressed in the basic strength of the plant and the early fresh beauty of the bloom, with its subsequent rapid collapse. This symbolizes the person who, although in total health, is also concerned about appearances. It also symbolizes a rapid aging and the fact that this essence influences the aging process. The withering of the bloom represents the various skin conditions that this essence treats. This remedy can be used externally.

"Many of the properties of mallow with people are transferred to animals, and they may eat this herb in the wild whenever it is provided. Animals may use this herb in its essence or raw forms to ease fears and difficulties with old age, and issues relating to a premature change of the reproductive system from spaying or neutering will also be eased. The emotional difficulty and some physical problems involved in this will be assisted.

"A great deal of energy associated with the seed-making process will be significantly accelerated by using this essence. However, this will be variable from one plant to another. At various times, particularly when the growing season seems to have the correct balance of sun, water, and a place of some quiet for the plant, this essence will have a more powerful effect in the formation of seeds. Greater life force energy is kept in the seeds, and they germinate more quickly and have greater resistance to disease.

"Positive aspects between Jupiter and Saturn are slightly strengthened. The ninth and tenth rays are made clearer for most, and the test point is the medulla oblongata or the achilles tendon."

MANGO
Mangifera Indica

This fruit tree, which is native to Burma, India, and Malaysia, produces pink, red, or yellow flowers in the spring.

Q What is the karmic background of this plant?
"This was the most popular fruit in Lemuria. There it was developed as a food staple and ethereal medicine. It coordinated the anatomical development of the Lemurians' bodies."

Q How is this tree now used as a flower essence?
"It is a universal tonic, similar to lotus essence, that everyone can benefit from. It should be ingested as a quick energizer rather than on a regular basis. Mango and papaya have similar properties to lotus; however, they are not as potent. Mango essence and fruit stimulate telepathy. Fasting on mango or papaya juice or essence for thirty to forty days dramatically increases telepathic abilities. Mango opens one to the level of his or her causal body, which helps the person harmonize telepathically with higher levels of consciousness.

"It stimulates and aligns the heart, pituitary, throat, tenth, and twelfth chakras, and all the meridians are cleansed. Any therapy involving the meridians such as acupuncture are more effective and immediate in clinical results.

"It has extremely stimulating effects on the pituitary gland, so stunted growth can be reversed. On the cellular level, it increases mitosis, it helps slow the aging process, and it rejuvenates neurological tissue. Mango eases the psora miasm, and it can be used externally.

"The meridian cleansing with animals may be stronger even than in people. This essence is utilized principally when energy flows are clearly out of balance from front to back or left to right. Such a rebalancing effect generally begins at the top of the head and moves slowly through the animal's body over approximately three days from one application of this essence. As a result of this, the animal will gradually gain greater strength. This is an excellent essence to use after a blow or injury that did not result in any serious harm but has seemed to disorient the animal or cause some minor difficulty. It is also useful in this alignment of subtle bodies for animals that appear to be too powerfully affected by using lotus. They may become listless or have difficulty listening where previously they gave you their full attention. This is indication for using mango.

"The ability to withstand greater heat will be noted in most plants when mango is applied. Times of conjunction between Neptune and Uranus will be eased and many messages made clearer for people when using this essence. The eleventh and twelfth rays are enhanced."

MAPLE (Sugar)
Acer Saccharum

This tall tree is the species that produces maple syrup. While this species of maple is the best one to use as a flower essence, other maple species are almost as good. It produces greenish-yellow flowers, and it is native to the Eastern United States.

Q What is the karmic background of this tree?

"In part, this tree was developed in early history to increase circulatory flow within the physical system to balance and regulate various moods. This was critical to develop ethereal and physiological control over the then developing ego structure. There is a difference between the personality and the ego. The personality is the personal correlated belief system of an individual; however, the ego extends strictly from the survival instincts of the individual. Both may function independently of each other. This essence was developed and used so that the biological structure would not imbalance the developing personality and ego structure."

This is another instance in which certain essences and plants were developed to shape the human form. As part of this process, there is a very special relationship between the blood and the ego. Rudolf Steiner often spoke of this connection in his discourses on esoteric anatomy and medicine.[1]

Q How is this tree now used as a flower essence?

"This essence has superior qualities to balance the humours or the yin and yang energies in the individual. You might call it a liquid acupuncture therapy. You can treat the person with a male or female flower essence from maple depending on which quality the person needs to restore a perfect balance in the yin/ yang energies.

"Acupuncturists, in some cases, may take this essence because it would enhance their own abilities of pulse diagnosis of the yin and yang energies. And it creates more empathy between practitioners and their clients.

"The effects of administering this essence are similar to actually giving an acupuncture treatment. It affects the red and white blood cells, and it aids in the absorption of blood sugars on the cellular level. It can be used externally in conjunction with realigning the meridians, which this essence induces.

"There is a complex technique to balance the yin and yang qualities that relate to the male and female flowers. This technique is similar in some ways to certain techniques called chigung in which the physical body moves through a series of ritualistic movements. These techniques are the basis for other important and well-known marshal arts including shaolin and tai chi. These balancing techniques are utilized in working with chigung energy, which is likely to become more accepted and understood in the world, particularly in China. They will first be observed in western medicine to create left-right brain balance. Flower essences can be utilized as part of this process. They can be added to incense or water, or they can be taken by the person before working in chigung techniques. They can also be massaged along the spine before the person works with these techniques. The specific techniques involve moving the arms in a circular fashion while the legs impart motion, particularly through the left and right thigh muscles.

"Its signature is the bisexuality of the flowers and the fact that this essence is used to balance the yin and yang or male and female qualities in an individual. The test point is the base of the feet and the right and left ear lobes.

"When an animal is ill, be it viral or chronic, and one is going to apply hands-on healing, acupuncture, or homeopathy, applying maple essence is of benefit. Wait about half an hour and then do this healing work. The animal will be more sensitized to it, and there will be a much easier balancing as a result.

"Use maple essence with plants around June 21st when the day and night are very imbalanced and the day is the longest for the year. Then plants begin new phases of growth. The other period to use this essence for plants that extend far into the growing season is around September 21st when these energies of night and day are more balanced.

"For most people easing of difficulties associated with squares between natal Saturn and Mars or Jupiter and progressed Mars or Jupiter, will be noted. The sixth and seventh rays are clarified."

1 Rudolf Steiner, *The Occult Significance of Blood* (London: Rudolf Steiner Press, 1967).
_____. *The Etherisation of the Blood* (London: Rudolf Steiner Press, 1971).

MORNING GLORY
Ipomoea Purpurea

This is a tropical American vine that has become a popular garden flower. Its sky-blue flowers usually bloom from early in the spring until the fall.

Q What is the karmic background of this plant?

"It was developed in early Lemuria to shape their forms of meditation in coordination with creative visualization. This ultimately became the Lemurian science of luminosity. The conical shape of the flowers made the essence effective in coordinating the subconscious and superconscious minds."

Q How is this plant now used as a flower essence?

"This is a good tonic for the entire nervous system, particularly the sympathetic nervous system. It helps one get up in the morning and maintain stamina and vitality throughout the day. This is primarily because it strengthens the mental body. With morning glory, one breaks nervous habits such as smoking or using opiates. This essence removes opiates from the sympathetic nervous system.

"Morning glory has some influence on the emotional body. Displays of nervous irritability, including grinding of the teeth and jitteriness exemplified by talking too much or restlessness at night to the point of insomnia are all states treatable with this remedy.

"It heightens the sensitivity of the practitioner to locate specific acupuncture or acupressure points. In each of these points, there is a spiral of energy. If the client took this essence, these points would be more sensitive or tender, and thus easier to locate. This is certainly a good essence to use externally. While it is best that the practitioner and client take this essence about one or two hours before treatment, it still works, but to a lesser degree, if only one party takes it. Taking this essence one or two hours before having a Kirlian photograph enhances the acupuncture points. It helps the practitioner find the most yin or yang part of the body."

Q With its hallucinogenic qualities, can this essence be used to treat people with advanced mental diseases?

"Because it strengthens all the meridians, it has some minor applicability here. What you are sensing is that the seeds of morning glory homeopathically prepared can treat advanced manic-depressive states or schizophrenia when the individual has lost complete touch with reality. This is the philosopher's stone of autism. These seeds also help bring people out of comatose states, particularly when this condition is caused by shock.

"The clingy vine and conical shape of the flowers implies the relationship the essence has to the nervous system. On the cellular level, it stimulates production of the endorphines. The test point is the spine, and it treats the syphilitic miasm. Many of these new flower essences have different clinical effects when prepared into homeopathic remedies.

"This is an excellent essence to use with animals immediately before proceeding with any healing method including drug therapy or traditional allopathic medical therapies as well as hands-on healing or acupuncture. There is greater sensitivity within the subtle bodies of animals, especially the emotional and etheric bodies, to absorb and utilize the healing components of whatever therapy is being applied.

"For plants exposed to diseased plants, when a contagious situation may develop as with certain plant viruses, there is benefit in using this essence as a preventative. Given alone, however, it will have little effect. It is useful to visualize the release of this negative thought form clearly, and it will focus positive healing energy within the plant when you give this essence and take it yourself.

"The most positive aspects of any transits of Venus through Scorpio will be greatly aided. The fourth and fifth rays are made clearer and the eighth ray is strengthened."

MULLEIN
Verbascum Thapsus

This tall biennial plant produces yellow flowers from mid-summer until early autumn. It is found in much of Europe, North America, and Asia. It is used for a wide range of respiratory problems, skin irritations, and digestive ills.

Q How is this plant now used as a flower essence?

"The key to using this essence lies in its signature. This is a biennial plant that produces flowers in its second and third years. The essences should be made and taken in two stages. It does not matter if the two essences are made from the same plant or from two different plants.

"The first year the plant blooms symbolizes the individual's need for nurturing, patience, and understanding to initiate projects. In a group project, an essence made from the first year the plant flowers creates a collective consciousness or group attunement on telepathic levels. As a by-product of initiating projects, mullein creates a vortex of collective energy which brings people together. But this essence does not enhance discipline in individuals or groups.

"An essence made during the second year that the plant blooms helps an individual or group maintain the momentum, persistence, and clarity of thought necessary to complete a project. This sense of fulfillment helps people enjoy the fruit of their labor.

"Another part of its signature is that the plant looks like the male sex organ, and it does invigorate male virility. This is a mild aphrodisiac for the male. Creative forces from the second chakra are released. Mullein has minor influences on the emotional body, and on the assimilation of vitamin E. The test point is the medulla oblongata.

"This is an excellent essence to use when long training periods for animals are required. This can take place in animal experimentation, training for seeing-eye dogs, or working with animals that are to assist humans in any fashion. Long training periods are made clearer and easier. Utilize the first stage of mullein during the animal's early childhood and the second stage as the midlife point is reached. For the animal it will be a time when they will reacclimate, in which they will even attempt to relearn in a new fashion. Learning patterns have been influenced by past patterns. As you begin to see signs of this, it is wise to follow the course the animal leads and help by training in the ways that the animal begins to present in this later life period.

"For plants it becomes easier to grow under conditions that were previously difficult. Each point of Saturn return where there is any difficulty will be eased by mullein. The second and eighth rays are enhanced."

NASTURTIUM
Trapaeolum Majus

This common garden annual is native to Peru. Orange, red, or yellow flowers bloom from June to October. Nasturtium is a disinfectant. It dissolves respiratory congestion during colds and aids in forming red blood cells.

Q What is the karmic pattern of nasturtium?
"This essence will ultimately provide greater levels of joy within individuals which will take root as courage within most people. This will, hopefully, bring greater awareness to all of mankind and unite it in a common purpose toward greater and more powerful spiritual awakening."

Q How is it now used as a flower essence?
"Psychological clues to look for include narrow-mindedness, compulsiveness, nervousness, or obsession with an issue. Hunger pangs during a fast exemplify this. It also broadens one's horizon and aids meditation.

"Color therapy is more applicable because individuals become more sensitive to colors. People even begin to see auras. Appropriately, the signature is that the blooms appear in a wide variety of colors.

"It influences the pituitary chakra, and it is a mild tonic for the entire endocrine system. Initiations received through the third eye or pituitary chakra make you a less narrow individual.

"When tiredness after meditation or channeling nasturtium may be indicated. A deeper connection to the center of the earth may result when using nasturtium flower essence. One's interconnection to the earth gets lost in the meditative process, and a sense of spaciness and tiredness develops.

"Nasturtium is applicable in deterioration of the nervous system, especially when the eyes are weakened. This essence mildly influences the meridians in strengthening the nervous system, assimilation of the B vitamins is enhanced, and the mental body is slightly stimulated. Conditions of square between Venus and Mars are eased. The third and fourth rays are strengthened. The test point is either arm pit.

"This essence has similar uses in animals as with people. Use it for nervous behavior, ticks of a facial or body nature, excessive muscular difficulty, difficulty in sleeping, inability to correctly absorb and utilize food as indicated in diarrhea, conditions of weight loss, or other indicators of nervous irritability. Some animals may manifest neurotic behavior as an obsession around a particular object, toy, or place. Also, birds have less pure territorial instincts with nasturtium. This is a good essence to add to any bird seed."

NECTARINE
Prunus Persica Var Nectarina

This popular fruit tree was first hybridized just over 100 years ago as a cross between peach and plum trees. Even today, it often comes from the seeds of peaches. The flowers are pink or red.

Q How is this plant now used as a flower essence?

"Nectarine has one purpose and that is to bring people into total spiritual balance on all inspirational levels, and to bring all the subtle bodies, especially the emotional body, into correct alignment with the chakras and nadis. This brings people into a correct psychological focus in this transitional period as the world enters the New Age of consciousness. This is a major flower essence for people of a New Age Consciousness.

"Nectarine flower essence represents a perfect merger between the peach and cherry plum, nectarine having expanded clinical effects to meet present-day needs. Any psychological imbalances discussed with peach or the Bach flower, cherry plum, can also be treated with nectarine, but nectarine is more broad, universal, and flexible in its application to these and other psychological states. For instance, cherry plum is very effective in treating people who experience religious fervor to a point of becoming emotionally imbalanced and perhaps even psychotic. Nectarine is effective in creating a state of clarity in any religious state or experience, not just in more extreme conditions.

"This essence is quite effective in treating schizophrenia, especially autism. If there is a tendency for poor absorption and low body weight, take nectarine essence with germanium.

"Some rebalancing of an animal's inner behavior system will be noted when the animal is subjected to significant dietary change based on New Age ideas, such as weaning an animal away from heavy meats into more vegetable-based products. If the animal fights, appears depressed or withdrawn, or has difficulty with digestion, this essence may help.

"Trines between Venus and Jupiter are slightly enhanced. The seventh and eighth rays are activated. It can be used externally, and the test point is the top of the head that is aligned with the area where the cranial plates close."

ONION
Allium Cepa

Onion is a biennial or perennial plant that produces greenish-white flowers in a round umbellate cluster from June to August. It originated in Asia but is now a common vegetable grown in many parts of the world with many cultivars. It acts as a digestant, it strengthens the heart, it restores sexual potency weakened by disease, and it is an expectorant.

Q What is the karmic pattern of onion?
"It is hoped that deeper insight and understanding throughout mankind will be transferred, and as a result of such transference other species—both extraterrestrial and those on the earth—will benefit."

Q How is onion now used as a flower essence?
"Look for a person who is undisciplined, illogical, or irrational. This essence is a liquid form of therapy that, during counseling sessions, slowly strips away barriers that may exist between the therapist and client. It aids the counselor in gradually removing barriers the mind has built around itself for protection. A skilled psychologist, of course, peels away these barriers one at a time, hopefully gradually reaching the root cause of the problems to release them. Onion is quite valuable in this process. This process is also connected to the signature. One peels away layer after layer of the skin to reach the sweet core of the onion.

"Another function of onion is the alleviation of emotional states in the sense that its volatile oils stimulate the eye ducts, which purges the emotions. As an interesting side-light, the body has its own degrees of homeopathy. If a person took this essence, then meditated on a particular emotional state, he or she could then squeeze an onion and tears directly connected to that psychological state would flow. This happens because the eye ducts are connected to the mid-brain. Then collect the tears maintaining that single thought and prepare a homeopathic potency or flower essence. With these tears you can remove psychological barriers and suppressed emotions. These tears can be mixed with onion essence or with a homeopathic remedy prepared from an onion."

Several years ago I met an individual who completed this process, although she did not use an onion. For some years she had been bothered by a particular emotional problem. During an episode of crying from this problem, she made some tears into a homeopathic remedy. Since taking that remedy she has not been bothered by this difficulty.

"Onion essence has these effects partly because it brings all the subtle bodies into a temporary state of alignment. This creates increased clarity and patience. Whenever a flower essence does this, it creates a more positive emotional outlook on life, and any toxicity that can block vibrational remedies from working are weakened or discharged from the system.

"For a few individuals onion will ease PMS. This will be for those who feel particularly spiritually attuned to the other properties described with onion.

"This essence influences the etheric body, opening the pores of the skin to receive more of the life force. On the physical and cellular levels it works mostly on the skin, increasing the capillary action there. It is a good essence to use externally. It also stimulates the liver. Onion can be used effectively in most skin diseases, and it eases the tubercular miasm.

"When it is difficult to achieve a deeper state of bonding or closeness to an animal, yet one feels that it is quite possible to achieve this, take this essence and give it to the animal. Use this essence for three days, during which time you could continue giving this essence as often as once every three or four hours. The animal will eventually present a new idea by a new form of behavior, some new way of reaching out to the human, as if seeking to allow this deeper bonding when it is possible. It is important that the human respond as if to acknowledge this, even if the person does not understand this new way. Over the three-day period, this pattern will slowly permeate more deeply into the human's consciousness to better under-stand the correct behavior and new bonding between the human and the animal. You might think of this as stripping away the layers of the onion.

"This essence has many effects with plants. The most important of these is that the plant is able to assimilate the human's idea of correct growing more easily, and the correct ways to utilize minerals to understand and work with humanity, machinery, and other things that people may apply to plants. Therefore, it is wise when using this essence that a clear picture be present in the person when the essence is given. This allows the plant's overall thought form to better acclimate and relate to the thought forms within a human. The devic order associated with most plants will be slightly assisted by this flower essence. This enhances the ability to continue the thought form you began with in your plants.

"The positive aspects of trines between Uranus and Mercury are enhanced. A conjunction between these planets is a time to consider using this essence. There is a strengthening of the fifth and seventh rays."

ORANGE
Cistus Sinensis

This common fruit tree produces fragrant, white flowers from February until April. While this species, which is native to China, is the best one to prepare into a flower essence, other orange trees with edible fruit can also be used.

Q What is the karmic origin of this tree?

"While orange was developed in Lemuria, its purpose was heavily debated in Atlantis, so intense positive and negative thought forms became associated with it, which is why it generates intense emotional states. A vestige of this is the recent sharply emotional debate between Anita Bryant and the homosexual community. At the time, she was promoting oranges in the media."

Q How is this tree now used as a flower essence?

"This is a rather versatile essence which brings clarity and calmness to almost any highly charged emotional state. It releases deep emotional tensions stored in the subconscious mind, so these problems can be faced and resolved, but this pro-cess should only be done with an experienced therapist. Orange essence releases emotional trauma and tensions associated with homosexuality in your society. An individual experiencing a fear of unknown origin upon taking this essence would often have a dream offering clues to the cause of this problem.

"In cases of obsession, orange essence and hypnosis can be used for the thera-pist to establish direct communication with the possessing entity. This would temporarily create an artificial form of mediumship, but again this technique should only be done by an experienced therapist. Fairly well balanced people can use this essence to develop their ability to experience conscious astral projections. In conjunction with this, orange juice can be taken just before going to bed, but orange flower essence should not be taken then because emotional tensions released from the subconscious mind might cause nightmares.

"Astral projection plays a role in using orange essence with hypnosis. Often the astral body is an important bridge between the possessing entity, vibrations allow-ing possession, and the person's difficulty recognizing possessive states. The astral body is brought into a state of greater harmony with the mental body, so that a person can understand some of this more easily, and have deeper visualizations. Deeper messages about the experience occur to achieve a more rational frame of mind. Certain emotional states associated with the astral body will naturally ease, and the individual will be able to clearly place the energy, largely unconscious, from the astral body into more conscious astral body phenomena, thus breaking the bridge and making possession very difficult.

"Orange has these effects partly because it balances the emotional and mental bodies, partly aligning them with the causal body. The eighth chakra is activated. It also assists in the absorption of vitamin C, and on the cellular level, the muscular system is relaxed. It can be used externally for sore muscles.

"The orange color of the fruit and the name of the plant signify its involvement with emotional entanglements. The color orange has traditionally been associated with emotions. The test point is the tip of the big toe or the tip of the thumb on either hand or foot.

"Deeper states of trust and relaxation between animals and humans will be enhanced by using orange flower essence. This extends into many different areas regarding behavior, new foods, and sexuality. Ways in which animals seek to learn from humans will be assisted if given with a great deal of love and at least half an hour of relaxation. These effects will be most profound and well absorbed by the animal. It is as if in some way the animal is reacclimating or becoming more used to civilization.

"Growing plants under conditions of civilization, such as in pots in the city in times and places that are not natural to the plant and are in fact very different from any growing conditions the plant is used to, are excellent indicators for using this essence.

"Most positive aspects of Jupiter are significantly enhanced. All of the negative aspects are reduced in their effect. The seventh ray is strengthened."

PAPAYA
Carica Papaya

This tropical fruit tree produces small yellow male, female, and hermaphrodite flowers. The flowers are funnel shaped with five separate petals. In the future, slight differences in the clinical effects of using the male, female, and hermaphrodite essences will be described. A digestive enzyme, papain, is extracted from the fruit.

Q What is the karmic background of this tree?
"It was originally developed in Lemuria to aid certain enzymatic and digestive processes to assimilate the life force into the colon. The development of the stomach and the eating of meat is relatively recent in the history of humanity. It was further used in Lemuria to regulate the yin and yang forces in the body. When the human race was divided into male and female in latter Lemuria extending into early Atlantis, a new application arose for this essence. Then it was used to negotiate new issues such as sexual morality between men and women.

"Ultimately, papaya will bring a greater sense of gentleness and assimilation to the understanding of basic spiritual principles in order to build upon such principles so that mankind as a whole will understand them."

Q How is this tree now used as a flower essence?

"Papaya focuses the mind to put people in touch with their higher selves and with higher spiritual planes. It increases memory retention and assimilation of information obtained on the higher planes, integrating it into daily life. Clairvoyant vision, telepathic ability, and most psychic skills improve.

"It creates a unity of mind and a clarity of consciousness between two individuals such as a married couple. In linking the minds of two people, clarity in the relationship increases. But this remedy is not good to use in groups.

"It resolves an identity crisis people have about their sexuality. This includes the problems society creates concerning homosexuality and lesbianism. Occasionally hermaphrodites are still born. Papaya helps such individuals decide if one sex should dominate emotionally, mentally, and perhaps even anatomically. Suppressed emotions and tensions are gradually brought to the surface to be examined and resolved.

"Sensitivity in the entire physical body increases. With hypnosis and perhaps creative visualization and meditation, different parts of the body become more or less sensitive. By focusing the individual's consciousness on specific parts of the body, pain can be eased or stopped.

"Some would consider papaya an aphrodisiac, but it is more a mild tonic to the sexuality of people. The breasts can slightly expand and become more sensitive, and other slight adjustments can take place such as in the shape of the pelvis. The male gets more fertile and the tip of the penis may get more sensitive. But as previously stated, for these things to happen this essence must be taken in conjunction with spiritual practices, including perhaps meditation, creative visualization, and chanting.

"There is a slight expansion of the pineal and pituitary glands' activities, but this is more a by-product of papaya's influence on the subtle bodies rather than the direct effect of the essence. It also alleviates problems associated with mixed-brain dominance. Various hormones are activated, including those associated with sexuality. Although it is not used to treat any miasms, it can be used to treat most sexual diseases. Breast cancer in transsexuals can be treated with papaya. Papaya eases the SV 40 virus, bovine leukemia, and aneurysms, particularly in the brain. It creates proper blood clotting and the correct utilization of vitamin K.

"Papaya alleviates tensions in the dream state. People are then more able to receive information from their higher selves. This cleansing of tensions in the subconscious mind also alleviates tensions in the physical body.

"Papaya has many of these effects because it aligns the mental, emotional, and spiritual bodies together to function more as a single unit. It stimulates the heart chakra to balance the yin and yang faculties in the body. The tenth and twelfth chakras are also stimulated. It is a mild tonic to the meridians, and the test point is the heart meridian by the physical heart.

"The papaya fruit is particularly powerful, so eating it increases telepathic harmony, improves astral projection, and brings more life force into the system, which increases longevity. If juice from the fruit or the flower essence were applied to the face, it would be a mild stimulant. There will be obvious softening effects with the female flower essence, certain strengthening effects with the male flower essence, and the hermaphroditic flower essence will bring greater insight as to the male half denied and female half denied within the person.

"Use papaya when one feels particularly close to an animal. This is not necessarily a close bond, but simply a way in which one is relating to one animal at a time. This essence does not work well with herds or large groups. When you have one animal that you are very close to and another is obtained, it is wise to utilize this essence with both animals and with oneself. This will assist in adjusting the overall relationship between these animals. This essence may also be very powerful for animals to understand themselves and humanity better and to better appreciate their purpose in working with humans. In easing fears of working with humans, those who train animals, particularly horses, may find that there is added assistance in using this essence with their animals.

"The ability of plants to assimilate negative thought forms from humans is reduced, and it is easier to assimilate positive ones. Times of square between Neptune and the sun will be eased for most people. The tenth, eleventh, and twelfth rays are made clearer."

PASSION FLOWER
Passiflora Incarnata

This hardy vine produces a blue, pink, or purple bloom from May until July. It is commonly prescribed for nervous conditions such as hysteria, insomnia, restlessness, and nervous headaches.

Q What is the karmic background of this plant?
"Originally it was formed by the priesthood in Lemuria. The fruit was then considered quite a delicacy. Because of this background, and the fact that Hawaii was an important part of Lemuria, with Honolulu being its capital, it is best to prepare this essence on these islands."

Q How can this plant now be used as a flower essence?
"This plant was given its name by certain Catholic priests when they discovered it in South America.[1] These priests accurately intuited the collective consciousness of the planet[2] because the flower essence does indeed help one attune to the level of Christ consciousness. This is because the essence has a direct link with the spiritual body, even circumventing all the other subtle bodies. Sharper visionary states result from this influence. The name of the plant symbolizes the association between the anatomical and numerical arrangement of the flowers and the crucifixion of Christ. Individuals will perceive the temporary period of sacrifice or difficulty in its true context and not see merely the pain.

"It creates equanimity in highly charged charismatic states so that people become stabilized and have easier access to higher levels of consciousness without becoming nervous or jittery. People in a religious frenzy are often too unstable to properly assimilate and apply the experience in their daily lives. Emotional confusion is gradually released and resolved in a balanced fashion.

"Passion flower opens the heart chakra, the throat chakra, and the chakra point in the upper side of the arch where the nail was driven into Christ on the cross. This minor chakra point on the foot stimulates compassion.

"Passion flower helps sleep. It creates self-regulating mechanisms in individuals who have trouble letting go of the day. This promotes sleep because it allows a deeper state of spiritual confidence within the person. Often these are people on a spiritual path who might learn a great deal from their dreams. It gives them greater courage to work with such energy. And nightmares are eased.

"Although this essence is primarily ethereal in its effect, it does strengthen the pituitary gland, and it eases the syphilitic miasm. It can also be utilized externally.

"The ability of animals to receive Christ consciousness is apparent but very different from the way humans receive this. Partly, it will be balanced by the human's ability, but partly it is a way animals come to understand this energy by a path of pure love, simple acceptance, and total surrender to the energies presented to them. These energies may involve certain ways people have had difficulty forgiving themselves and the animal kingdom. This essence can release all guilt and difficulties, and an allowance of Christ Love is discovered more easily within animals as a result of this. This is a gradual unfoldment, and passion flower could be given gradually but repeatedly throughout an animal's lifetime, particularly when those who guard an animal, work with it, or are close to it are people who have an affinity for Christ Consciousness, who see this as important and wish it in their lives.

"The ability of plants, particularly the devic order associated with plants, to absorb, utilize, and truly work at the deepest level with all aspects of Christ Love from humans will be enhanced. As one feels such energy and applies it to plants, and this essence has been given to your plants, they will also absorb and work with such an essence very powerfully. That the nature kingdom itself creates this embodiment of Christ in its signature form is a way by which this energy is transmitted. Thus, it is useful also to visualize the flower and the essence of Christ on the cross as you show this love for your plants.

"All aspects of Chiron in its most positive sense will be assisted. Thus, squares and oppositions will be eased in their intensity, lessons within them will be clarified, and trines, conjunctions, and other ways of positive interaction from Chiron to other planets will be strengthened. The tenth and twelfth rays are enhanced."

1 Ernst and Johanna Lehner, *Folklore and Symbolism of Flowers*, *Plants, and Trees* (New York: Tudor Publishing Co., 1962), p. 44.
2 Information from past civilizations resides on the level of the collective consciousness of the planet.

PEACH
Prunus Persica

While originally from China, this fruit tree now grows in many parts of the world. Soft, pink flowers appear in the spring. In some cultures, peach is used for respiratory and digestive problems.

Q How is this tree now used as a flower essence?

"This is a universal amplifier for all forms of healing. It can reduce by twenty-five to fifty percent the time that would otherwise usually be needed for healing to take place. While peach alone can accomplish this, it is an excellent catalyst to use in combination with other remedies.

"Peach activates the etheric body and ethereal fluidium, aligning them with all the subtle bodies, particularly the mental, emotional, and soul bodies. It brings the harmonics of these bodies into the physical body, so that emotional or mental diseases that would today be considered stress related can be alleviated.

"Actually, most degenerative diseases are usually associated with a deterioration of the etheric body's ability to assimilate prana or life force into the physical body and a weakening of the bond between the physiological cellular structure and the ethereal fluidium that surrounds each cell. In time, orthodox medicine will understand this. This will initially occur with skin diseases.[1] Peach strengthens the ethereal fluidium, so it acts as a screen against the sun's ultraviolet rays. This helps prevent skin cancer or cancerous states on the cellular level. This is a good remedy to treat the psora miasm, and it can be applied externally. It also helps assimilate air at high altitudes.

"Psycho-structural diseases including slipped discs and hypersensitivity to the sun, such as various forms of lupus, can be efficiently treated with this essence. Body builders could cut back on lifting weights without losing muscle tone. Chiropractors, osteopaths, massage technicians, and people accustomed to doing constant exercises will especially benefit from peach.

"Some balancing of metabolism will be noted, and there may be difficulty with the chronic fatigue syndrome, the Epstein-Barr virus. There will be some easing of difficult mood swings and a tendency toward depression. Some strengthening in the individual toward karmic purpose may be noted, and as a result of this, certain difficulties associated with the heart such as hardening of the arteries, mitral valve prolapse, and heart arrhythmia will be corrected.

"Peach strengthens the meridians, and there is increased coordination with the seventh, ninth, and tenth chakras. If there is a tendency for poor absorption and low body weight, take peach essence with germanium.

"This essence enhances a sense of joy, greater lightness, and ease in sleep. There is a general healing tendency, but for most animals this is borne from the sense of lightness and playfulness that is strengthened by using peach. A slight increase in life span and general longevity will also develop. And while there is no direct equivalent for laughing in the animal kingdom, the ability to be amused with humans and at themselves and not to take themselves too seriously is transferred into the animal kingdom. This can be especially important when animals are struggling under difficult environmental conditions or when their human owners or those who work with them are struggling in their lives and some of this is an emotional difficulty transfers to animals.

"Enhanced absorption of sunlight energy will be found for most plants, especially in the early morning hours. The best time to use this essence is as a mist about one to two hours before dawn. Then, in the time immediately following sunrise, the absorption of sunlight energy for most plants will be strengthened. These plants would be tall or short, but not plants whose primary component is beneath the ground, the root-producing plants.

"There is a strengthening of most positive aspects of trines, in particular between Jupiter and Venus. The fifth, seventh, and eleventh rays are strengthened, and the test point is about the area of the third eye on the forehead. Ultimately, this plant will provide a greater sense of combined force and gentleness for all people. It also allows this inner strength to be given greater direction in groups, so that a genuine understanding of purpose among many species will result."

1 Rudolf Steiner often spoke of the weak etheric body being a key factor in causing cancer.
Rudolf Steiner and Ita Wegman, M.D., *Fundamentals of Therapy* (London: Rudolf Steiner Press, 1967).
Victor Bott, M.D., *Anthroposophical Medicine* (London: Rudolf Steiner Press, 1978), p. 161-180.

PEAR
Pyrus Communis

This common fruit tree originated in Eastern Europe and Asia Minor. The flowers, which are white with violet-red anthers, appear in April. It is rich in nutrients, and it is used to treat various kidney problems.

Q What is the karmic background of this plant?
"In Atlantis, pear was used in early experiments combining quartz crystals with harmonics and sound structures amplifying the process of creative inspiration for musicians. Today, many New Age musicians would experience increased creativity with their music if they took this essence."

Quartz crystals were used in many Atlantean technologies. It is not by chance that, in these days, many are again experimenting with quartz crystals. In the esoteric literature on Atlantis, quartz crystal technology is often mentioned.[1] These techniques will be explained in a forthcoming book.

"Many powerful energies that are not only utilized through sound and vibration and healing techniques that will likely be discovered through sound, vibration, and music will also encourage deeper and stronger growth within pear. This will allow it to change into something that will provide many physical capacities to those involved in sound and vibration and in other healing disciplines. It is hoped that this will ultimately bring the final karmic purpose of this plant to bear, so that it achieves consciousness through vibration with a species other than the plant species."

Q How is this tree now used as a flower essence?
"Its main impact is to bring harmony to groups involved in conscious and spiritual endeavors. It would, however, be quite disruptive to a group involved in intellectual pursuits. It has these effects because it integrates the mental, emotional, and spiritual bodies, so the intellect is subdued and spiritualized. It forces one into a spiritual confrontation to put things in proper perspective. An atheist might reconsider his position.

"The expanded mental flexibility results in greater elasticity in the body; as a result, pear balances the spine and relaxes the muscles. But for the spine to be properly balanced, the aid of a health practitioner is required. Unlike many flower essences, pear will not create this effect on its own.

"Animals experiencing difficulty from heightened sensitivity will experience relief of such conditions. This can apply in particular to difficulty in the ears. In old age, deafness is sometimes a problem with animals. Pear helps when animals are formed into new units, when there is a loss from one family unit and it is taken up by another, or two distinct family units are pushed together due to outside circumstances. Some of the inner tensions and pressures of this are eased with pear.

"When hybridizing plants by mixing different species or different types of plants for five or more generations, sometimes for a few generations there is a significantly lowered yield. This yield may be compensated for or enhanced by pear flower essence. What happens here is that some of the merging that has not fully taken place at the plants' etheric body level are made more assimilable and intertwinable to each other, and the essential DNA exchanges are therefore enhanced.

"The clustered flowers express the influence this essence has on groups. Pear strengthens all the meridians, and the test point is the base of the spine. Negative aspects between Pluto and Mercury, in particular squares and oppositions, are eased. The fifth, sixth, and twelfth rays are clarified."

1 Hugh Lynn Cayce, ed., *Edgar Cayce On Atlantis* (New York: Warner Books, 1968).

Ruth Montgomery, *The World Before* (New York: Fawcett Crest Books, 1976).

PENNYROYAL
Hedeoma Pulegioides

This annual is found in the Eastern and Midwestern United States. The lavender or purple flowers appear from June to October. Medically it eases nausea, nervous conditions, and skin problems.

Q How is this plant now used as a flower essence?

"Pennyroyal is predominantly a repellent of thought forms, especially negative ones. Thought forms are semi-materialized ethereal forms or shapes the mind builds. They are ethereal energies translated to higher levels beyond the electromagnetic range into the subtle anatomies. In contrast, thoughts are activities projecting from the left and right brain hemispheres.[1]

"Pennyroyal also provides protection against psychic attack. It has these qualities because the essence strengthens the etheric body to such a degree that negative thought forms cannot penetrate the physical body or psyche. This impact also enables pennyroyal to permeate negative thought forms and push them out to the subtle bodies where they disintegrate into the ethers. It can be used in cases of alcoholism, heavy use of psychedelics, and mental illness such as schizophrenia, when holes are created in the etheric body. Such people are prone to being influenced by negative thought forms. Pennyroyal eases mental confusion, and it eases the constant barrage of negative thoughts that can take place during schizophrenia. Although it does not affect the pituitary gland, it does assist it in its role of unravelling thought forms."

Q How would this essence be compared with yarrow, which also can be used for psychic protection?

"Pennyroyal has superior impact in this area. This essence deals more with actual thought forms, while yarrow essence is more effective in blocking negative energy waves.

"It is a good remedy to prescribe for people dominated by a particular system of thought or people obsessed by a specific thought pattern. It also encourages hard workers to rest and take a vacation.

"It can be applied externally to the medulla oblongata, the entire length of the spine, and the base of the feet before meditation. In a highly diluted state, with very little brandy present, a few drops can be applied to the eyes. This awakens the telepathic abilities of the rods and cones in the eyes. These are heightened neurological points associated with features critical to anchoring the soul's forces in the physical body. Put a few drops of this essence in pure water and you can cleanse quartz crystal by dipping it into the water for a few minutes. Or add a few drops to sea salt that is being used to cleanse quartz. Both these techniques can also be utilized in conjunction with thyme essence.

"Rub pennyroyal over the medulla oblongata and spine, and use it as eye drops. In these areas, there is increased vibrational interactions between heightened etheric fluidium movement, magnetic field energy as presented by the earth, and the natural flows of such energies in the nerves. These are places where the nerve endings interchange powerful energies and also undergo etheric interchange. In the medulla oblongata, in particular, such nervous system interchange energies can easily be affected by poor flows through the etheric fluidium or by the influence of negative thought forms. Pennyroyal will naturally align and strengthen some of these flows as they come into alignment with earth's magnetic field.

"Pennyroyal is good to use as an atomizer spray about the head for psychic protection. In fact, utilizing atomizer sprays for many different flower essences is akin in many ways to using them in a bath. It provides another absorptive principle, especially to the etheric body."

Q As an herb pennyroyal can cause abortions. Does the flower essence have this ability?

"No, this herbal property is not transferred to the flower essence. The herb has this effect because it repels the soul from the physical body. This is related to its ability to strengthen the etheric fluidium, thus destroying negative thought forms. This creates a powerful energy current within a person which moves in resonance with soul energy. This gives the soul the capacity to move, and in this way, the choice of direction can be easily understood. The person may then be able to expel the soul easily or move it in any direction that might be desired.

"Pennyroyal energizes the emotional chakra, develops the ability of apportation, and treats the petrochemical and syphilitic miasms. Apportation is the movement of an object through the ethers from one location to another. This is usually accomplished by stabilizing the interior molecular dynamics of the object moved within the ethers. It allows forces which are primarily negative thought forms to dissipate more easily so that the natural ability that people might otherwise develop for apportation is far less hindered. The test point is the base of the spinal column and the medulla oblongata.

"For many animals pennyroyal is an excellent strengthener and tonifier, as it cleanses and strengthens the etheric body and repairs holes in the aura. Animals repeatedly exposed to human negative thought forms, whether the person is aware of it or not, may develop neurotic tendencies and some physical problems. Pennyroyal essence will also assist here. In many ways, pennyroyal is one of the best flower essences to use with animals, particularly when there is any difficulty observed in the animal for which there is no obvious organic cause.

"Pennyroyal as an herb has been used with animals for some time, especially to repel insects. When pennyroyal essence is taken internally, or is added to an insect repellent, or even just rubbed into the fur, some of it qualities are transferred to the animal. However, this will usually not repel insects that draw blood from animals such as fleas and mosquitoes.

"There is some assistance with plants that are being grown in an area not long after a fire or that was previously heavily infested with insects, oversprayed, or fertilized. The negative thought forms usually created by humans around fear in such areas will sometimes linger. Mixing one drop of this essence with ten gallons of water and applying it to the plant is sufficient to remove some of these negative vibrations.

"A significant balancing of several difficult aspects associated with the planet Mars will be noted. Consider using this essence when Mars is opposing or in square with Saturn and Pluto or just Pluto. The second, third, and seventh rays are made clearer and much more easily assimilable for most people."

1 Alice Bailey, *Ponder on This: A Compilation* (New York: Lucis Publishing Co., 1971), p. 410-415.
Annie Besant and C.W. Leadbeater, *Thought Forms* (Wheaton, IL: The Theosophical Publishing House, 1925).

PETUNIA
Petunia Hybrid

This popular garden flower is native to South America. The flowers come in mauve, pink, purple, white, or yellow colors, often speckled, striped, or veined in various shades.

Q How is this plant now used as a flower essence?
"Petunia helps reestablish proper psychological behavioral patterns by bringing in the activities of the higher self. It is an especially good essence for children, the aged, and for overly logical individuals. This does not necessarily mean it helps someone behave. It just puts one into a proper mental state to examine priorities. This essence eases mischievous behavior in children or in the aged. It is an antidepressant, and hyper-active children are calmed. The added spiritual courage and ability to face certain blocks and denials within an individual will yield insight into the source of depression for some people.

"While it influences the etheric and emotional bodies, its main impact is on the mental body to generate a proper mental attitude. When petunia, or any flower essence, stimulates the mental body, that information usually enters the person's consciousness through the left brain. This enables the person to eliminate what is unnecessary and to focus on or amplify the important. Other information from the mental body enters the physical body through the etheric body. This releases muscle tensions.

"Petunia increases blood flow to specific parts of the body, which assists healing. If rubbed on the forehead, it assists meditation or creative visualization. Anything that increases the blood flow to a region of the body stimulates that area, so petunia could be considered a mild aphrodisiac. It could be rubbed over erogenous zones.

"If taken internally or externally, it eases nervous tensions. Petunia is rapidly assimilated into the body through the skin. It is an excellent remedy to apply over bruises. Or apply petunia and pure water over recent scar tissue. Then massage the area with your hands perhaps also using a luffa, and this would stimulate the growth of new tissue. This is a good remedy for massage practitioners. But petunia is not very effective in inflammatory conditions.

"It can be used to treat speech impediments such as stuttering and most ailments associated with the left-hand portion of the brain. Public speakers would gain some benefit from this essence.

"The flower's conical shape symbolizes the fusion with the higher self that this essence creates. The pink, purple, and white flowers express the connection this essence has to the blood. It slightly strengthens the meridians, especially if you supplement your diet with blackstrap molasses. The iron in this food energizes the blood, which then influences the meridians. A person doing shiatsu or acupressure could put some blackstrap molasses on their fingertips. This increases the meridian activity and blood flow to that part of the body.

"Petunia has two important uses with animals. The first is when you are attempting to break bad habits by traditional means (those things that you have done before which have not seemed to work regarding reward, punishment) or showing the animal a new mode of behavior. Petunia will enable the animal to better absorb these techniques. For people, sometimes the message is that a different technique is necessary, one that uses some aspect intrinsic to the animal's behavior. Pose the question in your mind as to what the behavior is that you can work with and give petunia to the animal and take some yourself. Look for new inspiration around breaking these habit patterns. There will be a temporary mental body alignment between you and the animal, and what will likely result will be new patterns of behavior that you can work with with your animal to break them of old patterns and assist them in understanding the new ones.

"This flower essence helps when one is looking for inspiration in new gardening techniques, new ways to understand growth patterns, and questions that may be observed with plants such as why they grow in a certain area and not in another place when the mineral content of the soil or pH balance is the same in both locations. Take it at the same time as giving it to the plants.

"The most positive aspects of natal and progressed Mercury are enhanced. The fifth ray is strengthened for most people. The test point is the base of either palm or the center of the forehead."

PIMPERNEL (Scarlet or Red)
Anagallis Arvensis

This low-growing annual is found in Asia, Europe, and the United States. Starlike, red flowers with a purple center bloom from June until October. Blue, pink, brown, or white flowers appear. Medically, it alleviates nervous conditions, liver problems, and skin disorders such as sores.

Q How is this plant used as a flower essence?

"This remedy works mostly on the ethereal levels. When the awakened kundalini travels up the spine, pimpernel helps it penetrate and activate each main chakra. This process releases stored spiritual information and elevated emotions. This essence mainly assists people who are coordinating the kundalini energy, so this knowledge and emotional data can be released into the personality in an organized fashion. Pimpernel has this effect partly because it stimulates the crown, heart, and pituitary chakras and the mental, emotional, and spiritual bodies. People involved with meditative practices or who experience kriyas (sharp body movements from the awakened kundalini) would enjoy this essence.

"As kundalini amplifies within the physical body, it moves faster and faster. As it reaches certain critical velocities, this flow of energy will naturally take with it various other difficulties that may have stood in the way. These can relate to emotional blocks, so emotional energies may be released. This is what occurs when kundalini flows and people spontaneously cry out or make deep breathing noises or various sounds. This often occurs in meditation. The natural flow of such an energy up and down the spine allows the emotional releases to flow in patterns that are usually beneficial. The problem is that sometimes an emotional block will simply move from one area to another because the kundalini energy is not raised sufficiently."

Over the years, there has been some research on what information and emotions are released by the chakras when they are activated by the awakened kundalini. It has been discovered that when the heart chakra is awakened, controlled psychokinetic power and universal love for humanity can result.[1]

"This essence assists people who have trouble with their father image, men who have trouble relating to women, and people who have trouble developing a loving nature. Weakness in the pituitary gland and chakra cause a weakened sense of personal identity and even a fear of society. This, for some, causes difficulties in leadership or personal initiative. For such individuals, pimpernel affects a clarity in the person's spiritual philosophy.

"It creates harmony in the dream state. Prominent and disturbing nightmares or an inability to interpret recurring dreams can be treated. If the dreams keep recurring, a few drops of this might unlock from the subconscious mind the particular source of the emotions that the dream state is recounting. It can create a clarity of thought concerning the source of this tension. In some cases this essence is good for psychotherapists.

"The flowers are very sensitive; they close if rain even threatens. This symbolizes withdrawing into a meditative state after being overexposed to certain emotional stresses. The emotions are equivalent to the potential humidity. The various colors of the bloom represent the influence this essence has on the different chakras.

"This essence does not penetrate too deeply into the physical body, but it does vitalize the pineal, pituitary, and heart regions. The test point is the physical heart and the heart meridian. Pimpernel can be utilized externally to stimulate these organs.

"Nervous disorders in animals will be eased, particularly nervous tics or twitches, difficult sleeping patterns, or strange modification of behavior not seemingly based on outside events. Sometimes this is due to an inability to assimilate and work with subtler forms of information which are made more available to the animal by this essence.

"Many negative aspects of Neptune are eased, as if greater clarity is made available to the person. When progressed Neptune is in square or opposition to key natal planets such as Venus or Jupiter such clouding effects may be apparent for individuals. The ninth and tenth rays are enhanced."

1 Dr. Hiroshi Motoyama, *Science and the Evolution of Consciousness* (Brookline, MA: Autumn Press, Inc., 1978).

_____. *Theories of the Chakras: Bridge to Higher Consciousness* (Wheaton, IL: The Theosophical Publishing House, 1981).

POMEGRANATE
Punica Granatum

This fruit tree is native to Western Asia. The flowers are red, leathery, and bisexual. Parts of the plant have been used to treat fevers, leucorrhoea, and throat problems.

Q What are karmic origins of pomegranate?

"In Lemuria, the plant was developed partly so that its flowers would create a powerful symbolism for people at deep levels relating to the ultimate purpose of the root chakra, particularly its highest spiritual nature. It is as if the spiritual purpose of the root chakra is deeply locked within the seeds. This has largely been lost. Many of its other capacities, its ability to provide important spiritual energies were mainly developed by the Atlanteans. This is what is currently noted with pomegranate. These are also important, but its ability to provide energy for transition is what will ultimately come out.

"It is to provide the ability to tap into deep levels of courage and strength whenever necessary, particularly towards the end of what might be termed the thousand year glory period soon to come on the earth. Pomegranate will then be very important in allowing this transition to flow easily and smoothly. And pomegranate itself will change as a result of this transition."

Q How is this tree now used as a flower essence?

"This is a remedy primarily for women. It can be universally applied for any emotional problems, but particularly for problems women are experiencing. It is a love potion for women, and if they have trouble accepting their femininity, pomegranate helps them overcome such insecurities. This essence creates a sense of nurturing or a recognition of a need for nurturing within the individual. The source of many insecurities and over-compensating or false bravado in the personality lies in a lack of love as a child. Men who have trouble developing the maternal aspect of their personality would also benefit from pomegranate.

"Pomegranate can be used to treat all female problems in the physical body. This includes childbirth, an ability for a woman to become multi-orgasmic, and an increase or loss of fertility. A woman could even conceive sextuplets with this essence. It has some beneficial effects on the cardiovascular system. It increases blood flows to the cervix, clitoris, fallopian tubes, ovaries, uterus, and vaginal lining. It is a marvelous remedy for treating tumors or cysts in these areas. The detailed information given for fig flower essence can be applied here. But meditation and creative visualization should be used in conjunction with taking this remedy. Leucorrhoea, ammenorea, irregular menstruation, constipation, root chakra energy problems, yeast infection in the vaginal tract, and excessive dryness in the entire physical body in women are also assisted.

"Pomegranate brings all the subtle bodies into a temporary state of alignment, which pushes toxins out of the system, so that vibrational remedies work better. It influences the spiritual body, giving one the wisdom to use this essence properly. There is a tendency for energies to proceed from the spiritual body in a natural integrated fashion into the other subtle bodies. These energies, as received by each of the subtle bodies, are not generally utilized or understood by most people under normal circumstances. As these interconnections become more clear and conscious under the influence of pomegranate, it is easier to establish the model within oneself for not just mental, etheric, and emotional bodies but also the understanding of their relationship to the integrated spiritual body.

"Its influence on the etheric body regulates blood flow. Its influence on the mental body increases acids in the physical body by directing the mental attitude into the body. And it balances the emotional body.

"As with the banana essence, there is a sweetness and metallic or astringent taste in the fruit, expressing the fact that this essence balances the yin and yang qualities in people. The thickness and redness of the bloom are associated with the influence on the blood flow, particularly in the vaginal lining.

"Certain boundaries of communication between cells weaken. This can sometimes be useful for individuals experiencing residual difficulty from psychotropic drugs such as LSD or MDA. Such drugs sometimes disrupt communication boundaries between cells. These boundaries are often necessary. You see this in the interesting compartmentalization within the fruit of pomegranate as an important signature.

"Sometimes when spiritual principles and meditation are at work, difficulties with diabetes, particularly relating to insulin absorption and production, difficulties of correct nerve growth as in multiple sclerosis, and difficulties in the brain relating to nerve interconnections as in Alzheimer's may be aided by this flower essence.

"This remedy assists in assimilating vitamin E, iron, and zinc. Iron is particularly strengthened during menstruation, which gives a woman more stamina. It opens and stimulates the sexual chakra, the nadis are invigorated, the psora miasm is eased, and it can be used externally. It occasionally aligns the eighth, tenth, and twelfth chakras. The test point is the area around the ovaries, including the clitoris.

"When an animal has become pregnant consider using this flower essence. Pomegranate assists in the animal's assimilation of new information beginning to come through about the animal fetus—nesting instincts and the ability to work with new energies will be enhanced. About one year after birth, animals may have some difficulty in seeing their young grow up, in seeing change occur with them. These changes may relate to certain nurturing aspects within the animal. Giving pomegranate then will assist.

"The period immediately following fertilization, just after flowering, is a good time to give this essence. It may strengthen seed yield for some plants, and it is likely to increase vitality and health within most plants then, as it deepens the connection to Mother Earth.

"Many of the most positive aspects relating to Venus are strengthened. This association runs fairly deep, so when Venus is prominent in an individual's natal chart, they are more sensitive to this flower essence. The second and eighth rays are made clearer."

PRICKLY PEAR CACTUS
Opuntia Vulgaris

While native to Brazil, Northern Argentina, and Uruguay, prickly pear cactus is now widely grown in the United States. It produces large golden-yellow or reddish flowers about three inches across.

Q What is the karmic background of this plant?

"Originally, before spirit fell onto the earth plane, this plant was formed in dry desert regions, including the Southwestern United States. The plant had to develop self-sufficiency in such a climate. It was felt that people in the future could use this as a conscious vehicle to develop more self-confidence and self-sufficiency."

Q How is this plant now used as a flower essence?

"If a couple took this essence at the same time, emotional compatibility and objectivity between them would increase. Normally volatile issues can be resolved partly because the essence relaxes the emotional body. However, this essence alone is not a charm that can settle bitter arguments between couples. There must already be a degree of emotional compatibility between a couple for this essence to work.

"It alleviates lung and kidney congestion, and it oxygenates the system, especially the brain. The lungs in esoteric anatomy are associated with emotions. The flat shape of the prickly pear plant looks somewhat like the lungs. And this essence can be applied as a spray.

"This essence is connected to the Kachina devas, which have a relationship to the Hopi Indians in the Southwest. The Kachinas have traditionally been involved in certain Hopi mud baths and dance ceremonies. In a related issue, this flower essence is excellent to take with mud baths to remove negative emotions caused by emotional arguments.

"The chakras on each wrist just to the left of where the pulse is tested toward the hand are stimulated. These chakras ease hidden fear and anxiety. Positive aspects relating to Pluto will be enhanced. There is a strengthening of the sixth and tenth rays.

"Greater patience between animals may be noted, as well as the ability to withstand longer periods of loneliness. Thus, if you have an animal that you must leave during the day for long periods of time and see that the animal appears to be upset by this, this is a good essence to apply. It is also useful in times of stress between animal mates. This can occur sometimes when food is scarce or when the babies they bring into the world die. Such deep stress is difficult for animals to communicate, but it is a shared loss between them.

"When plants are grown without deep understanding and at the same time they show new patterns such as new colors or new ways of growing, give this essence to yourself and to the plants to have a deeper affinity with the plants and to form a stronger bond to understand some of these new patterns."

QUEEN ANNE'S LACE
Daucus Carota

Wild Carrot is native to Europe, West Asia, and North Africa. It is botanically related to the cultivated carrot. The white flowers in compound umbels, usually with one purplish flower in the center, appear from June to September. Medically it is used for many digestive problems and kidney stones.

Q How is this plant now used as a flower essence?

"It helps one develop inner sight so that auras can be seen and telepathic abilities can be developed. Physically it strengthens the eyes; it can be used for treating all eye problems.

"People who are confused in their spiritual patterns, agnostics, individuals who over-intellectualize, or people overburdened with visionary states that might be incorrectly diagnosed as schizophrenia can benefit from this essence. These visions are usually of a religious nature.

"It activates the pineal gland. In doing this, it helps a person analyze the highest thought among various thoughts. It is an excellent tonic for the spine, especially the atlas. It may assist individuals to understand the process of diabetes and provide more inner nurturing, but it will probably not directly affect insulin production. Queen Anne's lace opens the crown chakra, the petrochemical miasm eases, and the assimilation of vitamin A increases. The test points are the atlas, crown chakra, and medulla oblongata.

"This essence temporarily suppresses or calms the mental body. This means that the constant activity of the mental body such as with people who over-intellectualize is lulled. The spiritual body is cleansed and brought closer to the physical body so that decisions are made from a more spiritual perspective. If you had many choices to make at a seminar, this essence would help you decide from a point of higher consciousness."

Q Why does the spiritual body need to be cleansed?

"The spiritual body and all the different levels are still the activity of consciousness and still are part of the known periphery of the ego in the sense that it is even possible to possess that which is termed a spiritual ego.

"There is a relationship between nearsightedness and the subtle bodies. In many cases, when nearsightedness occurs it is difficult for the mental body to focus on larger issues. This is a way the physical body reminds one of the particular problem. Queen Anne's lace helps because one gains a more general understanding, the bigger picture becomes clearer, and gradually some of the difficulties associated with the physical body are no longer necessary.

"The signature is most fascinating. Most types of carrots with their basic root stock look like the rods and cones in the nerve endings of the eyes that lead to the mid-brain. Queen Anne's lace strengthens these rods and cones. When individuals turn their eyes upwards and backwards, such as in states of ecstasy, this bars much of the light and decreases the normal activity of the eyes. These impressionable rods and cones become telepathic antennas highly sensitive to electromagnetic frequencies, that allow the individual to become more telepathic by tuning into the delicate frequencies along which telepathy functions.

"The root stock of the plant looks like the rising of the spinal column. Finally, the plant has white flowers with a purple flower in the center. White symbolizes various spiritual affairs and the ability to focus them, while purple represents spiritual activities, which are also practical on the earth plane.

"Most animals today are exposed to significant quantities of fluoride in the water. This is today present in most tap water and even in most rivers or spring water. Queen Anne's lace stimulates the pineal gland in humans, and this effect can be especially apparent with animals. Here the psychic gifts tend to be unconscious and difficult for the animal to assimilate. The addition of fluoridated water to an animal's diet affects various psychic abilities making them harder for an animal to work with and understand. This essence alleviates some of these effects. It is wise to also increase magnesium in the diet when you are attempting to help animals when they become ultrasensitive. This may be noted when the owner of the animal or those close to it appear to develop psychic abilities, either in a harmonious or disharmonious way, and yet the animal appears to be negatively affected by these new things. It is the animal also tuning in, but largely unconsciously, to these new abilities.

"There is a strengthening of the energy that brings a plant's purpose into existence. Use this essence when deciding what plant will be grown in a certain area before a plant is actually placed there. The positive thought form of that plant and its purpose is held in the mind as it is applied to the ground. This effect can last in the ground for quite some time. Be sure, however, that you are actually able to plant that particular variety, species, or type of plant in that location. If a different plant is chosen, repeat the procedure, only this time visualize the new plant that is to go there.

"Positive aspects between Mercury and Mars are slightly strengthened. The seventh and eighth rays are enhanced."

Q Would these effects also apply to the cultivated carrot?
"To varying degrees this would be true."

ROSA WEBBIANA

This is a wild rose native to the Himalayas. This shrub produces pink flowers.

Q What is the karmic background of rosa webbiana?
"This rose was developed for the ability to expand consciousness into many areas. While these energies were focused into the plant in Lemuria, it was primarily used in Atlantis for the developing psychic faculties.

"Ultimately, this essence will find its way into earthly life. It is hoped that rosa webbiana will be understood that it can be used in food production, in taking other flower essences, and in general assimilation so that the resulting strengthening, mixed with the ability to incorporate many psychic faculties will become an important part of daily life."

Q How can this plant now be used as a flower essence?
"There is an attunement to the earth's crown chakra, which stimulates superconsciousness and rapport with spiritual masters in angelic realms. One can transfer energy and information to and from multidimensional levels. This does not mean that one just receives information from subtle levels; one is also able to transmit it. Energy can be taken from life and created as simple life experience, as in visualization. Understanding one's purpose, working with others and conceptualizing what one has learned also develop. This energy, under the influence of rosa webbiana, can then be transferred as if to an etheric bank. This information will be available at a later time. It can be created with other

information, integrated, and understood. This is an ability by which energy assimilated through the channeling process, or through the ability to work with subtle forms of information, is made available to others and then taken back into the individual at the appropriate time.

"There is a release of an inability to work with channeled information. Certain blockages around channeled information that is difficult for a person to receive can lead to deep depression, struggles with understanding what one is capable of, and other difficulties in assimilating the psychic faculty. Psychic abilities, especially channeling, develop.

"There is a strengthening of the arms and legs. Greater attunement to earth energy increases the ability of the physical body to absorb energy through the feet, and the knees are slightly stimulated. This is at the level of muscles and bones. The energies associated with the earth become more absorbed and assimilable, and they rapidly move through the physical body to be released through the crown chakra.

"The energies in the cells will be connected and attuned with earth's vibrations very temporarily, less than half an hour after taking this essence. These will rapidly move through the cells and coordinate all of them so that some memories of the past and patterns associated with the cells may be released to consciousness.

"Some diseases eased include many nervous disorders associated with psychic openings that occur too quickly. Certain states of schizophrenia and an inability to assimilate information gained through psychic experiences will be eased. And the gonorrhea miasm is slightly eased. Enhanced absorption of B_6 and B_{12} will be noted. Some release of the heavy metal cadmium and an increased intake of zinc, chromium, and selenium occur.

"The rapidly growing plant, which assimilates earth energy through the etheric body, brings a glow at the etheric level throughout the plant. This glow, which may be noted by those with etheric sight, concentrates in the plant so that it will grow under varying conditions and extend rapidly into new areas.

"The fourth, fifth, and sixth chakras are stimulated. The sixth chakra may awaken to such a level under repeated use of this essence that an easy blending of energy from the eighth to seventh and then to the sixth chakra may result, leaving a deeper understanding of one's life and circumstance. The seventh chakra is opened to become a bridge to the higher chakras. The minor chakras in the backs of the knees may be stimulated.

"There is a strengthening of the gall bladder and stomach meridians. Energy flows throughout the gall bladder meridian may be temporarily accelerated after taking this essence, and the nadis in the feet and fingers are stimulated. Coordination of the integrated spiritual body, the soul body, and the causal body with the mental body may result, bringing through new levels of information and understanding.

"Animals may respond to this essence by finer attunement in meditative state to a human near the animal. This may release some emotions from the animal and allow it to experience joyous ecstasy while the human is meditating. For animals that experience difficulty while people are channeling, working in intuitive states, or changing their consciousness, this essence is suggested. Some plants will respond negatively to powerful levels of psychic energy. This essence applied to the plant will gradually shift that energy until it is assimilable by the plant.

"The beneficial aspects, trines, and conjunctions, primarily between Chiron and slower moving Pluto in both progressed and natal aspects, are enhanced by this essence. Some negative effects felt lifelong from natal Pluto will be eased. The fifth and tenth rays are enhanced, and the test point is the third eye center."

ROSEMARY
Rosmarinus Officinalis

This evergreen shrub produces pale-blue flowers that bloom in April and May. Its aroma is pine-like. This popular herb has been prominently used as a medicinal plant since ancient times. Heart problems, female ailments, nerve disorders, and skin problems are resolved with this herb.

Q What is the karmic background of rosemary?
"The plant was observed to provide soothing energies, particularly to children. This was developed in the flower until some of this energy became available vibrationally in the flower essence. However, much of this was misunderstood until the mid-Atlantean period when many the other properties were strengthened in rosemary."

Q How is rosemary now used as a flower essence?
"Rosemary stimulates the pineal gland and crown chakra. It is a liquid ambrosia because one experiences a state of inner peace or ecstasy. It brings out a person's creativity; for instance, someone having difficulties writing can be helped by this essence.

"It does not bring clarity to visions, but it does bring clarity to the person's state of mind. This is a good remedy for a philosopher. It allows individuals to learn who they are from their own level and range of perception. Take rosemary when you have to negotiate with someone.

"Rosemary transforms surly, withdrawn individuals into happy, sensitive, and sentimental people. This is partly because it brings order to the emotional body. It creates a practical form of balance in the individual. This may be a balance that a juggler would have, not a steadfast balance, but a juggling to keep things moving. People going through inner cleansing often experience this state of poise.

"While it is not an aphrodisiac, it does increase the body's sensitivity on the physical and cellular levels. It can be applied externally. The lavender-colored flowers denote some qualities of the crown chakra. The thorniness and shrub-like qualities of the plant, with a bloom in it, symbolizes the blooming of higher forms of thought in tangles of activity.

"The essence's property of balancing the emotional body extends into the animal kingdom, producing many effects similar to those described for humans. However, for animals it will often involve a strong release of energy, so it is wise after giving rosemary that a time of playfulness or energy release be experienced by the animal, followed by a period of rest. During that period, peaceful and soothing thought forms created by the human may deeply affect the animal and be well absorbed. Therefore, with such a program, difficult animal behavior such as extra aggression, effects of overcrowding, or difficulty absorbing negative thought forms from humans or other animals is significantly eased by rosemary.

"In plants, the effects of overcrowding and poor assimilation of soil nutrients due to a low quantity of such nutrients will be eased by this essence. Most negative aspects of Saturn are slightly relieved, and the seventh and eleventh rays are strengthened."

SAGE
Salvia Officinalis

This common garden perennial is native to the Mediterranean region. The blue, purple, or white two-lipped flowers grow in whorls that form terminal racemes. The flowers bloom in the summer. Sage is utilized for excessive perspiration, nervous conditions, and digestive problems.

Q What is the karmic background of this plant?
"Sage was as formed in Lemuria to stimulate higher states of consciousness not only as through meditation but also to treat and be in accord with the then existing collective consciousness. In the phases of Lemurian society, some individuals needed more balance as they traveled in harsh climates. When they traveled beyond the Lemurian society, there was, with sage, increased ability to tune into the collective consciousness of Lemuria in order to survive in severe climates."
Beyond the Lemurian civilization the climate was quite harsh. This plant was developed to keep some individuals in tune with the collective consciousness of Lemuria. Sage still has properties to help people harmonize with the current collective consciousness of the planet.

Q How is this plant now used as a flower essence?
"Sage aligns the mental and spiritual bodies. If the spiritual body is activated with no influence from the mental body, you may become a religious fanatic. If the mental body is vitalized with no influence from the spiritual body, you may become an atheist. The spiritual body stores energy that influences the psycho-spiritual dynamics of the individual. Sage aligns the spiritual body, so the psycho-spiritual dynamics of individuals can flow more freely.
"There are certain differences between the personality and psycho-spiritual dynamics of people. The psycho-spiritual accord is when spiritual inspirations integrate with the psyche or the personality. The personality is at times highly functional without necessarily entering into the spiritual realms. Such people usually govern their lives by strict materialism, or they lean toward atheism.
"As the psycho-spiritual dynamics of people are activated, they become philosophically more active, an interest in spiritual matters is awakened, psychic faculties, especially mediumistic abilities, may be awakened, and laughter is stimulated. Attuning to future lives may also develop. Laughter develops from a release of tensions in the body.
"The etheric body is also activated because when the spiritual body is augmented it usually strives to decisively influence the physical body. To do this, the etheric body must first be influenced. The spiritual body is rarely used by most people, so it often atrophies. When it is activated, there is a natural tendency for it to strive to influence the individual mentally, emotionally, physically, and spiritually.

"Sage has a complex signature associated with the Book of Revelations. Many of the capacities within individuals for releasing through fire, through destroying what is in the way, providing the path towards revelation (as is described both metaphorically and in the predictions of events in the Book of Revelations) are similar in their essential vibration to many capacities of burning sage. This allows the spiritual quest deep within an individual, the understanding that what stands in the way may be that which is to be developed, worked on, and finally released, so that what is underneath, the deeper revelation, the deeper message of God on earth as it relates to all people in harmony, may be revealed. The powerful and penetrating nature of this essence is such a bridge. Those who wish to understand the truer nature of the Book of Revelations should consider using sage.

"Sage is especially good for jet lag. It is best taken while still on the plane and then within two or three hours after landing. Corn can be useful, particularly when there is overcrowding on the airplane. With such stress, many negative thought forms may also accumulate around people immediately after landing. If this occurs, also use pennyroyal. These three essences make a good combination for jet lag. Lotus and clear quartz could be added for those with a deeper understanding of the subtle bodies or spiritual understanding of any kind.

"Sage augments the digestive system, not so much from the cellular level, but from the assimilative level in the production of certain enzymes. It can be used as a laxative, and it stimulates autolysis. This is a good essence to take while fasting, particularly when drinking tomato juice because that encourages autolysis. This essence awakens the heart and abdominal chakras, it is a tonic and cleanser of the meridians, and, the test point is the temple.

"Many of the subtle properties of sage will gradually transfer into most subtle bodies in animals as a cleansing of the circulatory system. This can be useful in difficulties relating to the heart, poor blood, or other circulatory system problems. Also, when an animal has developed poor circulation to a particular limb, this essence can be rubbed into the limb and taken internally. The effect of sage will be a gradual one, in that over three to six weeks this gradual vibrational effect will build within the animal. This is good, because it creates natural self-governing mechanisms within the animal to transfer some of the new energies and cleansing into the circulatory system.

"Increased ability to absorb water occurs in plants given sage. And when it is given in the fall, as a mist or added to the water, plants may show a slightly extended life span. This is because the absorption of certain thought forms saying the end of the season is at hand may be released and eased for plants so that some of the shock of the change of season does not contribute to the plant's natural cycle.

"Many astrological aspects are eased by sage. These relate to cyclical happenings, those things that happen to individuals regularly. These patterns are often predicted in astrology. Therefore, grand alignments, grand trines, and other important movements of the planets will be eased for all people, and progressions towards natal aspects will be eased when these line up in powerful modes. This can relate to, for instance, conjunctions or programmed alignments of three or more planets in a given sign within a person's chart. The fourth, eighth, and ninth rays are clarified."

ST. JOHN'S WORT
Hypericum Perforatum

This shrubby, perennial plant is native to Europe and Western Asia. The bright-yellow flowers appear from June to September. As an herb, it eases burns or wounds when applied externally, and it relieves digestive or respiratory problems. In homeopathy, it is often used for injuries to the nerves.

Q How is this plant now used as a flower essence?
"This essence is universally applicable as a tonic to release any hidden or obvious fear or paranoia, including fears from past life experiences. St. John's wort is an invaluable remedy in psychoanalysis. When the emotional and mental bodies become too fused together, there is an inability to separate emotional feelings and mental constructs. This leads to frustration and ultimately to fears, especially of an unknown quality.

"St. John's wort aids the individual having astral projections and soul travel beyond the lower astral planes to experience visionary states. Cluttered dreams and nightmares are eased when the soul's forces properly separate from the physical body during sleep."

Q Does this essence help when a person has trouble getting up in the morning?
"No, that is more a problem with vitality. St. John's wort relates to the soul's forces leaving, not returning to, the physical body.

"It influences the assimilation of zinc, magnesium, and phosphorus. It has a slight enhancing effect on the RNA, which slightly improves the memory. While this essence has little direct effect on the physical body, it is effective in treating the psora miasm. It can be used externally.

"When this is given as a flower essence, animals better understand pain, but this may relate to deep-seated fears. Animals cannot verbalize the way a human does, but they may come in touch with such fears and be more able to release them. The way an animal releases is comparable to the way a human speaks about such fears; they act them out. This may involve dramatic shaking on the animal's part, or odd behavior such as running around or barking in the middle of the night, or doing something that is completely out of the animal's usual behavior pattern.

"When you can accept this, be with the animal but do not stop it, simply observe this release of fears and difficulties, and some of these problems will be eased. This can be especially important immediately after an accident, injury, or operation that is performed on an animal. Some of these effects will last for two months after such difficulty if the the problem has not been released on psychic levels.

"Trauma to plants may be relieved by this essence. In particular, vines or plants that reproduce by runners may experience dramatic difficulty when such runners are cut. It may be necessary to trim back the plants. That is a good time to apply this essence. This also reduces the possibility of disease within plants.

"Some positive aspects of Jupiter are enhanced. The fourth and fifth rays made clearer. The test point is the lung or kidney meridians, particularly the kidney alarm point."

SHOOTING STAR
Dodecatheon Media

This wild flower is found in the Central and Eastern United States. Its flowers are magenta to lavender or white.

Q How can this plant now be used as a flower essence?
"This essence is totally ethereal in its effects, and it is universally applicable. It heightens consciousness and the body's frequencies to become more sensitive to the celestial position and movement of different planets. Many already understand that specific parts of the body are influenced by various astrological configurations. Astrologers could use shooting star in conjunction with various remedies, psychotherapy, or just general counseling for better clinical results. This is an excellent essence to take if you are studying astrology. The experienced astrologer would benefit from this essence by experiencing a heightened intuition and understanding of various astrological configurations.

"There are entire realms of thought regarding various uses of astrological energies on subtle levels. Many teachers, guides, helpers, and angels understand a great deal about astrology. Much of their information and understanding is available to people, and this is enhanced by this essence. However, even people who do not understand astrology may be able to receive more information and understand it better, particularly some of its technical aspects, when using this essence. Shooting star is a booster whenever another essence of any type is utilized primarily for its astrological effect. Therefore when taking such an essence, consider taking shooting star along with it, and some of these inner abilities will be strengthened.

"Shooting star aligns the mental, emotional, and causal bodies. This essence activates the causal body to be more sensitive to planetary movements. This is crucial because the causal body is the key to attunement with astrological influences. The causal body is the web or pattern of telepathy that you hold in your electromagnetic field. It links you with the magnetic and gravitational fields of the earth and other planets and stars. Your linkage to various planets and stars is from their tremendous vibration and energy, as well as their gravitational influences, which travel in waves at approximately the speed of light. These influences reach the earth in varying degrees of time depending on the distance the planets and stars are from the earth. This is an important cause of error in some astrological predictions.

"Shooting star also enhances the study and practice of astronomy. Astronomy is but as a projection of the physical study and physical movement of astrology. Protection against radiation from the earth and outer space is another benefit of shooting star. It offers protection in areas where there is increased background radiation such as with naturally bound uranium ores. This essence provides protection against most environmental pollutants. When technology develops so scientists can take a holograph of the gravitational waves between planets and stars, it will look like this flower. Its name suggests the stellar influence of this essence.

"Shooting star strengthens all the meridians, it is a good tonic for all the nadis, and the properties of all the chakras are magnified. The seventh, eighth, and twelfth rays are enhanced.

"The main properties that transfer to most animals relate to the lunar cycles. When you notice difficulties with animals concerning phases of the Moon, consider using this essence. It also makes it easier for animals that have difficulty living around astrologers or understanding some of the energies that they create. The animals better attune, though certainly at a secondary level, to these subtler energies.

"Use this essence with plants only when aware of the various astrological aspects regarding planting and harvesting. There are traditional characteristics and aspects associated with these from earth's past. Much of this relates to planting just before the new Moon or harvesting during the full Moon. These are ancient traditions based partly on the tides, gravity, and periods of light and dark. Yet these only partly explain the subtle energies associated with how various astrological aspects affect plants. Therefore, in attuning to these yourself and growing plants, it is useful to use this essence. Utilize it in the planning period for yourself, and spray it upon the seeds in a light mist at least a week before the seeds will be planted. Then some of the thought forms associated with astrological energies will also be strengthened within the plants. Do not use this essence without such inner knowledge, that is, thinking that this in and of itself will attune the plants to these astrological aspects. It will not matter when during the lunar cycle that you plant. Just the opposite is the case. Without such knowledge, some difficulties may develop with the plants."

SKULLCAP
Scuttellaria Lateriflora

Skullcap is a North American perennial from one to three feet tall that produces axillary, two-lipped flowers pale-purple or blue from July to September. It alleviates headaches, convulsions, and nervous conditions such as insomnia and restlessness.

Q What is the karmic background of this plant?

"This particular plant form was, in part, developed when there was finally as settled within the Lemurian community the existence of a soul passing from the physical anatomy of the cranial capacity. This occurred during the first quarter of the Lemurian civilization, when there was the final physical settlement of the crown chakra into the pineal gland."

In early Lemuria the crown chakra, with its special link to the soul's forces, was connected to the cranial area through the pineal gland. It was during this period that the Lemurians accepted the existence of the soul. In early Lemuria, there was a debate, not unlike today, concerning the possible existence of the soul.

Q How is this plant now used as a flower essence?

"This essence is primarily for massage practitioners, for people doing psychic healing and psychic analysis, and for their clients. A person receiving the treatment becomes more attuned to accept the healing. A dab of this essence massaged over the medulla oblongata increases the psychic healing ability within each person. Healers should use an essence from the light-blue flowers over their medulla oblongata while the essence from the duller or purple flowers is for the person who receives the treatment. The brighter the blue the greater the healing properties of the essence. Massaging this essence over the medulla oblongata enables the healer to establish a deeper sympathetic bond with the client.

"These properties occur partly because the pituitary gland is stimulated, which activates the neurological system and then the meridians. The emotional and etheric bodies are aligned, thus sensitizing and merging the emotions with the spiritual forces. This is notably because the crown chakra is activated, which stimulates the pineal gland and the neurological processes.

"Some of the herbal properties of skullcap that stimulate the neurological system are transferred to the essence. This also extends to the pineal gland, which is neurologically stimulated by a greater bioelectromagnetic process. In other words, the activated crown chakra stimulates the synapses, which are the junctions or relay point between the nerve cells. This awakens the pineal gland and the entire nervous system. Some natural morphines are stimulated, which engenders a sense of physical and emotional relaxation. As an external salve, it relaxes the nervous system.

"Skullcap alleviates general deterioration of the nervous system such as from the long-term effects of the heavy metal miasm, caffeine, or morphine. This essence alleviates the extremes of morphine addiction and withdrawal by mitigating the intense cravings. The essence lessens some of the classical symptoms associated with drug addiction. This includes low self-esteem, stress, anxiety, and feeling an inability to cope with life. This is not synonymous with low self-esteem outside of addiction, but it does parallel that state. For skullcap to have these clinical effects in addiction, it should generally be associated with depression withdrawal symptoms from addiction.

"Runners experience exhilaration by the release of endorphines in the brain or sometimes depression if the endorphines are not released. Skullcap balances each state. Concerning the signature, there is a vague resemblance in certain parts of the plant to the entire spinal column.

"Hands-on healing with animals is enhanced, animal massage becomes easier, and certain nervous system disorders are assisted. These relate to systemic disorders—those that affect the entire body of the animal, as in undue shaking or odd times of waking and sleeping. Skullcap is sometimes useful in cranial readjustment with animals. Animals are often able to do this by themselves. As you give this essence, massage the animal, moving its head around. It may be better able to relax and allow you to touch it on the head. This assists the animal and brings energy into the pineal and pituitary glands to create an inner strengthening.

"Thought forms relating to growth patterns, particularly periods when extra spurts of growth are needed in plants, are enhanced by skullcap. It is useful here for the person working with plants to have a clear picture of the necessity for such growth. This is also true in governing growth patterns that are either too long or too short or those of too much energy or too little. Use of this essence by both the person and plant is recommended to enhance communication between humans and plants.

"Positive aspects between Venus and Saturn are strengthened, and clearer insight and understanding with the fourth and sixth rays develop. The crown chakra is the test point."

STINGING NETTLES
Urtica Dioica

This species of nettles is native to Europe and Asia. The small, greenish male and female flowers grow in axillary clusters from July to September. The entire plant is covered with stinging hairs that irritate the skin if touched and damage the kidneys if eaten uncooked. Medically, nettles stimulates digestion, treats urinary tract problems, and eases rheumatism. Its juice is used as a hair tonic.

Q How is nettles today used as a flower essence?
"It eases all emotional stress associated with a broken home. This essence is good for adopted children, parents who have adopted children, and divorced people. Sibling rivalries and other problems in an existing family unit can also be eased with nettles.

"The signature is that the flowers are male and female. Usually only one sex blooms on a plant, but if they appear together on the same plant it is often in a somewhat broken pattern. The flower essence integrated with male and female flowers is the most potent.

"Nettles is a tonic for the kidneys, lungs, and nervous system. Asthma, neural inflammations, and scarring in the inner lung tissues can be treated with this elixir. It can be used externally as a salve for skin problems.

"Calcium, potassium, zinc, vitamin A, and all the B vitamins are better assimilated with nettles. And it creates a state of calm in the emotional and etheric bodies. The test point is the kidneys.

"This is an important cleanser for most animals. It increases etheric flows and the transfer of energy from the etheric to the physical body. This is an herb that animals sometimes seek in the wild. This seems strange because it can sometimes harm them when eaten. However, stinging nettle does have some benefit when given as a flower essence, and the many ways this can cleanse, heal, and assist animals can be fairly powerful. This can be especially useful when applied to aching or tired limbs or when utilized with sore feet. Also, if an injury has taken place and the animal has lost excessive blood, assistance and added inner strength will be created by this essence.

"The ability of plants to strengthen and create new and positive thought forms, particularly associated with the devic kingdom, will be noted with this essence. If you have a powerful love, caring, or affinity for your plants and wish this to be transferred to them, particularly when it is necessary as when you are growing a rare species or there is trouble with environmental conditions, this is a good time to use this essence.

"Positive aspects between Venus and Neptune are strengthened. Some negative aspects between Venus and Pluto are alleviated. The third and tenth rays are enhanced."

SUNFLOWER
Helianthus Annus

This annual herb grows to twelve feet. Its large, golden-yellow flowers are composed of small tubular flowers arranged compactly on a flat disk. It originated in Mexico and Peru. Medically it is prescribed for rheumatism and numerous respiratory problems.

Q What is the karmic background of this plant?

"Although developed in Lemuria for the express purpose of attunement with higher spiritual forces, it had a peculiar karmic development in the latter days of Atlantis when Egypt existed as an Atlantean colony. It was then used by the priesthood, an independent faction in the Atlantean community, to amplify qualities of spiritual leadership in the personality. But this quality was carried to an extreme and was an abuse of sunflower's attributes."

Q How is this plant now used as a flower essence?

"Sunflower tempers and spiritualizes the male ego. Lessening the impact of the overbearing male ego awakens the male's maternal instinct and desire to have children. This draws the individual closer to a sense of androgyny within the self. It also aligns the superconscious mind's spiritual values with the heart chakra; thus, the heart chakra is cleansed, which causes increased caring and sensitivity in the male and female. Sunflower balances the yin and yang energies, and attunes people to higher wisdom. This is an interesting essence for atheists. People demonstrating anger or hostility toward their father experience increased understanding with this essence.

"The subtle body most affected is the spiritual body, and the soul body is also moderately influenced. Sunflower aligns all the other bodies closer to what the spiritual body is perceiving. When people have trouble with their intuition, and want to know if their perception is correct, or if it is just the idle chatter of the material mind, sunflower essence resolves this problem. Or if the person had the emotional, causal, and astral bodies misaligned from, for instance, a weak heart chakra, sunflower realigns them.

"Osteopathic and chiropractic adjustments are augmented. It stimulates the kundalini and aligns it properly along the spine, so the chakras associated with the spinal column are awakened. On the cellular level, absorption of vitamin D increases.

"Poor posture, strains in the spinal column, spinal degeneration, and heart diseases can be treated with this remedy. Sunflower also eases sunburn, particularly if there is heat exhaustion or toxicity in the skin from an excessive discharge of uric acid. It also alleviates the radiation miasm caused by overexposure to the sun or exposure to nuclear fusion involving hydrogen, and skin cancer eases.

"Sunflower dissolves fatty tissue. This is one of the more powerful effects of sunlight energy that is easily bridged into a person. It is particularly useful to take this upon wakening and concentrate the effect by creative visualization in the physical body.

"All sunflower seed nutrients are transferred to the flower essence.[1] Thus, taking this essence increases these nutrient properties in the system. It can also be applied externally.

"The signature is mostly astrological since sunflower looks like the sun and astrologically the sun is associated with the father, the male ego, and spiritual knowledge. The height of sunflower symbolizes its influence on the spinal column. The devic orders connected to this plant include the Kachinas and some associated with the Vedas—the holy scriptures of India.

"Greater attunement of the entire animal kingdom to the sun's energy will be created by this essence. This attunement can assist with obvious cases of sunburn or excessive exposure to heat, but it can also assist the animal to attune to the positive healing qualities of the sun. When male animals show too much aggression or passivity there is a self-balancing effect here. Many animals naturally gravitate towards and will eat sunflower seeds. When there is seen a strong tendency or repeated desire to eat such seeds, this is also a good flower essence to provide. Sometimes animals will seek the seeds for the higher vibrational effects of transferring sunlight energy rather than the direct nutritional effects.

"The ability of plants to receive the afternoon or evening sun will be enhanced. Plants grown in shady areas may need more sunlight energy and respond better to bright sun. Sunflower essence may be applied to give some compensation.

"Many direct associations with Leo are noted; for instance, the ability of individuals to work with energies of progressed planets moving through Leo will be intensified and strengthened. But do not take sunflower if planets one has undue sensitivity to are moving through Leo so that such negative effects will not be strengthened. There is a strengthening of the first, seventh, and eighth rays."

1 Nutrients in sunflower seeds include: albumin, betaine, calcium, chlorine, copper, fatty oil, histidine, iron, lecithin, niacin, and vitamin B_1.

SWEET FLAG
Acorus Calamus

This perennial herb is native to much of Asia, but it is now found in most of Europe and the Eastern United States. A strong flower stalk bears a cylindrical spadix covered by minute greenish-yellow flowers. It alleviates gastritis, hyperacidity, pyrosis, and stomach problems. In a bath, it calms the nerves and eases insomnia.

Q How is this plant now used as a flower essence?
"The signature is somewhat complex and esoteric. The entire plant breaks down into threes and sixes. These numbers are numerologically associated with the mind, body, and spirit, which is what this essence clinically treats. This occurs on many different levels, not only with the number of petals, but in the branching of the plant, the way various spores form, and there is an etheric counterpart. In each case, when the threes and sixes occur, the overall summation will also be present.

"The division of this group of nine into threes and sixes will often symbolize the ways in which the God reality—the essential triangle of being—relates very highly to an understanding of relationship as personified in the six. This way always adds up to these nines, which tends to give change as their basic overall characteristic. These things can be taken to esoteric levels, but you may notice that there are vortex energies at the etheric levels under which the interference patterns created by the threes and the sixes create powerful energies within the plant. These are independent inner currents and are the source of much of the energies drawn from the earth into the flowers.

"There is a remarkable resemblance between the human aura and the stamen and ovaries of this plant. A person who could see auras would acknowledge this relationship.

"This essence primarily integrates the mind, body, and spirit by merging the mental, emotional, and etheric bodies. In many ways, they represent the three basic units in people: the physical, the emotional, and the mental. The etheric is the physical, the emotional is the spirit, and the mental is the mind. This activity makes sweet flag an enhancer for other flower essences. Use this essence in combination remedies and in certain difficult cases such as schizophrenia.

"Consider applying this essence for extreme anxiety, stress, or fear such as when confronted with physical passing. Practitioners involved in the hospice movement will find this an excellent remedy, especially if utilized with other essences.

"It slightly stimulates capillary action as it penetrates the ductless gland system. Some strengthening of positive aspects between Uranus and Mars develop, and the sixth ray is strengthened. The test point is the medulla oblongata and the center of the forehead.

"This flower essence can prepare animals for periods of extreme stress such as when a long period in an automobile or a move to a new location is imminent. It is wise to use the essence two or three days before moving the animal and then just before the move. This can assist in preventing anxieties and fears of the unknown. This essence is also useful for airplane travel. Most animals are not used to this. They have a deeper affinity and understanding of their relationship to the earth than do most people, and this is significantly disrupted in such movement. Give the essence for as long as three days after airplane travel.

"This is also true for the transportation of plants from places where they may have grown for many generations into a new location. This mainly refers to plants not the movement of seeds. Seeds have already disconnected from the earth and will attempt to reconnect to the devic order of a general nature in whatever location they arrive. But plants being transplanted from one location to another, especially those moved by airplane, would benefit from this essence before, during, and after such transportation, even for three days after the trip."

SWEET PEA
Lathyrus Latifolus

This climbing perennial is native to Southeastern Europe. It is a wild flower now common in many parts of the United States. The rose-red or purple flowers appear on elongated peduncles in July and August. While this is not used in herbalism, in homeopathy it alleviates nerve disorders such as polio.

Q How is this plant now used as a flower essence?

"Sweet pea creates a sense of social responsibility, so certain adolescents need it. Anyone exhibiting antisocial behavior could benefit from this essence. People experience the present and therefore develop a social commitment to life. If they are always daydreaming this can be a difficult process. Sweet pea draws people out of their fantasies.

"This essence is valuable in physically tight group situations such as people living in big cities. Scientists have already proven that congested living conditions cause antisocial behavior. Families having trouble living together, especially from overcrowded conditions, benefit from sweet pea.

"Sweet pea augments the meridians. It creates emotional stability because it calms the emotional body, and it awakens the chakra connected to the pancreas. This minor chakra balances the pancreas and calms the emotions, thus inspiring inspiration. It strengthens the body and ethereal fluidium because it extends into the cellular level of the system. It stimulates the nervous system on the physical level, and mitosis on the cellular level. It also eases the gonorrhea miasm.

"The influence of the essence on tight living conditions is expressed by the numerous pods bound tightly together in the pea. The pod looks somewhat like the colon, which this essence also augments.

"Use sweet pea when an animal is moving from the adolescent phase into adulthood or when an animal is having nervous difficulty resulting from loss of a limb and is attempting to somehow understand and work with this. Give this essence from one or two weeks after loosing a limb for up to one year. This helps the animal assimilate new information. Also, animals subjected to new environmental conditions and overcrowding may respond well to sweet pea.

"Plants being experimented with for companion planting will benefit from this essence. There will be an easing of certain characteristics that might be in opposition to each other. The plants will grow together more harmoniously and will combine their forces to assist the plants that they naturally work with. This is especially true when companion planting gets fairly complicated, as when a dozen or more plants are placed together.

"When Venus passes through Scorpio consider using this essence. A strengthening of the fourth and eleventh rays will be felt for most people."

THYME
Thymus Vulgaris

This species of thyme is the common garden variety. It produces small bluish-purple, two-lipped flowers whorled in dense, head-like clusters. It blooms from May until September. Thyme is a powerful tonic and antiseptic commonly used in liver, digestive, and respiratory illnesses.

Q What is the karmic pattern of thyme?

"In Lemuria, this plant was developed partly for use in ritual because of the aroma and to develop its flower essence so that a full understanding of the energetic principle of time might be known to people. This was obviously seen in the way energy was transferred between the roots and people as the plant grew. However, no direct development of this energy was seen as important for people. It was simply understood that the nature of time was a gift that could provide the essential understanding of sequential events to people in the sense that patience, development, and natural expression would be the result.

"However, much of this was abused in Atlantis in that some of the energies relating to the ability of this plant to mutate and change energy flows were developed. Many of these continue to the current day, and thyme has a powerful penetrating ability to strengthen people. Its ultimate karmic purpose in providing such strength may be that which mankind will develop. Thyme itself is requiring such direction, and that is why it is likely to be closely united with people for use as an herb and flower essence for some time."

Q How is this plant now used as a flower essence?

"It primarily is used to amplify the effects of other flower essences. It should generally be utilized in combination remedies.

"A dab of this essence on any part of the body amplifies the time flow in that part of the anatomy. Doing this localizes the effects of thyme, so healing works faster. Quickening the time flow allows for penetration beyond the speed of light thus projecting one into the past or future.[1] One can attune to future lives. Although the tendency is to quicken the time flow, thyme is neutral in effect. The only reason it tends to speed up the time flow is because that is the general direction in which people look.

"Thyme can be utilized in past-life therapies. Under the guidance of a skilled therapist, such past-life recall releases stored tensions and traumas. Another interesting result of this ability to accelerate the time flow is that by putting a few drops of this essence in pure water you can cleanse quartz crystals by dipping them into the water for a few minutes. A few drops can be mixed with sea salt that is being used to cleanse quartz. These two processes can be done with pennyroyal essence. Such quartz can then be used for scrying or seeing into the future."

Q What is the exact connection between thyme affecting the time flows and it having these influences such as being a general amplifier for any flower essence?

"In seeking to quicken the time flow, the properties of flower essences already work with ethereal patterns functioning just beneath the speed of light, yet they still somewhat integrate with the ethers that travel beyond the speed of light. In accelerating the time flow you are increasingly integrating the properties of flower essences with the ethers that travel beyond the speed of light and with the dimensions that exist beyond the three known ones.

"The complex signature of thyme relates to the ways energies that change the factoring of time are observed to flow, particularly between the roots and people. The body's natural metabolic processes tend to be better governed with this flower essence. It can be externally applied to each of the chakras. This creates a temporary balancing effect in that the balancing between anabolic and catabolic processes will result. This essence has a slight influence on the thymus gland, which is also the test point. The plant slightly resembles the thymus gland. Many difficult aspects associated with Uranus are eased. The seventh ray is better understood.

"For most animals the ability to enhance and assimilate information obtained in dreams will be felt. Animals often journey on the astral level in the dream state. Some of this experience is made more available. Often animals do not understand time. They do not work with it in the usual way that most humans do. They do not understand blending the past, present, and future and the distinctions which humans have artificially constructed for themselves. Sometimes, individuals are struggling with time or have times that are hard for them based on deadlines, yet their animals appear to be calm and not affected by such tension. Some energy of assimilation and relaxation may be observed to be transferred to the person when thyme flower essence is applied to both the animal and the human. It is a way by which animals teach people.

"If an animal in such periods maintains calmness, take the essence yourself in the morning and just before going to bed. Invite a dream in which you journey with your animal, and note the symbols that may occur. Many of these may be symbols of deep relaxation for you. It can be useful in periods of stress. Lastly, when animals approach old age and appear to drift off as if they are not concentrating, as if they are in a reverie state and yet they are fully awake, they will gain greater concentration and enhanced physical stamina if the essence is applied shortly after such a reverie state.

"Greater affinity in plants for seasonal change will be noted with thyme. This can be important when a plant is moved from one location to another very different in latitude, so that the plant is exposed to extremely different seasonal change. This can be especially important when a plant is moved from the Southern Hemisphere to the Northern, or vice versa. Under such circumstances, a seasonal reversal takes place. The ability of the plant to accommodate and work with such energy is usually enhanced by thyme. This is even true for seeds that are transplanted from one hemisphere to another. Spray them with this essence right after the movement and again just before planting."

1 Larry Dossey, M.D., *Space, Time and Medicine* (Boulder, CO: Shambhala Publications, 1982).

TUBEROSE
Polianthes Tuberosa

This small perennial is native to Mexico. It produces waxy, funnel-shaped, white flowers from July until frost. It is one of the most fragrant flowers in the world; thus, it is used as a perfume.

Q How is this plant now used as a flower essence?

"Its intense fragrance symbolizes the fact that it stimulates the crown chakra. Most flowers with a strong scent have this ability when prepared as a flower essence. They also augment the subtle bodies. It realigns the nadis in all the chakras for the proper distribution of the chakras' energies. But in doing this, except for the crown chakra, its direct effect is on the nadis, not the chakras. It is likewise a general tonic for the meridians.

"Tuberose can be used in conjunction with aromatherapies. This is partly because it augments the body's membranes and tissues. Sometimes intense or synthetic smells such as perfume or camphor block homeopathic remedies from working. Tuberose prevents or overcomes these problems. The karmic purpose of this is to create functions of uniting between individuals so that many abilities in all plants can be strengthened.

"On the cellular level, mitosis and capillary action are strengthened because the ethereal fluidium is tightened about the cells. The etheric and spiritual bodies are stimulated. The impact on the spiritual body aligns the emotional body, which creates increased sensitivity in the emotions and physical body, especially the neurological system. The test point is the forehead.

"Energy flows within the animal's subtle bodies are strengthened. When acupuncture is attempted with animals and there is no direct results, tuberose will help. Animals will find it easier to assimilate and work with acupuncture, massage, and movement of a physical therapy nature. Hands-on healing will be slightly enhanced with animals, but enhanced even more if movement is a part of the process. This means that you may move with the animal, carry it, or in some way move your hands around the animal. Such energy is created in etheric tubes of a temporary nature and will last for a few minutes. These are formed by the movements of the biofields of the person's hands near the biofields of the animal. Thyme will strengthen the transfer of energy during such movements.

"Better assimilation of water in poor soil will take place for most plants. Some easing of difficult aspects between Mars and Saturn will be noted, and the eighth ray is enhanced."

WOOD BETONY
Stachys Officinalis

This is a perennial herb with spicate whorls of red or purple flowers, which appear from June until August. Medically, it is used for asthma, heart problems, nervous troubles, and kidney or bladder problems.

Q How is this plant now used as a flower essence?

"This is an enhancer. It works primarily in balancing attitudes in the conflict of sexual energy and the desire for higher principles. One gains insight into whether or not celibacy is the correct path. This essence enhances the higher philosophies and the necessary sacrifices that transpire with abstinence. Celibacy should be an abstainment and inner calmness, rather than an agonizing struggle and suppression of sexual desires. Wood betony duplicates this inner calm without suppressing the sexual appetite. It just helps a person resolve the issue. An absence of the sexual drive for a long period of time allows the individual to concentrate more on higher goals and principles.

"A person embracing tantric practices in which the sexual energies are channeled into higher philosophies could use this essence. It helps some oversexed people exert more self-control. Wood betony also helps people who have certain types of diseases such as herpes in the genitals to adjust to being celibate, so they will not spread the disease to others.

"The signature relates to the red and purple flowers. The red bloom should be used in the immediate phase of the struggle with celibacy and sexuality. Once the individual becomes celibate, the purple flower essence strengthens his or her higher goals and principles.

"The emotional, mental, and spiritual bodies are strengthened as is the sexual and crown chakras. The pineal gland is also enhanced. This is generally the only part of the physical body that is affected by this essence. Some of the medical properties of the herb are transferred to the flower essence but only in a rudimentary form. The test point is the tip of the index finger.

"A balancing of sexual energies takes place with an animal, but it is often best to use this essence immediately before and after spaying or neutering. This procedure is psychically extremely difficult for an animal but, as most humans have noted, is fairly temporary and the overall benefits to the animal population are clear. However, the karma associated with this is generally unresolved between the person who elects to have the animal neutered and the animal's own karma and association with its soul.

"There must always be an energetic interaction, particularly for releasing karma and balancing cause and effect between the animal and the human responsible for neutering that animal. This interaction has certain aspects of fear and difficulty associated with it. But the higher aspects, that of seeing the sexuality as it is released, being allowed by the person to transform into the essence of sexuality and relationship at an intimate, loving, and spiritual level is transferred back to the animal.

"Sometimes as a result of this neutering a disturbing dream takes place, and the person will want to help the animal, perhaps bringing it extra love. It is wise to work with such an energy, as this finer attunement to the higher spiritual principles governing sexual functioning that are now no longer available to the animal now come to the human.

"Many aspects of sexual functions have their roots in the physical level. But at the higher level, sexual functioning comes not from physical interaction but from higher levels of understanding. It is for people to understand this to transcend the animal state. Many animals have the ability to learn from humans about this. It is not done by interaction with the animal, but rather by the conception of the entire thought form, and that this functioning of sexuality on a higher level will eventually be transferred to other animals is inevitable.

"Gradually, over a period of three months after such neutering, the animal will reaccommodate to its physical body, and there will be no lasting result. But the gift shared of the animal's inner sexuality now released to the human and expressed will reflect back to the animal's soul and will help it better understand and work with humans. It is as if it enhances the forgiving that animals naturally have with most humans.

"Many forms of reproduction are enhanced in plants. This essence can also be applied near or around insects that are utilized for fertilization such as bees. However, use this essence when you wish your plants to be fertilized, when they are in the flowering season.

"Transits of any planets through Scorpio will have some of their energies increased. Excellent times to use this essence are when Chiron or Pluto move through the sign of Scorpio. The second and eleventh rays are strengthened."

YARROW
Achillea Millefolium

This perennial herb flowers from June to September. The small, umbrella-shaped flowers are white and pink. Yarrow is used for digestive, kidney, lung, and vaginal illnesses.

Q How is this plant now used as a flower essence?

"Yarrow offers protection from negative influences such as radioactive fallout and thought forms from psychic attack or extreme emotionalism. It does this by enhancing the aura. It balances the upper and lower poles in the body.[1] The umbrella-shaped yarrow flowers disrupt radiation waves because radiation travels at those same peculiar angles and is dispersed when it meets a similar field. Pink yarrow essence is more for protection against negative emotions, while white yarrow essence offers better protection against radiation.

"Negative emotions being projected toward someone can be stopped by yarrow. It stabilizes a person working with emotionally disturbed people, so that they do not become too empathic with those people."

Q In our society with so much background radiation would it be wise to take yarrow every so often as a preventative?

"Yes, take a few drops once every six months."

Q Does yarrow ease the radiation miasm?

"No, this is an unusual case. Although this essence offers protection against radiation, it does not penetrate to the level of that miasm. Again, miasms reside on the cellular level, and yarrow does not penetrate to that level."

Q When you state yarrow offers protection against negative thought forms such as psychic attack, would this include the use of radionic instruments? Some believe the Russians are psychically attacking the United States using radionics instruments. Radionics involves the use of an instrument and an operator for sending vibrations to a person some miles away. It has been used as a modality in healing and agriculture for many years.[2]

"It is true that the Russians are doing this. After all, it has been proven that they bombarded the American embassy in Moscow with microwave radiation; thus it is not so esoteric for them to also work with enhanced thought forms.[3] But to be susceptible to psychic attack, one must believe in it. Without that empathy, on a conscious or subconscious level, you will not be influenced. Many around the United States are somewhat superstitious and are indeed susceptible to these forms of enhanced thought forms.

"Telepathy and levitation can gradually develop when yarrow is ingested over a period of time. If applied externally, it stimulates the aura, and it is a good tonic for the meridians.

"Animals exposed to humans in a relationship undergoing difficulty such as struggles, anger, or fighting, particularly when it is verbal or when direct emotional impacts are felt by the animal, will be alleviated and assisted. This, however, is difficult because under many such circumstances humans will not be aware of the stress they are causing their animals. Thus they would not readily choose this essence. There may be decreased appetite, difficulty sleeping, strange physical or nervous conditions where the animal, for instance, picks at itself or scratches excessively. These problems often take place when the human working near the animal is experiencing emotional distress. Animals that experience a deep sense of fear around their human owners then may have some of these effects eased.

"Plants will also experience stress around people experiencing emotional difficulty. Again, the energies are largely unconsciously transferred. Again, it is a somewhat difficult condition to note. But if you experience emotional difficulty, particularly in a relationship, be on guard for difficulty in the plants around you. Exposing them to this essence at such a time will generally increase their ability to release energies that may flow through them as a result of energy that is exuded by your subtle bodies.

"There is an easing of squares between Mercury and Mars and between Mercury and Venus. The fourth ray is strengthened. The test point is either ear lobe."

1 As depicted by Rudolf Steiner, there are three poles in the body. The upper pole relates to sensory and nervous activity, the lower pole to metabolism, and the middle pole to rhythmic activity such as breathing.

Rudolf Steiner, *Spiritual Science and Medicine* (London: Rudolf Steiner Press, 1975).

2 Edward Russell, *Report on Radionics* (Sudbury, Suffolk, England: Neville Spearman Ltd., 1973).

3 Thomas E. Bearden, *Excalibur Briefing* (San Francisco: Strawberry Hill Press, 1980).

Robert Beck, *Extreme Low Frequency Magnetic Fields and EEG Entrainment, A Psychotronic Warfare Capability?* (Los Angeles: Biomedical Research Associates, March, 1978).

YERBA SANTA
Eriodictyon Californicum

This shrub is native to Northern California and Oregon. The flowers appear in clusters lavender to white. Medically it is prescribed in a variety of digestive and respiratory illnesses.

Q How is this plant now used as a flower essence?
"The conical shape of the plant symbolizes the fact that the life force extends through the subtle bodies in a conical shape, and this essence brings into the system information from the higher self to resolve emotional issues. For instance, it almost immediately ends hysteria. If hysterics will not ingest the essence, apply it to the medulla oblongata. A person who rambles on would experience increased perspicuity with this remedy. It strengthens the life force and distributes information throughout the anatomy, easing emotional stress in the body.

"Yerba santa is a general tonic for the meridians, it calms the emotional body, and it has some attunement with the causal body, which is one of the doorways to the higher self. It slightly influences magnesium and zinc, which increase clarity of thought. It eases ulcerous conditions resulting from mental stress, and it eases the tubercular miasm. Use it externally to relax the individual for deep tissue work.

"Sometimes, after long periods of playfulness, animals collapse as if extremely tired or find themselves in conditions of extreme stress. As a result of this, certain behavioral patterns or problems may occur. This essence can be applied before such playful periods with such animals on a regular basis to alleviate such conditions, so that they will notice the approaching time of fatigue and stop their playfulness before they reach it. Also, the ability to relieve hysterical states may be noted in animals, though such states are much rarer. Usually, this will occur with overcrowding. Animals may be exposed to new animals that they have difficulty being around, or may experience acts of aggression from other animals. With primates, hysterical states are sometimes noted that seemingly have nothing to do with environmental conditions or neighboring animals. Squares between natal Mars and progressive Uranus ease. The fourth and eighth rays are clarified."

ZINNIA
Zinnia Elegans

This popular Mexican annual flowers from early summer until late autumn. The single or double flowers appear in large heads that are crimson, orange, red, violet, white, or yellow.

Q How is this plant now used as a flower essence?

"This remedy teaches people that laughter is a superior form of medicine.[1] Zinnia restores humor by uplifting the person's outlook on life. It creates this effect by aligning the etheric and emotional bodies. This is partly the source of humor.

"Zinnia is useful for people who need to laugh, which includes agitated, depressed, or hypersensitive individuals. It gets people in touch with their child-like properties. Many adults have trouble communicating with children because they do not relate to their child-like nature. Zinnia can also be applied for marital problems, parental image troubles, and unfulfilled parental or maternal instincts. General tensions in the system are alleviated.

"Viral, bacterial, and degenerative diseases are mildly relieved by zinnia. But zinnia does not have a pronounced impact on the physical body. The heart and abdominal chakras are stimulated. The intensity of the flower's colors expresses the nature of festivity, which this essence engenders. The shape of the plant is similar to the vortexes of energy in the subtle anatomies and aura. This essence mildly augments the meridians, and the test point is the joy of life meridian above the elbows. Much orgone energy is concentrated here.

"In old age, animals sometimes benefit by being around young animals. In order to bridge the gap that sometimes occurs here, zinnia could be applied. Also, sometimes the point of a playful state between people and animals is not well taken by the person. Then if the person takes this essence at the same time as the animal, there is better communication of the inner feeling of this playful state. This is sometimes very important for people, and it is one of the important lessons that animals can teach. In addition, after experiencing stress due to work overload or difficulty of any kind, humans may find that using this essence while playing with a pet or an animal one feels close to will enhance the playful period and add greater joy and love. Afterwards, the human will actually feel rested and the animal replenished.

"Certain inner messages of plants, particularly where they are growing under harmonious conditions and flowering and reproducing profusely, are indicative of inner joy within the plant. This is magnified by zinnia flower essence. Also, in the germination period, when there are repeated signs of such joy being available in both the human and in the environmental conditions around the plant, using this essence will speed up the process of germination, bringing more energy into the plant, enhancing the yield, and increasing the connection between the human and the devic order associated with this plant.

"Positive aspects of a trine, conjunction, or sextile will be enhanced by this essence, particularly between Venus and Jupiter. The third, fifth, and sixth rays are made clearer for most people."

---

1 For a fascinating story of how someone was cured of a serious disease through laughter read:
Norman Cousins, *Anatomy of an Illness as Perceived by the Patient* (Los Angeles: Cancer House, 1979).

Section III

Chapter I

Trends in Using Flower Essences

In the coming years, the use of flower essences will become much more popular. Current trends in medicine and the growing popularity of natural healing therapies exemplify this movement.

"The development of flower essences for holistic therapy is a system of the future because it is an advanced system of healing with energy. The dominant system of medicine in thy society is moving toward ways, means, and applications of energy, with energy being the healer. Examples of this are as follows: the healing of bone tissue through stimulation of activity from electrical application for treating pain and tissue regeneration, the application of electricity to stimulate the body physical's endorphins, the use of sound and ultrasonics in massage, and the stimulation of circulatory flow from electrical application. Other areas and principles of healing are that, of course, energy has been used in diagnostic principles such as with X-rays, sound, heat, and illumination. In addition, heat is used in treating cancer, lasers are used in surgery, and radiation is a form of energy. These are some of that which is attempted in the orthodox systems of medicine. All these activities represent graduations toward a system of purely using energy in healing.[1]

"In many ways flower essences are the aspect of the future, already existent within the cognizant knowledge of mankind but not within the practicing knowledge. The future development of healing with energy, particularly those strictly of the ethereal accord, is that there shall be continued progression working toward biofeedback, visualization, homeopathy, flower essences, and other natural systems eventually as supplementing and perhaps even replacing, in combination with other systems of diagnostic tools, the entire content and full range of orthodox medicine in the various systems of radiations, chemotherapies, and other applied drugs. Possibly those things which shall remain are the system of immunologies, antibiotics, and various diagnostic properties contained therein. Surgeries of an orthodox physician would only remain in cases of immediacy being applied to same. With the application of flower essences as an activity of energy, eventually their total study and clinical application shall evolve to wherein you begin to witness these changes and applications within the orthodox structures."[2]

Q Why do you feel orthodox practitioners will, as these changes develop in the future, still use certain antibiotics on occasion?

"It shall only be the accordance that this is a graduating falling aside of the structure, and there shall be the legitimate development of immune systems applied on the physical level, which shall be as drawn naturally from the system of immunology. These may continue to be wise in practice, for indeed, they are part of the natural biological cycle; engineered, but still as portions of the natural cycle."

New technologies will be introduced in the coming years that will greatly reduce the need for surgery as currently practiced, but still there will remain a need for surgery in some emergency situations. Many of the more traditional and safer diagnostic procedures of orthodox medicine will continue to be used for many years. Some of these techniques, however, are quite dangerous and, as many now feel, can of themselves cause serious problems.[3]

In recent years, numerous books have been published on what has come to be termed 'new physics.' One of the basic themes of this philosophy is that matter is really a condensed form of energy, and this theory is increasingly being applied in medicine.[4] Flower essences are, of course, another form of energy healing that can, in part, be studied and understood in the science of 'new physics.'

"The increased development of using flower essences as a science shall probably, in early spectrums, be dominated by its application to psychological and behavioral changes, and it shall as gain some forms of prominence and study in early psychological studies at first, as though it has as a form of benevolent placebo-like effect upon individuals of theological and philosophical background. Its original scrutinization shall be suspiciously investigated by the orthodox structure, in that its impacts will not be able to be denied."

Q In other words, they will see changes that cannot be denied, and they will claim it is from the placebo effect, not because the remedy could be causing an actual change?

"Correct. These shall probably be some of the first rudimentary explorations in the coming years. This shall as bring these forces more into the popular play of consciousness.

"There shall then be an evolution perhaps over fifteen to twenty years wherein homeopathically prepared psychotropic flower essences, independent of other medical portions of the plant, shall also be as used in the treatment of various mental diseases. Flower essences fully recognized in their whole and spiritual principles in reeducating the individual to spiritual endeavors are yet to be found in the activity of the time spectrums except for an approximation of the holistic practicing community, which shall rise more so into prominence towards the close of the fifteen to twenty year cycle spoken of, in its full issuance, application, and acceptance as both a spiritualizing force and an entity recognizing its principles of merger of mind, body, and spirit.

"There shall be as large advancements made in this particular field when instruments, that are approximately in current levels of development and shall be of more popular level and knowledge in the public consciousness in approximately three to five years, for measuring the existence of the ethereal anatomies, come into focus and play. For these shall eventually be the instruments that are used to evolve and isolate through scientific method and practice the impact of various forms of vibrational therapies, including flower essences, homeopathic remedies, and gem elixirs upon the subtle anatomies. When these become an accepted isolated science, it is then that these ethereal properties will reach the greatest level of appreciation.

"Some of these instruments are, in part, in use, such as those which measure the activities of brain waves, those which measure the capacities of neurological points relative to acupuncture, galvanic skin response, and above all those that measure the pulsation of biomagnetic energy from cellular division.[5] These machines allow for measuring the physiological responses of the body physical when essences are prescribed. They will likewise allow for the scrutinization in laboratory tests the potency of flower essences and their fields of effect in same.

"As is given, the subject material on flower essences is as staggering in its implications, particularly if they were as to become the complete medicine. The content and nature of using them as medicine in these days would reintegrate man's focus upon his link vibrationally with nature through a particular area of study, concentrating on healing. Eventually, the entire emphasis must become reintegrated with the entirety of these energies."

There obviously has been a major shift toward holistic health in recent years in the United States and Europe. Many will not be surprised to hear John's statement that natural healing will become much more popular in the coming years. The recent widespread acceptance of acupuncture, biofeedback, and visualization techniques in orthodox medical circles exemplify this trend. In the coming years, using flower essences will become even more popular in the holistic community and will be increasingly used by orthodox medical physicians, partly as an extension of the growing interest in homeopathy and energy forms of healing. Indeed, Bach flower essences have already been used by thousands of people for some years.

The equipment developed by Dr. Voll, a German neurosurgeon, exemplify the new inventions John discussed. His electroacupuncture machine, which in certain ways represents a merger of some principles of homeopathy and acupuncture, has been available for several years and is now utilized by thousands of physicians, especially in Europe.[6] Various devices are now available that use Kirlian photography to measure the human aura.[7] Many have studied the works of Harold Burr, Ph.D., a Yale Medical School professor, on the electrodynamic properties of life.[8] William Teller, Ph.D., of Stanford University, is now studying the ovation, a Burr-type electronic ovulation detector. Numerous doctors have used the pendulum to analyze the physical and subtle bodies.[9] In England today, there is the Psionic Medical Society, a group of doctors and dentists using homeopathy and the pendulum to diagnose and treat people.[10] In addition, radionics has been used for many years as a modality to analyze and treat subtle imbalances in people.[11]

"The public consciousness is now ready for this material. It is basically a fairly acceptable healing form as it is. Holistics is gaining in popularity, even to the point of influencing legislatures, such as with laetrile. It is freedom of choice more than anything and the fact that flower essences work."

Q Can you name some areas especially valuable for flower essence research in the future?

"Areas of importance include Santa Barbara, Hawaii, Cambodia, Nepal, Israel, and Egypt, especially that which was historically called Nubia or South Egypt. Other areas include the Southwest, especially New Mexico, the Superstition

Mountains in Arizona, and Red Rock by Sedona, Arizona. Areas where there is a concentration of any pure mineral structure, especially those in Mexico, are also important. The plant forms on Easter Island, which was part of Lemuria, should likewise be studied. Seek many of the plant forms along thy eastern and southern United States that were occupied by the Cherokee nation. Their historically sacred spots have peculiar properties. And study the areas of the midwest mound builders. These are as found throughout Pennsylvania, Ohio, Illinois, Indiana, Missouri, Kentucky, and Tennessee, extending even to the Dakotas. Study the plants in Ireland, Scotland, and the Netherlands. Isolation of other spots can be accomplished either through intuitive art forms or studies of further plant forms sacred to native areas.

"Many of the plants from Mexico and South America are psychotropic, and they include a large concentration of the original plant forms from Lemuria. These areas are a sanctuary for the deva-like properties and it is still in some forms the evolutionary force put into the activities of the flower essences and their workings. There shall be the nature of botanical research from Mexico and South America, concerning as crop studies and the abilities of multiharvests. These areas shall be developed as fully for their food resources in same. There shall also be hybrid plant forms coming from direct botanical research and new species that have taken the next step in evolution. This is partly because of the concentration of deva properties stored in those areas. This is also a by-product of Lemurian past ethereal influences. Most of these plants shall be of a medical accord. It shall be one of the first areas where there shall be the merger of the coming forth of the holistic botanical medica approach. This process has already begun."

Q Can you say exactly where in Latin America this is happening?
"In Mexico and the ancient lands of the Incas, Toltecs, Olmecs, and Mayans. Also, in Brazil, Argentina, Peru, Costa Rica, and Nicaragua."

Q Could you now discuss in detail the historical background and special value of the flower essences in several of these areas?
"The first area, that of Santa Barbara, was originally part of the continental shelf of Lemuria. Historically, this was as a position of many of the original botanical researches accomplished in Lemuria. Therefore, there remains many of the vibrations to that particular area; even though it is in an arid environment, vibrationally and somewhat to the degree of climate, there is the enhancement of much growth and many various forms of flowerings as such.

"Herein is where there was the content of seeking to integrate more fully the conscious processes of mental and gardening principles, as well as the use of essences from the area of Santa Barbara for their spiritual progressions. This was as considered a sacred spot to the areas of Lemuria, sacred in the sense of spiritual principles, more so than religious structure. This particular principle has been reenacted in that it became a central horticultural center during the latter 19th and early 20th centuries, and still carries the impacts of same. Many exotic plant forms have been brought here from many levels as across the planet. Thus, a high degree of concentration of unusual botanical studies has taken place here. Their properties are perhaps some of the most heightened upon the planet. This could be as a central area involved in principles of genetic engineering, and their properties are more so immediate to perhaps a system of testing the remedies on people."

In the late 19th and 20th centuries many wealthy people, especially from Japan, moved to Santa Barbara. They brought into the area many tropical plants and trees. During this period a good deal of botanical research took place. This research proved that even plants not native to Santa Barbara and not used to its particular climatic conditions could grow quite well in that area. This is partly because of the influence of the devic orders in that region and from the vibration of past botanical research done in Lemuria.

"The second area would be greater San Francisco. In this particular continental portion of land mass there were activities for studies as one of the major points of debate concerning the application of psychic forces between Atlantis and Lemuria. This was as a special city-state that gathered and became a particular point of focus and research for the original principles of genetic engineering. These were, again, the negotiations between Atlantis and Lemuria in those days, for it was desired that the information that emerged from Atlantis and Lemuria would not become a functional part of either civilization. This became as a central point of research in rediscovering the principles of those properties, not so much as an enhancement of any peculiar properties of the essences gathered in this area, but more so specific to the location of research in this area of thought. Flower essences from this area can especially enhance the intellectual processes. They are as unique and distinct in this particular area, and their properties are heightened in same."

Q So those flower essences were of special value in the communication between the Lemurian culture, which was more 'right brain' with a focus on intuition and a close relationship with nature, and the Atlanteans, who were more 'left brain' and focused on technological and intellectual endeavors?

"Correct. Flower essences native to the San Francisco area have a special value in establishing a proper balance between the left and right brain.

"That which arose in Atlantis was more so a colony of Lemuria, and was not so much as an opposing system of thought but a development of technologies made and based upon material sciences. In these accords, it was desired that the emergence of both these systems of information could as merge and become a focus or a spiritualizing focus in same so that the spiritual advancements obtained in Lemuria could then proceed also in Atlantis, but would evolve rather than being assimilated only into that civilization. But above all, it was desired that the materialistic Atlantean influences would not penetrate into Lemuria."

There was a fundamental and profound difference in the outlook on life by the Atlanteans and Lemurians. It was like comparing a traditional native culture today with a very technologically advanced and sophisticated western nation. A key difference, however, is that the Atlanteans had much respect for the wisdom of Lemuria; we in the west today rarely have such respect for the teachings of more traditional societies.

When people from the two ancient civilizations intermingled, stress and even disease sometimes developed. Thus, research was carried out in the San Francisco area with various native flower essences to deal with these kinds of problems. Similar difficulties are sometimes seen today when people move between rural and very urban areas. It is interesting that San Francisco is again a center for research in the holistic health movement, including both left and right brain functioning.

"The third area is that of Hawaii, which was the capital of Lemuria. It was the central seat of the original principles of discovery, even as Athens was the activity of the central most degrees. And indeed, Hawaii is perhaps the central most activities of wherein the stable and unshifting environment is such that the quality level of flower essences, particularly those which enhance the spiritual qualities of the individual, is perhaps the highest which can be as discovered on the planet. It is desired to give no further information, for this as creates a perfect triad in the essences almost as in locations of a triad effect of mind, body, and spirit."

Q The spirit is Hawaii, the mind is the San Francisco area, and the body is Santa Barbara?
   "Correct."

Q When Lemuria rises from the Pacific Ocean will there be flower essences rediscovered and old records found?
   "While portions of Lemuria are having an aspect of resurfacing, Atlantis will be more so the rising element. There may be some records of essences as flowers to be found but there is no particular connection with current subject materials. Some can already be obtained in the preservations of pyramids and Egyptian kings' tombs and burial urns. These are currently confused as only being grains preserved in same."

Q Which kings' chambers are involved here?
   "This information cannot be given at this time."

Q In other words, some of these seeds found in Egypt are ancient plants that became extinct and were buried under the Atlantic and Pacific Oceans?
   "Accurate."

Q Would you now suggest some laboratory tests that would prove the validity of flower essences?
   "Take a common toxin like streptococcus, or use one of the bacterias that are commonly used in laboratory experiments. Or if you want to work closer to the human condition, take some bacteria in the intestinal flora, certain skin tissues, or blood. Put this in a nurturing culture, so this life form will continue to multiply. The idea is to show that the life force in the flower essence will support some of these cells under adverse conditions.

"Use lotus and other essences associated with the crown chakra, or that are good tonics for the meridians, or that are enhancers for the ethereal fluidium. These work closely with the life force.

"Divide the cultures from a given life form and put a drop of the Lotus flower essence, for instance, in half of them. Freeze them all for the same amount of time. When they are thawed out, it will be found that the untreated ones tend to have no life force left, and the ones treated with lotus will still be quite alive. In a similar fashion, expose the cultures to a form of extreme heat or sonics. Again, the untreated ones would be mostly dead, and the treated ones would be mostly alive. The main difference in these experiments would be the amount of time it takes under adverse conditions to kill the tissues.

"Another test would be to take pictures of a person's aura through some of the various devices that are now available.[12] The subject, while not moving from his position, ingests a flower essence that notably affects the etheric body. Then over the next few minutes to an hour take more pictures of the person's aura and compare them to the photo taken just before the subject ingested the flower essence. In each case, you should find an increase in the life force from the initial photos. For instance, there would be an increased brightness in the pictures."

Q Can you suggest a format for compiling and documenting case histories with a questionnaire, so clinical data can be gathered on the effectiveness of flower essences?

"While many of the essences work with behavioral modification and symptomatic changes, others work directly on organic illnesses. Work especially with essences that create noticeable physical changes that are easily observable. It is usually much easier to gather and explain clinical data on observable physical changes than on psychological or spiritual changes. The exact contents of the questionnaire can be drawn from traditional sources where similar testing has been done. In this testing, it would be wise to gradually identify the best species to use with each flower essence. This kind of exactness will interest the scientific community more in this work."

Q Can you describe the different categories of flower essences that will be channeled in the future?

"Some will be involved in healing the spirit, not the soul, but the spirit. This includes past-life therapies, spiritual attitudes, and some degrees of psychism. There are also flower essences for dissolving crystallizations of unhealthy karmic patterns within the self. There are some related to psycho-dynamics, including a group of flower essences for treating mental illness. Certain flower essences relate to spiritualizing the intellect. There are some specifically for the subtle bodies, the seven ethers, the seven dimensions, the nadis, the meridians, and the chakras. Some will enhance learning, such as in the study of astrology and mathematics. There are some related to going more deeply into the physical, just barely touching the ethereal levels. Specific essences will be given for chiropractors and for people doing 'body work.' Others will be provided for use in acupuncture and for people using essential oils. There will be a complete system of flower essences from buds for prenatal care and treatment. In addition, flower essences with similar properties will be compared to each other. Then there are the flower essences relating to treating the body, which, of course, separates into the various organs, certain specific physical diseases, and nutrient requirements. Roses are not specifically a breakdown of healing properties. They are a specific range or closed system unto themselves in the study of flower essences. Some of these categories have, of course, already been touched upon. Much more will be provided in the future."

Forthcoming volumes on flower essences will tend to be divided into these areas for people doing work in different modalities. There will be at least one book on just clinical case studies of the new flower essences, and many combination remedies will be presented. In some instances, flower essences will be combined with herbs, homeopathic remedies, essential oils, and gem elixirs. Specific combination remedies to release past-life information stored in the genetic code will likewise be offered. Other combination remedies will bring the soul's forces directly into the daily activities of physical, mental, and emotional life. And more information will be presented on the relation of flower essences to tissue regeneration, androgyny, and nature spirits.

Q How valuable are physical level flowers as a food substance?

"They can be taken internally for certain nutritional and ethereal properties; however, fruits, in part, contain many similar properties. Violets in particular have potency in the preservation of the skin tissue, the lymphatics, and the basic cleansing tracts as such, even to the degree of reversing the aging process. The bloom remains as such a potent force because of the concentration of the life force."

There is already a long tradition of using certain blooms in herbal teas. Chamomile is an excellent example of this, and it is not unusual for rose blooms to be eaten.[13] It is felt that these flowers have nutritional and medicinal value. While fruits are beneficial in this area, flowers are more potent. The custom of eating flowers will become more common in the coming years, and gradually a science will develop using physical flowers to treat various physical and psychological illnesses.

The *East West Journal* recently had an article about the growing popularity of eating flowers.[14] Paradise farm in Carpinteria, California has been doing a thriving business as interest in flowers as food increases.

There is also a long tradition of studying the meaning of flowers. The technical name for this study is "florigraphy." There are numerous books written on the folklore of flowers, and some of them are listed in the bibliography.[15]

It is only a matter of time before these new steps manifest with flower essences. They have already begun! Some experiments are being carried out to scientifically document the validity of flower essences. The Bach flowers have already been successfully used for many years by thousands of people. In recent years, a growing number of individuals have, on their own, begun preparing and using locally grown flower essences. Ingesting flower essences for various imbalances is a very simple form of therapy, which anyone can learn to do. This is not a system to be used exclusively by physicians.

Q Is it true, that with flower essences and gem elixirs, their more spiritual effects will become more common in future years as consciousness expands?

"Correct."

Q Is this a key reason why people now rarely experience the keen spiritual effects you quote and why such preparations should be amplified with various quartz crystal and pyramid technologies?

"Yes, as has often been stated, it is the consciousness of the individual that is the final phenomenon. Spiritual qualities grow in the pattern of each individual. If individual psychological or behavioral studies were done, people would find their consciousness enhanced by flower essences and gem elixirs with a radical spiritualization of behavioral patterns taking place, more than would be the case with others not taking these preparations. It would also be found that these effects would be independent of any placebo-like influences."

When it is noted, for example, that passion flower helps one experience Christ consciousness, very few people today will experience such exalted states. Yet as the respiritualization of society takes place, gradually a small but growing number of individuals will experience these states. Ultimately, we will again experience a state approaching the consciousness of Lemuria so that almost all people using vibrational preparations will innately understand and experience the total effects of these preparations in mind, body, and spirit.

Well over one hundred individuals have told me that they could tell that vibrational preparations amplified with quartz crystals and pyramids work faster and stronger in them and their clients than has been their experience with other vibrational preparations not receiving this amplification. These individuals happen to have the sensitivity to understand the effect that such techniques have on vibrational preparations. Yet most people today do not have the sensitivity to detect this in vibrational preparations. In the coming years, more and more people will have the sensitivity to tell almost immediately if a flower essence, gem elixir, or homeopathic remedy has been amplified and if it has been done properly. It is inevitable that all manufacturers of such preparations will use quartz crystals and pyramids to amplify such products.

"Today, people often take flower essences without really understanding their role in the process. Flower essences will work better when people understand that it is not just the taking of a vibrational essence. Activating one's consciousness through techniques such as creative visualization are very important in this work. For instance, many people wrongly assume that taking pennyroyal flower essence by itself will dispel negative thought forms. That will not be sufficient for most individuals; the essence increases your interaction with negative thought forms. The ability to understand and work with negative thought forms appropriately can develop as you actively and consciously work with the process.

"There has been the growth of many individuals in this process as each person becomes a student to this work. Vibrational remedies advance and enhance the concept of thyself as energy. Energy is unified with spirit and consciousness and so ye enlighten thyself to the great accord to wherein you merge the total concept of mind, body, and spirit, even though you have divided these things into perhaps various sciences and various art forms. Indeed, these begin to approach the level of that integration known as the Christ principle, for the Christ principle is the manifestation of God's nature on this plane and the merger of mind, body, and spirit.

"God is love and love is harmony and harmony begets peace. It is harmony that ye seek to begin to make in thy own personal endeavors through interrelationships with each other. For indeed, life is interactivity with thy fellow beings and fellow souls, be they incarnate or discarnate, or in the various accords that ye seek to bring them to harmony with. This accord is consciousness.

"Take all this information and know that there are many techniques and there are many concepts, but none must supplement the content and nature or even be as given as the higher priority, than to know that God is within you. These things that are given forth are teachings, then as applied teachings, then as to stimulate more that each and every one of thee may as make progressions and evolve toward that which ye already are which is God's love, which is within thee, which begets harmony and peace."

1 Alice A. Bailey, *Telepathy* (New York: Lucis Publishing Co., 1980), p. 140.

2 _____. *Esoteric Healing* (New York: Lucis Publishing Co., 1980), p. 280, 482.

Aart Jurriaanse ed., *Prophecies* (Craighall, South Africa: World Unity and Service, 1977), p. 132-137.

3 Robert Mendelsohn, M.D., *Confessions of a Medical Heretic* (New York: Warner Books, 1979).

4 Fritjof De Riencourt, *The Eye of Shiva: Eastern Mysticism and Science* (New York: William Morrow & Co., 1981).

Michael Talbot, *Mysticism and the New Physics* (New York: Bantam Books, 1981).

Larry Dossey, M.D., *Space, Time and Medicine* (Boulder, CO: Shambhala Publications, 1982).

5 Ian L. Pykett, "NMR Imaging in Medicine," *Scientific American*, CCXLVI (May, 1982), 78-88.

Alcestis Oberg and Daniel Woodard, "Anti-Matter Mind Probes and Other Medical Miracles," *Science Digest*, XC (April, 1982), 54-62.

6 James F. Scheer, "Electroacupuncture: New Pathways to Total Health," *Bestways*, X (June, 1982), 40-47, 119.

7 Kendall Johnson, *The Living Aura* (New York: Hawthorn Books, 1976).

Daniel Rubin and Stanley Krippner ed., *The Kirlian Aura* (New York: Doubleday & Co., 1974).

8 Harold Burr, *Blueprint for Immortality* (Sudbury, Suffolk, England: Neville Spearman Ltd., 1972).

9 H. Tomlinson, M.D., *The Divination of Disease: A Study of Radiesthesia* (Saffron Walden, England: Health Science Press, 1953).

W. Guyon Richards, M.D., *The Chain of Life* (Rustington, Sussex, England: Leslie J. Speight, 1974).

10 J. H. Reyner, *Psionic Medicine* (York Beach, ME: Samuel Weiser, Inc., 1974).

11 David Tansley, D.C., *Radionics and the Subtle Anatomy of Man* (Saffron Walden, England: Health Science Press, 1980).

_____. *Dimensions of Radionics* (Saffron Walden, England: Health Science Press, 1977).

12 Oscar Bagnall, *The Origin and Properties of the Human Aura* (York Beach, ME: Samuel Weiser, Inc., 1975).

Walter Kilner, *The Human Aura* (Secaucus, NJ: University Books, 1965).

13 Julie Clements, *Treasury of Rose Arrangements and Recipes* (Nashville, TN: Heartside, 1959).

Eleanor Rohde, *Rose Recipes* (Danby, PA: Arden Library, 1979).

14 Bill Thomson, "From Mushroom Mania to Flower Power," *East West Journal*, (December, 1988), 46-52.

15 Barbara Coyner, "Flower Talk," *Bestways*, XI (November, 1984), 84-85.

Cross Reference Tables

Minor Chakras Chart	Apricot	Blackberry	Bo	California Poppy	Chamomile (German)	Chaparral	Daisy	Dandelion	Garlic	Lavender(French)	Madia	Marigold (French)	Passion Flower	Prickly Pear Cactus	Rosa Webbiana	Saguaro	Snapdragon	Sweet Pea	Yerba Mate
Arm Pits		•																	
Base of Arch of Feet							•												
Behind Each Knee				•															
Both Heels															•				
Breast Bones						•													
Center of Ears									•										
Elbows																			•
Feet		•																	•
Hands																			•
Knees																•			•
Liver										•									
Medulla Oblongata											•								
Palm of Hand-Venus area																	•		
Pancreas																		•	
Shoulders																			•
Spleen									•										
Tip of Index Finger	•			•															
Upper Arch													•						
Wrists														•					

Diseases Chart

Disease	Almond	Aloe Vera	Amaranthus	Angelica	Apricot	Avocado	Bells of Ireland	Bleeding Heart	Bloodroot	Bo	California Poppy	Camphor	Cedar	Centuary Agave	Chaparral	Clover (Red)	Coffee	Comfrey	Corn (Sweet)	Cosmos	Daffodil	Daisy	Dandelion	Date Palm	Dill	Eucalyptus	Fig	Forget Me Not
Addiction Withdrawal																												
Aging Diseases																												
Aging Slowed																								●				
AIDS														●														
Allergies																												
Alzheimers														●														
Anemia																												
Anorexia Nervosa																												
Appendicitis				●																								
Arteriosclerosis			●											●														
Arthritis																												
Asbestos Problems																												
Asthma									●													●				●		
Athlete's Foot																												
Atonic Dyspepsia									●																			
Autolysis																												
Bacterial Inflammation		●																										
Balance Off										●																		
Bell's Palsy																												
Birthing																											●	
Blood Sugar					●																							
Body Tensions																							●					
Brain Imbalances		●												●				●								●		
Breathing Trouble																								●		●		
Bronchial Conditions																			●									
Bubonic Plague								●																				
Caffeine Problems				●							●						●											
Cancer	●	●			●	●		●			●			●	●				●	●			●					●
Candida			●																●									
Cerebral Palsy																										●		
Circulatory System		●			●			●	●					●	●									●				
Colon Spasm																												
Common Cold										●																		
Connective Tissue						●																						
Constipation																												
Cranial Inflammation		●																										
Cyst, Female Organs																												

Green Rose	Hawthorne (English)	Hyssop	Jasmine	Khat	Koenign Van Daenmark	Live Forever	Lotus	Mallow	Mango	Manzanita	Mugwort	Nectarine	Onion	Pansy	Papaya	Paw Paw (American)	Peach	Pomegranate	Redwood	Sage	Saguaro	Self Heal	Skullcap	Snapdragon	Spiderwort	Spruce	Squash	Star Tulip	Stinging Nettle	Sugar Beet	Sunflower	Tuberose	Wisteria (Chinese)	Yerba Mate	Zinnia
																							•												
								•																											
				•	•				•									•									•								
					•									•							•														
•																							•												
								•									•																		
										•						•																			
																•																			
								•								•	•																		
																							•												
																										•									
•																												•							
																						•													
																•			•																
		•		•																				•				•		•					•
																								•											
											•																								
																														•					
											•																							•	
			•																					•											
						•	•				•	•	•				•	•				•									•	•	•		
	•	•		•										•			•	•	•					•	•		•			•	•				
																	•																		
																					•														
														•			•				•						•								
•																																			
															•																				
																	•																		
																	•																		

Diseases Chart

Diseases Chart	Almond	Aloe Vera	Angelica	Apricot	Banana	Blackberry	Bleeding Heart	Bloodroot	Bo	Cedar	Centuary Agave	Cosmos	Cotton	Daisy	Dandelion	Date Palm	Dill	Fig	Garlic	Ginseng	Grapefruit	Green Rose	Harvest Brodiaea
Dehydration																							
Diabetes			●																	●			
Diaphragm Deterioration																							
Digestive Imbalances	●									●						●							
Diseases from Guilt																							
Diseases from Sun																							
Diseases when Tongue Coated																							
Dryness, Entire Body																							
Dwarfism	●																						
Dysentery									●														
Eczema			●	●					●														
Epilepsy			●																				●
Epstein-Barr										●					●								
Esophagus Imbalances																							
Excessive Acidity																							
Eye Problems																							●
Face Lift																					●		
Fatigue									●														
Female Problems						●											●						
Fevers															●				●				
Gallbladder Stones				●																			
General Detoxification																							
Genetic Diseases							●																
Genitals																					●		
Hair Loss										●			●										
Headaches										●												●	
Hearing Loss										●													
Heart Disease						●	●			●	●					●							
Hemophilia																							
Hemorrhoids																							
Herpes																							
Hiccups															●								
Hirsutism										●			●										
Hormone Imbalance																					●		
Hypoglycemia				●	●																		
Inflammations																	●		●				
Inner Ear Problems																							

Hawthorne (English)
Henna
Hops
Hyssop
Jasmine
Lemon
Luffa
Macartney Rose
Mallow
Mango
Manzanita
Marigold (French)
Nasturtium
Pansy
Papaya
Paw Paw (American)
Peach
Pomegranate
Queen Anne's Lace
Redwood
Saguaro
Snapdragon
Spruce
Squash
Star Tulip
Sugar Beet
Sunflower
Watermelon
Wood Betony

Diseases Chart

Diseases	Almond	Aloe Vera	Amaranthus	Angelica	Apricot	Avocado	Banana	Bells of Ireland	Blackberry	Bloodroot	Bo	Bottlebrush	California Poppy	Cedar	Celandine	Centuary Agave	Chamomile (German)	Coffee	Comfrey	Corn (Sweet)	Dandelion	Date Palm	Dill	Eucalyptus	Fig	Four Leaf Clover	Garlic	Ginseng	Green Rose
Immune System Diseases		●																											
Impotency & Infertility					●			●	●																●				
Jaundice																								●					
Jet Lag																				●									
Kidney Diseases																●								●					
Laryngitis																													
Laxative															●														
Left-Right Brain Imbalance						●																							
Leprosy																													
Liver Imbalance									●						●									●				●	
Lowers Pulse									●																				
Lung Imbalance										●														●					
Lymphs Imbalanced																													
Malaria																								●					
Menieres Disease																													●
Menopause																													
Menstruation																													
Migraine																													●
Motion Sickness																													
Mucous Colitis																													●
Multiple Sclerosis												●	●																
Muscular Diseases				●									●								●								
Nasal Passages		●																						●					
Nausea																													
Nerve Diseases		●		●								●	●			●			●	●		●				●			
Obesity					●		●																						
Opiates Discharged																													
Overexposure																													
Pain Eases																													
Pancreas Imbalances																													
Parasites																											●		
Periodontal Diseases							●																						
Phantom Limb																			●										
Physical Growth Helped	●																												
PMS																													
Pregnancy Helped									●																●				
Progeria (Aging Too Fast)																						●							
Psychosomatic Illnesses																				●									
Radiation Problems	●																							●					

Hawthorne (English)															●																								
Henna																								●							●						●		
Hyssop															●																								
Jasmine																	●											●											
Khat			●																																				
Koenign Van Daenmark																																							
Live Forever			●																																				
Loquat																●					●																		
Lotus																																				●			
Mallow																								●														●	
Manzanita																												●											
Marigold (French)										●								●																					
Morning Glory													●																										
Mugwort																															●						●	
Nasturtium															●																								
Onion					●																																		
Orange																		●																					
Pansy																														●									
Papaya				●							●																					●							
Paw Paw (American)												●		●																									
Peach																																							
Pennyroyal																																				●			
Petunia															●			●														●							
Pomegranate				●																			●																
Redwood														●																	●								
Rosa Webbiana															●																								
Sage																																	●			●			
Saguaro																											●												
Skullcap															●																								
Snapdragon																																		●					
Spice Bush											●				●																								
Spiderwort	●																																						
Squash				●																			●															●	
Stinging Nettle															●													●											
Sugar Beet	●																																						
Watermelon				●																																			
Yarrow	●																																						
Zinnia																																							

Diseases Chart	Aloe Vera	Amaranthus	Angelica	Apricot	Avocado	Banana	Bloodroot	Bottlebrush	Cedar	Centuary Agave	Comfrey	Corn (Sweet)	Cosmos	Cotton	Daffodil	Dandelion	Dill	Eucalyptus	Fig	Four Leaf Clover	Ginseng	Grapefruit	Green Rose
Scalp Problems									•				•										
Senility																							
Sexual Diseases																							
Sickle Cell Anemia			•																				
Sinus Congestion																							
Skin Conditions	•		•		•	•										•	•		•				
Skin Ulcers	•		•																				
Slipped Discs																							
Smallpox																							
Smoking																							
Solar Plexus Imbalance																							•
Spinal Degeneration																							
Spinal Inflammation																							
Starvation																							
Stroke										•													
Subluxation of Bones						•																	
Sun's Ultraviolent Rays Blocked																							
SV 40 Virus																							
Testosterone Imbalance																							
Tetanus																							
Throat Disease																			•				
Throat Sore												•					•						
Tic Douloureux																							
Tics							•																
TMJ Problems						•																•	
Tonsilitis																•							
Torn Tissue Rejuvenated			•																				
Toxemia																							
Typhoid Fever																•							
Ulcers (Internal)	•			•			•			•					•	•	•						•
Uric Acid Removed																							
Vagina																							
Varicose Veins																							
Viral Inflammation		•										•											
Weakens All Diseases																							
Weight Control				•																			
White Corpuscle Imbalance												•											

Hawthorne (English)	Henna	Jasmine	Koenign Van Daenmark	Lemon	Lilac	Luffa	Mallow	Manzanita	Marigold (French)	Morning Glory	Onion	Orange	Pansy	Papaya	Paw Paw (American)	Peach	Petunia	Pomegranate	Redwood	Saguaro	Self Heal	Snapdragon	Squash	Stinging Nettle	Sunflower	Yerba Santa	Zinnia
							●																				
														●									●				
																			●								
		●						●																			
	●			●		●	●				●						●		●	●							
						●																		●			
	●															●											
										●																	
								●	●														●		●		
					●																						
															●												
																●											
														●													
																							●				
																						●					
																						●					
		●											●									●					
												●										●					
								●														●					
																						●					
																			●								
																										●	
																					●						
																		●									
							●												●								
●		●	●						●				●									●					●
			●																								
																					●						

Psychological States Chart	Aloe Vera	Amaranthus	Angelica	Avocado	Banana	Bells of Ireland	Bleeding Heart	Borage	Bottlebrush	Celandine	Century Agave	Chaparral	Corn (Sweet)	Daffodil	Eucalyptus	Forget Me Not	Four Leaf Clover	Garlic	Ginseng	Grapefruit	Harvest Brodiaea	Hawthorne (English)
Adapt to Hard Environment	●		●																			
Adults and Children																						
Adults-Maternal Instinct																						
Agnostic																					●	
Agoraphobia																						
Alcoholism			●																			
Androgyny											●							●				
Anger										●						●						
Anorexia Nervosa																						
Anti-Depressant																						
Anxiety						●		●							●							
Aphrodisiac				●																		
Arguments														●								
Autism		●	●		●			●														
Bad Luck																●						
Birthing																						
Bitterness																					●	
Broken Love Affair							●															●
Cannot Link Issues																						
Cannot Make Decision																						
Clarity of Thought											●	●	●	●		●	●		●	●	●	
Claustrophobia																						
Compassion Increases																						
Completes Projects																						
Compulsive Gamblers																	●					
Compulsiveness																						
Confusion																						
Couple During Pregnancy																						
Courage							●															
Crippled People-Attitude																						
Cut Off From Community																						
Cynicism																						

Helleborus (Black) | Iris-Blue Flag | Jasmine | Khat | Lavender(French) | Lemon | Loquat | Luffa | Macartney Rose | Madia | Mallow | Marigold (French) | Mullein | Nasturtium | Nectarine | Onion | Papaya | Passion Flower | Paw Paw (American) | Pennyroyal | Petunia | Pimpernel | Pomegranate | Prickly Pear Cactus | Rosemary | Saguaro | Self Heal | Skullcap | Spice Bush | Spiderwort | Squash | Sweet Flag | Tuberose | Watermelon | Zinnia

Psychological States Chart

Psychological States Chart	Almond	Amaranthus	Angelica	Avocado	Banana	Blackberry	Bo	Borage	California Poppy	Carob	Celandine	Centuary Agave	Chamomile (German)	Chaparral	Comfrey	Corn (Sweet)	Cosmos	Cotton	Daffodil	Date Palm	Dill	Eucalyptus	Fig	Forget Me Not	Garlic	Green Rose	Harvest Brodiaea	Hawthorne (English)	Helleborus (Black)	Hops	Hyssop	Iris-Blue Flag
Daydreamers																•																
Depression								•	•													•										•
Desire to Raise Children																																
Develop Loving Nature																																
Develop Social Responsibility	•												•																			
Disorientation		•	•			•																										
Dreams		•				•		•	•							•	•									•			•			
Drug Addiction Symptoms																																
Eccentric Genius																													•			
Ego Problems	•			•																												
Emotional Cleansing			•						•							•	•	•						•		•	•					
Express Inner Feelings																																
Family Pressures																						•										
Fear From Past Lives																																
Fear of Aging	•																				•	•										
Fear of Dying									•													•							•			
Fear of Food																																
Fear of Religious Sects																		•														
Fear of the World																																
Fear of Unknown Origin																									•	•						
Fear Someone Will Die						•																										
Fears In General																										•						
Feels Life Against Them																																
Frustrated										•									•													•
Grief																						•										•
Grief-Death of Beloved																						•					•					
Grinds Teeth																																
Group Process Affected									•																							•
Guilt								•														•										•
Hallucinations	•																															
Handle Details																																
Hard to Express Oneself																						•										

Khat | Lavender(French) | Live Forever | Loosestrife | Madia | Mallow | Manzanita | Maple (Sugar) | Marigold (French) | Morning Glory | Mugwort | Mullein | Nectarine | Onion | Orange | Passion Flower | Paw Paw (American) | Peach | Pear | Pennyroyal | Petunia | Pimpernel | Pomegranate | Redwood | Rosemary | Saguaro | St. John's Wort | Self Heal | Skullcap | Snapdragon | Spiderwort | Spruce | Squash | Star Tulip | Stinging Nettle | Sugar Beet | Sunflower | Sweet Flag | Sweet Pea | Watermelon | Yerba Santa | Zinnia

Psychological States Chart

Psychological States	Almond	Avocado	Banana	Blackberry	Celandine	Centuary Agave	Chamomile (German)	Chaparral	Coffee	Cotton	Daffodil	Daisy	Date Palm	Fig	Four Leaf Clover	Grapefruit	Harvest Brodiaea	Henna	Khat	Lemon
Helps One Get Up																				
Hidden Fears Eased													●							
Hidden Talents Released																				
Homosexuality																				
Hostility																●				
Humility											●									
Hyperactive Children																				
Hypochondria												●								
Hysteria																				
Identity Crisis			●											●			●			
Illogical																				
Immaturity	●					●														
Impatience						●														
Inability to Cope with Life																				
Indecisiveness									●											
Initiates Projects																				
Inner Peace																				
Insomnia							●	●												
Intellectual Capacity Low											●									
Intuition Improved			●		●					●	●	●			●					
Irrational																				
Joy																				
Juvenile Delinquents	●					●														
Known Fears Eased														●						
Lacks Humor																				●
Lacks Vision in Life																			●	
Laughter																				
Laughter As Medicine																				
Leadership Problems																				
Lesbians																				
Lethargic				●															●	

Live Forever	Luffa	Madia	Mallow	Marigold (French)	Morning Glory	Mullein	Nasturtium	Onion	Orange	Pansy	Papaya	Paw Paw (American)	Petunia	Pimpernel	Prickly Pear Cactus	Rosemary	Sage	St. John's Wort	Shooting Star	Skullcap	Snapdragon	Squash	Sunflower	Sweet Pea	Yerba Santa	Zinnia
					●																					
															●			●								
		●																								
									●		●								●							
●													●													
																										●
		●								●	●	●		●												
								●											●							
																							●			
						●		●																		
																	●									
						●																				
																●										
					●																					
●				●						●								●				●				
									●																	
							●																			
																							●			
															●			●								
																	●									
																										●
													●													
											●															
	●																									

Psychological States Chart	Almond	Aloe Vera	Amaranthus	Angelica	California Poppy	Celandine	Centuary Agave	Chaparral	Clover (Red)	Coffee	Comfrey	Corn (Sweet)	Daffodil	Dill	Fig	Forget Me Not	Four Leaf Clover	Green Rose
Long Range Planning												●						
Loquacious																		
Loss of Attention Span		●	●		●							●						
Lower Astral Plane																	●	
Male Ego Balanced																		
Manic-Depressive													●	●				●
Maturity	●																	
Memory Influenced									●	●		●			●	●		
Men Develop Maternally																		
Men-Trouble With Women																		
Mental Calmness										●								
Mental Clarity										●						●	●	
Mental Diseases																		
Mental Stimulation																		
Mentally Upset																		
Mischievous																		
Moodiness of Artists																		
Narrow-Minded																		
Needs Love																		
Negative Thought Forms					●													
Negativity Eased																		
Negotiating Skills Helped						●												
Nervous About Appearance																		
Nervousness												●						
Night Terrors, Nightmares																		●
Objectivity and Detachment												●						
Obsession		●																●

Iris-Blue Flag	Luffa	Madia	Mallow	Manzanita	Morning Glory	Mullein	Nasturtium	Nectarine	Papaya	Passion Flower	Pennyroyal	Petunia	Pimpernel	Pomegranate	Saguaro	St. John's Wort	Self Heal	Spiderwort	Star Tulip	Sunflower	Watermelon	Yarrow	Yerba Mate	Yerba Santa
					●																			
	●		●																				●	
																			●					
																				●				
									●							●	●	●					●	
													●											
												●												
			●														●							●
				●																			●	
																		●						
							●																	
											●													
●																								
							●																	
		●				●							●											
				●				●	●												●	●		
																	●							
		●																						
				●																				
									●			●		●										
																					●			

Psychological States Chart

Psychological States Chart	Aloe Vera	Amaranthus	Angelica	Apricot	Banana	Blackberry	Bo	Bottlebrush	Cedar	Chaparral	Coffee	Corn (Sweet)	Cosmos	Daffodil	Dill	Fig	Forget Me Not	Four Leaf Clover	Garlic	Ginseng	Grapefruit	Green Rose	Harvest Brodiaea	Hawthorne (English)	Henna
Older People Helped																									
Over-Aggressive									●																
Over Analytical Mind											●														
Overly Logical																									
Paranoia																●	●								
Past-Life Problems	●					●			●		●						●								●
Patience																									
People In Crowded Cities								●					●												
Persistence																									
Personal Initiative Problems																									
Poor Father Image																									
Precancerous Emotional State																	●							●	
Procrastinate													●												
Protection-Psychic Attack		●																							
Psychological Problems of High and Low Blood Sugar			●	●																					
Puberty																									
Purpose in Life Increases																	●		●						
Relax-Difficult Therapy																		●							
Resourceful																				●					
Restlessness								●																	
Schizophrenia		●	●			●				●													●		
Self-Centered																								●	
Self-Confidence		●										●													
Self-Critical														●										●	
Self-Esteem												●									●			●	
Selfishness																								●	
Self-Nurturing																				●					
Self-Righteousness																									

Hyssop	Iris-Blue Flag	Jasmine	Live Forever	Loosestrife	Lotus	Macartney Rose	Madia	Mallow	Manzanita	Marigold (French)	Morning Glory	Mullein	Nectarine	Paw Paw (American)	Pennyroyal	Petunia	Pimpernel	Pomegranate	Prickly Pear Cactus	Queen Anne's Lace	Redwood	Rosa Webbiana	Saguaro	St. John's Wort	Self Heal	Skullcap	Sugar Beet	Sunflower	Sweet Flag	Sweet Pea	Thyme	Yarrow	Yerba Mate	Zinnia
																●																		
									●																									
																●																		
																								●										
●	●				●			●																●							●			
																					●										●			
																														●				
												●																						
																	●																	
																	●						●					●						●
															●																	●		
																											●							
								●																										
											●																							
			●	●		●				●			●		●				●		●								●				●	
	●						●												●			●	●											
	●	●												●												●								
																	●																	
									●																									

Psychological States Chart

Psychological State	Almond	Aloe Vera	Amaranthus	Angelica	Banana	Bells of Ireland	Blackberry	Borage	California Poppy	Carob	Cedar	Celandine	Centuary Agave	Chamomile (German)	Clover (Red)	Comfrey	Corn (Sweet)	Cosmos	Daffodil	Daisy	Dandelion	Dill	Fig	Forget Me Not	Garlic	Ginseng	Grapefruit	Green Rose	Hawthorne (English)	Helleborus (Black)
Self-Sufficiency		●																												
Sense of Festivity																														
Sense of Practicality																														
Sense of Relaxation																●														
Sense of Stability																														
Sensitive and Caring																														
Sex Drive and Spirituality																														
Sex-During Pregnancy																														
Sexually Insecure						●																				●				
Share Work with Others																														
Shy																		●												
Sleep Disturbed																							●							
Sluggish Response			●																											
Stage Fright																									●					
Stress		●	●		●		●			●			●	●		●	●		●		●							●	●	●
Stubborn												●																		
Stuttering																														
Subconscious Mind Cleansed																●								●						
Sulking													●																	
Surly and Withdrawn																														
Tantra												●																		
Think Clearly in Emergencies																								●						
Thought Form Amplification							●			●						●	●							●						
Too Extroverted																														
Too Introverted																	●													
Transference of Information								●			●		●						●											
Unbending Rigid People																						●								
Understand Problems Better			●																									●		
Undisciplined																														
Universal Emotionalism															●															
Will-Power Balanced	●																													
Will-Power Weak																														
Wisdom of Aging Process									●																					●
Women Accept Femininity																														

Henna | Iris-Blue Flag | Jasmine | Lemon | Live Forever | Lotus | Luffa | Macartney Rose | Madia | Mallow | Manzanita | Morning Glory | Mugwort | Nasturtium | Nectarine | Onion | Orange | Passion Flower | Paw Paw (American) | Peach | Petunia | Pimpernel | Pomegranate | Prickly Pear Cactus | Redwood | Rosa Webbiana | Rosemary | Saguaro | Skullcap | Snapdragon | Spice Bush | Squash | Stinging Nettle | Sunflower | Sweet Flag | Watermelon | Wood Betony | Yerba Mate | Yerba Santa | Zinnia

Physical Parts of the Body Chart

Physical Parts of the Body	Almond	Aloe Vera	Apricot	Avocado	Banana	Bells of Ireland	Blackberry	Bloodroot	Borage	California Poppy	Camphor	Cayenne	Cedar	Century Agave	Chamomile (German)	Chaparral	Clover (Red)	Coffee	Comfrey	Cosmos	Cotton	Eucalyptus	Fig	Forget Me Not	Garlic
Abdomen																						•			
Acids in Body																									
Adrenals	•								•										•						
All Senses Activated																									
Alpha State																									
Anesthetic																									
Antibodies																									
Appendix			•																						
Arms																									
Assimilation of Sugars					•																				
Balances Left & Right Brain					•								•						•						
Body Changes																									
Brain		•		•																					
Breasts			•																						
Capillaries																									
Cervix																									
Circulatory System	•	•				•	•	•		•			•		•	•	•		•			•			•
Cleansing																									
Coccyx																									
Colon													•												
Color Sensitivity Improves																									
Connective Tissues						•																			
Conscious Mind-Immune System																									
Control of Glands Improve																			•						
Cranial Plates																									
Digestive Enzymes																									
Digestive Tract	•												•		•										
Ear										•															
Electricity in Brain Increases																							•		
Electromagnetic Attunement																									
Eliminative Processes				•																					
Endocrine System	•							•	•						•	•	•		•						
Esophagus																									
Estrogen													•								•				

Grapefruit																									●									
Harvest Brodiaea				●																														
Hops																	●																	
Iris-Blue Flag											●																							
Jasmine															●					●						●								
Khat													●						●													●		
Koenign Van Daenmark											●												●						●			●		
Lemon																		●								●								
Lilac							●																											
Loquat																										●								
Macartney Rose											●																		●					
Madia										●																								
Mallow																	●															●		
Manzanita													●				●								●									
Maple (Sugar)																	●																	
Mugwort					●						●		●																					
Nasturtium																					●											●		
Pansy													●																					
Papaya														●												●	●							
Petunia																	●																	
Pomegranate		●														●	●																	
Redwood																	●															●		
Rosa Webbiana									●																									
Sage																											●							
Saguaro														●				●																
Self Heal																	●			●													●	
Shooting Star																														●				
Snapdragon																									●								●	
Spice Bush																					●						●							
Spiderwort													●				●																	
Squash																●																		
Star Tulip						●																												●
Sugar Beet																	●																	
Watermelon												●					●																	
Wisteria (Chinese)																	●																	
Yerba Mate											●																							

Physical Parts of the Body Chart

Physical Parts of the Body Chart	Almond	Aloe Vera	Amaranthus	Angelica	Apricot	Avocado	Banana	Blackberry	Bleeding Heart	Bo	Borage	Bottlebrush	California Poppy	Camphor	Cedar	Celandine	Centuary Agave	Chamomile (German)	Chaparral	Coffee	Comfrey	Corn (Sweet)	Cosmos	Cotton	Dandelion	Date Palm	Eucalyptus	Fig	Four Leaf Clover	Garlic	Ginseng
Eyes													•								•										
Face																															
Fallopian Tubes																															
Fatty Tissue					•																										
Feet	•																														
Female Sex Organs																												•			
Gravity Attunement																															
Hair															•						•										
Hara																															
HCl Acid																															
Heart									•	•									•			•	•								
Hemoglobin																											•				
Hormones																															
Immune System		•																	•		•										
Insulin																															
Intestinal Tract																•															
I.Q.																															•
Jaw						•																									
Kidneys						•		•				•					•		•												
Knees																															
Knocks Out Items Blocking Vibrational Remedies				•										•				•													
Kundalini									•																						
Larynx																													•		
Left Brain																													•		
Legs																															
Lips																															
Liver						•		•																	•					•	
Longevity	•																•									•					
Lower Intestinal Tract						•																									
Lungs								•									•										•				
Lymphs						•																									
Male Sex Organs																													•		
Medulla Oblongata																						•									
Metabolism	•										•					•							•								
Mother's Milk																															

255

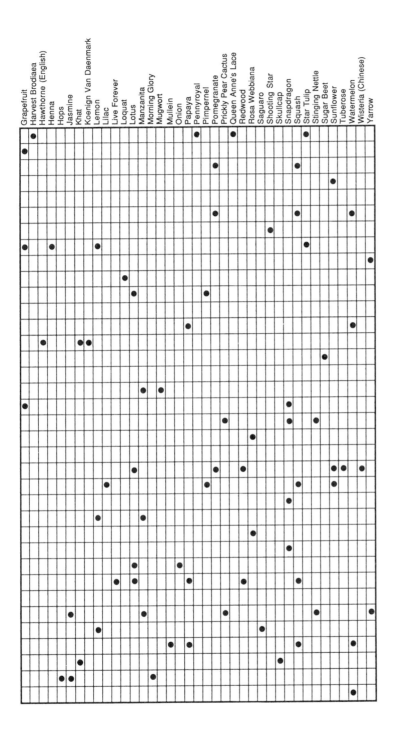

Physical Parts of the Body Chart	Almond	Aloe Vera	Amaranthus	Angelica	Apricot	Avocado	Banana	Bells of Ireland	Blackberry	Bleeding Heart	Borage	Bottlebrush	California Poppy	Camphor	Cedar	Centuary Agave	Chamomile (German)	Coffee	Comfrey	Cosmos	Cotton	Dandelion	Date Palm	Eucalyptus	Fig	Forget Me Not	Four Leaf Clover	Garlic
Mucous Regulated																												
Muscular System						●				●		●							●		●							
Nails																●												
Nasal Passages Cleared																					●							
Natural Hallucinogens																										●		
Natural Morphines																		●										
Nerve Ganglion—Throat																												
Nervous System	●		●									●	●			●	●	●	●	●		●			●	●	●	●
Nose	●																											
Ovaries							●																					
Pancreas					●																		●					
Pelvis																												
Physical Flexibility Increases		●											●						●		●				●			
Pineal Gland							●						●			●										●	●	
Pituitary Gland	●	●			●								●															
Posture Poor																						●						
Pulses Stabilized					●																							
Pylorus																												
Reflex Responses Increase																			●								●	●
Respiratory System																	●						●					
Retina																												
Rhythmic Processes in Body									●																			
Scalp																												
Scar Tissue																												
Sense of Hearing																												
Sense of Physical Relaxation																												
Sense of Smell																												
Sense of Touch						●														●								
Sensitivity of Body																												
Sinuses																												
Skeletal System							●					●																
Skin		●																			●		●		●			

Grapefruit, Green Rose, Harvest Brodiaea, Helleborus (Black), Henna, Hops, Hyssop, Jasmine, Khat, Koenign Van Daenmark, Lemon, Lilac, Loquat, Lotus, Luffa, Macartney Rose, Mallow, Mango, Marigold (French), Morning Glory, Mugwort, Nasturtium, Onion, Papaya, Passion Flower, Pear, Pennyroyal, Petunia, Pimpernel, Pomegranate, Queen Anne's Lace, Redwood, Rosemary, Saguaro, Self Heal, Skullcap, Spice Bush, Star Tulip, Stinging Nettle, Sunflower, Sweet Pea, Wood Betony, Yerba Mate

Physical Parts of the Body Chart

Physical Parts of the Body Chart	Almond	Aloe Vera	Amaranthus	Banana	Bells of Ireland	Blackberry	Bleeding Heart	Bo	Borage	California Poppy	Camphor	Cedar	Celandine	Centuary Agave	Chamomile (German)	Chaparral	Coffee	Comfrey	Corn (Sweet)	Cosmos	Cotton	Daffodil
Small Intestines																						
Solar Plexus										●												
Spinal Fluid																						
Spine			●	●							●						●	●	●			
Spleen																		●				
Stomach		●														●					●	
Strengthen							●															
Sweat Glands							●															
Teeth				●																		
Testicles																					●	
Testosterone											●										●	
Throat																						
Thymus	●		●		●																	●
Thyroid												●		●						●	●	
Time Flow Influenced																						
Uterus																						
Vagina				●																		
Vitality Increased						●			●		●	●		●							●	
Vocal Cords																						

Miasm Chart

Miasm Chart	Almond	Apricot	Banana	Bells of Ireland	Blackberry	Bloodroot	Bottlebrush	California Poppy	Camphor	Celandine	Chamomile (German)	Chaparral	Clover (Red)	Coffee	Comfrey	Cotton	Daffodil	Dandelion	Eucalyptus	Fig	Four Leaf Clover	Garlic	Grapefruit	Green Rose	Hops	Hyssop	Iris-Blue Flag	Jasmine	Lemon	Lilac	Live Forever	Lotus
Gonorrhea																		●													●	
Heavy Metal						●													●											●		
Petrochemical	●	●											●								●											
Psora								●										●	●	●		●	●							●		
Radiation						●															●									●		
Syphilitic			●	●			●	●		●	●	●		●								●					●	●				
Tuberculosis				●										●		●		●							●	●					●	
All Miasms																																●

	Dandelion	Date Palm	Eucalyptus	Four Leaf Clover	Ginseng	Grapefruit	Jasmine	Koenign Van Daenmark	Lemon	Lilac	Live Forever	Loquat	Lotus	Madia	Manzanita	Marigold (French)	Morning Glory	Papaya	Pear	Pomegranate	Queen Anne's Lace	Redwood	Saguaro	Snapdragon	Squash	Star Tulip	Sunflower	Thyme	Tuberose	Yerba Santa
	●																													
									●							●													
									●										●	●						●			
																								●					
												●						●												
					●	●													●		●					●			
											●																			
																									●					
																										●				
								●																						
			●						●								●													
				●																										
																												●		
																				●					●					
																				●					●					
	●	●										●		●		●	●			●	●								●	●
																								●						

	Luffa	Mango	Morning Glory	Onion	Pansy	Passion Flower	Peach	Pennyroyal	Pomegranate	Queen Anne's Lace	Rosa Webbiana	St. John's Wort	Skullcap	Snapdragon	Squash	Star Tulip	Sunflower	Sweet Pea	Watermelon	Wisteria (Chinese)	Yerba Mate	Yerba Santa
											●							●				
													●									
							●			●												
	●	●		●		●		●			●											
														●		●	●					
	●			●		●	●						●						●		●	
			●																	●		●

Nutrients Chart

Nutrients Chart	Angelica	Apricot	Avocado	Banana	Bells of Ireland	Blackberry	Bleeding Heart	Bloodroot	Bo	Borage	Bottlebrush	California Poppy	Cedar	Centuary Agave	Chamomile (German)	Coffee	Comfrey	Cosmos	Cotton	Dandelion	Dill	Eucalyptus	Fig	Four Leaf Clover	Hawthorne (English)	Henna	Hops	Hyssop
Albumin																												
All Minerals		•			•	•														•								
All Nutrients					•	•				•		•										•	•					
All Vitamins																												
Aluminum Eliminated																												
Betaine																												
Cadmium Eliminated																												
Calcium			•							•			•	•											•			
Chlorine																												
Chlorophyll		•																										
Cholesterol													•															
Chromium																												
Copper																												
Fatty Tissue																												
Germanium	•												•															
Gold												•	•															•
Histidine																												
Hospital Food																												
Iodine										•						•	•											
Iron										•			•	•								•	•					
Iron Oxide			•																									
Lecithin																												
Magnesium													•															
Manganese										•																		
Niacin																						•			•			
Oxygen																						•						
Phosphorus			•										•															
Potassium																												
Protein		•	•										•						•							•		
Raw Food Diet																									•			
Selenium																												
Silica													•				•											
Silicon																												•
Silver																												
Sulphur																												
Vitamin A												•		•														
Vitamin B							•						•	•	•	•								•	•		•	
Vitamin C		•											•													•	•	
Vitamin D																											•	
Vitamin E		•			•	•							•						•					•	•			
Vitamin K								•																				
Zinc			•						•					•								•						

Jasmine
Khat
Lemon
Lilac
Live Forever
Loquat
Lotus
Madia
Manzanita
Mugwort
Mullein
Nasturtium
Orange
Papaya
Paw Paw (American)
Pomegranate
Prickly Pear Cactus
Queen Anne's Lace
Redwood
Rosa Webbiana
Sage
Saguaro
St. John's Wort
Self Heal
Snapdragon
Spice Bush
Spiderwort
Spruce
Squash
Stinging Nettle
Sugar Beet
Sunflower
Watermelon
Wisteria (Chinese)
Yerba Santa

Professions Chart

Profession	Almond	Aloe Vera	Angelica	Avocado	Banana	Bells of Ireland	Blackberry	Bleeding Heart	Bloodroot	Borage	Bottlebrush	California Poppy	Camphor	Carob	Cedar	Celandine	Chamomile (German)	Chaparral	Clover (Red)	Coffee	Comfrey	Corn (Sweet)	Cosmos	Cotton	Daffodil	Dandelion	Date Palm	Dill	Eucalyptus	Fig	Forget Me Not	Four Leaf Clover	Garlic	Ginseng	Grapefruit	Green Rose	Hawthorne (English)	Helleborus (Black)
Acupressurist		●	●	●			●		●		●	●				●	●	●	●	●		●		●						●	●			●			●	●
Acupuncturist		●	●	●			●	●		●	●	●				●	●	●	●	●	●	●		●						●	●			●			●	●
Adoption of Children																																						
All Healers Use	●																																					
Aromatherapy		●										●		●																●				●				
Artistic Creativity			●				●			●												●								●				●				
Astrologers																																						
Athletes										●											●																	
Biofeedback Practitioners		●							●								●				●	●	●							●	●							●
Body Weightlifters																																						
Children Helped																																						
Chiropractors			●																		●									●								
Client-Practitioner Relations			●										●																									
Colonic Therapy													●																									
Color Therapy				●																																		
Crystal Balls Cleansed																									●		●											
Dancers			●																																			
Dentists				●																															●			
Dowsers																							●	●														
Enhances Flower Essences													●								●	●						●							●			
Fasting													●												●													
First Aid Remedies		●																												●								
Homeopaths			●								●									●																		
Hospice Movement					●																																●	●
Hypnotist			●												●																							
Insect Spray																																			●			
Laboratory Tests	●																																					
Lecturers													●								●					●					●	●						
Light Therapy				●																																		
Marriage Counselors																																						
Massage Practitioners			●				●		●												●						●								●	●		

Henna · Hops · Hyssop · Iris-Blue Flag · Jasmine · Khat · Koenign Van Daenmark · Lavender(French) · Lemon · Lilac · Live Forever · Loquat · Lotus · Luffa · Madia · Mallow · Mango · Manzanita · Maple (Sugar) · Morning Glory · Mugwort · Mullein · Nasturtium · Nectarine · Onion · Orange · Pansy · Papaya · Paw Paw (American) · Peach · Pear · Pennyroyal · Petunia · Pomegranate · Prickly Pear Cactus · Redwood · Rosemary · Sage · Saguaro · Self Heal · Shooting Star · Skullcap · Snapdragon · Spice Bush · Squash · Stinging Nettle · Sunflower · Sweet Flag · Sweet Pea · Thyme · Tuberose · Watermelon · Wood Betony · Yarrow · Yerba Mate · Zinnia

Professions Chart

Professions	Almond	Aloe Vera	Amaranthus	Angelica	Avocado	Banana	Blackberry	Bleeding Heart	Bo	Borage	California Poppy	Carob	Celandine	Chamomile (German)	Chaparral	Comfrey	Corn (Sweet)	Cosmos	Cotton	Daffodil	Dandelion	Dill	Eucalyptus	Fig	Forget Me Not	Four Leaf Clover	Garlic	Grapefruit	Green Rose	Harvest Brodiaea	Henna
Mathematical Professions																															
Mega-Vitamin Therapy																															
Midwives																							●								
Monks																															
Musicians								●																							
Negotiators											●					●						●									
Optometrists											●																			●	
Osteopaths									●						●														●		
Past-Life Therapy		●						●		●			●			●									●						●
Philosophers																		●	●												●
Primal Scream Therapy																															
Prison Reformers																															
Psychic Abilities		●		●	●					●	●	●					●	●	●	●	●			●					●		
Psychotherapy			●	●		●	●			●		●					●	●	●						●	●	●			●	
Reflexology		●																													
Refugee Camps																	●														
Reichian Therapy	●							●				●	●																		
Rituals																															
Runners										●																					
Singers												●																			
Spiritual Healing											●																		●		
Stop Smoking								●																							
Students Cramming																	●														
Tai Chi Chuan																															
Teacher-Student Relations											●	●																			
Theologians																															
Touch Therapy				●																											
Travelers																															●
Vegetarians																															
Yoga Teachers											●					●															

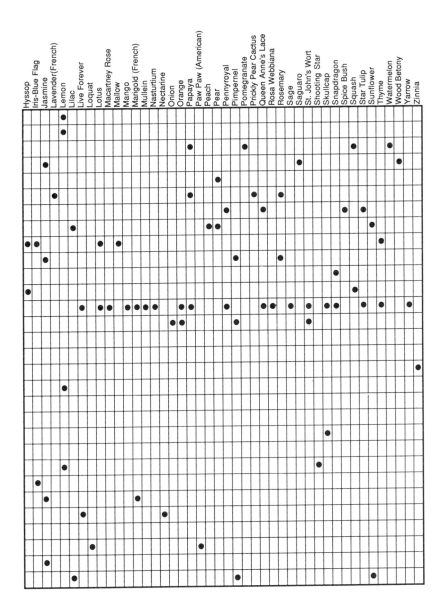

Cellular Level Chart	Almond	Amaranthus	Angelica	Avocado	Bells of Ireland	Blackberry	Bloodroot	Bo	Bottlebrush	California Poppy	Cedar	Centuary Agave	Chamomile (German)	Chaparral	Clover (Red)	Coffee	Date Palm	Eucalyptus	Fig	Four Leaf Clover	Garlic	Ginseng	Helleborus (Black)
Blood Sugar Assimilated																							
Brain																							
Capillary Action																		•					
Cell Communication																							
Cholesterol										•													
Circulatory System									•				•	•							•		
Connective Tissue																							
DNA	•		•														•		•				
Electrical Charge Stabilized																							
Endocrine System																						•	
Estrogen										•													
Fatty Tissue Removed																•							
General Strengthening							•										•						•
Immune System																						•	
Interferon		•																•					
Joints																							
Larynx																							
Liver																						•	
Lungs								•															
Male Fertility																							
Mitosis					•																	•	
Morphines in Body												•											
Muscles			•					•															
Nerve Tissue																							
Ovaries																						•	
Oxygenates the Body																		•					
Pancreas																						•	
Pituitary																						•	
RNA	•									•						•			•				
Skin																		•					
Slows Cell Aging																							
Spinal Fluid																							
Spleen																							
Sweat Glands							•																
Teeth Enamel																							
Testicles																						•	
Testosterone											•												
Thymus																						•	
Tissue Regeneration					•					•						•	•						
Vitamin D																							

Henna	Hyssop	Jasmine	Khat	Lemon	Lotus	Luffa	Macartney Rose	Mallow	Mango	Manzanita	Maple (Sugar)	Morning Glory	Mugwort	Orange	Pomegranate	Redwood	St. John's Wort	Self Heal	Snapdragon	Spice Bush	Spiderwort	Spruce	Sugar Beet	Sunflower	Sweet Flag	Sweet Pea	Tuberose	Wisteria (Chinese)	Yerba Mate
											●																		
							●					●								●									●
																									●		●		
															●														
																●							●						
																	●												
●	●							●							●													●	
							●																						
				●														●			●								
																			●										
																			●										
		●																											
									●							●										●	●		
														●															
							●		●																				
							●						●				●				●							●	
						●		●																					
										●																			
									●																				
																								●					
																		●											
			●		●		●	●								●							●						●
																								●					

Psycho-Spiritual States Chart

States	Amaranthus	Angelica	Blackberry	Bloodroot	Bo	Borage	California Poppy	Carob	Celandine	Centuary Agave	Chamomile (German)	Chaparral	Clover (Red)	Coffee	Comfrey	Corn (Sweet)	Cosmos	Cotton	Daffodil	Daisy	Dill	Eucalyptus	Fig	Forget Me Not	Grapefruit	Green Rose	Harvest Brodiaea	Helleborus (Black)	Henna	Hops	Hyssop
Agnosticism																											●		●		
Angels-Attunement		●																													
Astral Projection											●									●											
Atheist																															
Chanting																															
Christ Consciousness																															
Concentration Improved				●																											
Debate Over Religion																													●		
Ecstasy																															
Future Lives																		●													
Higher Self	●					●	●	●		●	●		●				●	●	●							●	●	●	●		
Karmic Problems							●									●					●										
Intellectual Seekers																													●		
Meditation Helped		●	●	●	●						●	●		●				●						●							●
Mind Body and Spirit																		●													
Nature Attunement			●	●												●									●						
Organized Religion Rejected For Spirituality																		●													
Psycho-Spiritual Balance																		●													
Religious Experience																															
Soul Travel																															
Spacy New Agers																		●													
Spiritual Balance						●																									
Spiritual Confidence																															
Spiritual Courage																															
Spiritual Group Balanced						●																									
Spiritual Growth				●														●												●	
Spiritual Leadership																															
Spiritual Quest				●																											
Spiritual Stability																		●													
Spiritualizes Emotions												●				●															
Spiritualizes Intellect				●														●									●				
Superconscious and Subconscious Minds																															
Understand God																															
Visions	●	●																					●	●							
Wisdom							●		●	●																			●		

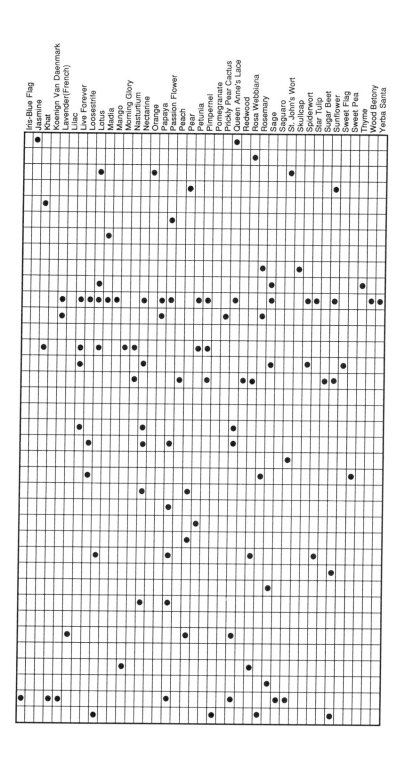

Meridians and Nadis Chart

	Angelica	Banana	Bleeding Heart	Bo	Borage	California Poppy	Camphor	Celandine	Chamomile (German)	Chaparral	Clover (Red)	Coffee	Corn (Sweet)	Cotton	Eucalyptus	Fig	Garlic	Ginseng	Grapefruit	Green Rose	Hops
All Meridians	●				●	●	●	●	●	●	●	●	●	●	●	●	●	●	●	●	●
Gall Bladder Meridian					●																
Heart Meridian						●															
Lung Meridian																					
Stomach Meridian																					
Yin-Yang Qualities				●																	
All Nadis	●					●	●					●								●	
Feet Nadis					●																
Finger Nadis																					
Hand Nadis					●																
Heart Nadis				●																	
Throat Nadis								●													

Major Chakras Chart

	Almond	Aloe Vera	Amaranthus	Angelica	Avocado	Banana	Bleeding Heart	Bloodroot	Bo	Borage	California Poppy	Celandine	Centuary Agave	Chamomile (German)	Chaparral	Coffee	Comfrey	Corn (Sweet)	Cosmos	Daffodil	Date Palm	Dill	Eucalyptus	Fig	Forget Me Not	Four Leaf Clover	Ginseng	Green Rose	Harvest Brodiaea	Helleborus (Black)
First Chakra																		●									●			
Second Chakra																											●			
Third Chakra			●	●		●		●	●					●	●					●					●	●				
Fourth Chakra		●	●			●			●		●	●		●			●			●				●		●	●			●
Fifth Chakra	●								●	●				●				●						●		●	●			
Sixth Chakra			●											●										●		●		●	●	
Seventh Chakra																					●					●		●	●	●
Eighth Chakra																											●			
Ninth Chakra					●			●																			●			
Tenth Chakra																											●			
Eleventh Chakra																						●					●			
Twelfth Chakra									●													●					●			
All Chakras			●						●						●															

Table 1

	Hyssop	Iris-Blue Flag	Lavender(French)	Lemon	Lotus	Mango	Manzanita	Maple (Sugar)	Morning Glory	Mugwort	Nasturtium	Papaya	Peach	Pear	Petunia	Pomegranate	Rosa Webbiana	Sage	Saguaro	Self Heal	Shooting Star	Skullcap	Squash	Sunflower	Sweet Pea	Tuberose	Watermelon	Wisteria (Chinese)	Yarrow	Yerba Santa	Zinnia
	●	●	●	●	●	●		●	●	●	●	●	●	●	●			●	●	●	●	●			●	●	●	●	●	●	●
																●															
							●																								
																●															
								●	●			●				●						●	●								
					●					●						●				●	●				●						
																●															
																●															

Table 2

	Hops	Hyssop	Iris-Blue Flag	Khat	Koenign Van Daenmark	Lavender(French)	Lilac	Live Forever	Loosestrife	Lotus	Madia	Mallow	Mango	Mugwort	Nasturtium	Orange	Papaya	Passion Flower	Peach	Pennyroyal	Pimpernel	Pomegranate	Queen Anne's Lace	Redwood	Rosa Webbiana	Rosemary	Sage	Shooting Star	Skullcap	Spiderwort	Squash	Star Tulip	Sunflower	Tuberose	Watermelon	Wood Betony	Zinnia
								●														●									●				●		
		●						●	●													●									●				●	●	
		●	●					●									●									●		●	●		●				●		●
		●	●					●				●			●	●		●				●			●		●			●				●		●
								●				●					●			●				●													
	●			●				●				●		●								●		●	●												
				●		●		●										●			●	●		●	●		●			●			●				
														●								●															
												●						●																			
												●						●	●																		
												●										●							●								
												●						●				●															
					●				●			●										●						●		●				●			

Subtle Bodies Chart

	Almond	Aloe Vera	Amaranthus	Angelica	Apricot	Avocado	Banana	Bells of Ireland	Blackberry	Bleeding Heart	Bloodroot	Bo	Borage	Bottlebrush	California Poppy	Camphor	Carob	Cedar	Celandine	Centuary Agave	Chamomile (German)	Chaparral	Clover (Red)	Coffee	Comfrey	Corn (Sweet)	Cosmos	Cotton	Daffodil	Daisy	Dandelion	Date Palm	Dill	Eucalyptus	Fig	Forget Me Not	Four Leaf Clover	Garlic	Ginseng	Grapefruit	Green Rose	Harvest Brodiaea	Hawthorne (English)	Helleborus (Black)	Henna	Hops	Hyssop	Iris-Blue Flag	Jasmine
Ethereal Fluidium		•								•				•										•						•	•	•															•		•
Etheric Body	•	•														•	•	•	•					•					•	•	•	•	•							•			•		•	•	•	•	
Astral body		•														•	•						•								•	•		•															
Emotional Body			•		•	•							•	•						•		•	•	•						•	•	•	•	•	•	•												•	•
Mental Body			•	•		•			•	•				•	•	•	•	•	•	•	•	•	•	•		•	•		•		•	•	•			•	•	•	•	•	•	•		•		•		•	•
Causal Body							•		•			•		•							•	•	•						•	•																			
Soul Body							•		•					•									•																										
Spiritual Body		•						•	•	•	•		•			•															•		•								•					•			
All Subtle Bodies			•											•								•								•																			
Aura		•																													•																		
Odic Force																•															•																		
Thermal Body																																																	
Permanent Atom																																																	•

Twelve Rays Chart

	Almond	Aloe Vera	Amaranthus	Angelica	Apricot	Avocado	Banana	Bells of Ireland	Blackberry	Bleeding Heart	Bloodroot	Borage	Bottlebrush	California Poppy	Camphor	Carob	Cedar	Celandine	Centuary Agave	Chamomile (German)	Chaparral	Clover (Red)	Coffee	Comfrey	Corn (Sweet)	Cosmos	Cotton	Daffodil	Daisy	Dandelion	Date Palm	Dill	Eucalyptus	Fig	Forget Me Not	Four Leaf Clover	Garlic	Ginseng	Grapefruit	Green Rose	Harvest Brodiaea	Hawthorne (English)	Helleborus (Black)	Henna	Hops	Hyssop	Iris-Blue Flag	Jasmine	Khat	Koenign Van Daenmark	Lavender (French)
First Ray					•					•																									•													•			
Second Ray	•	•				•													•														•													•				
Third Ray		•			•				•	•				•								•			•			•		•		•												•						
Fourth Ray			•			•			•	•		•	•					•				•			•						•				•	•				•		•									
Fifth Ray			•	•		•								•	•					•			•		•						•	•					•			•		•									
Sixth Ray			•		•									•															•		•							•		•			•		•	•					
Seventh Ray			•											•			•			•								•		•	•			•					•												
Eighth Ray								•					•																	•			•							•					•	•					
Ninth Ray								•														•						•			•									•					•			•		
Tenth Ray			•																•												•						•			•										
Eleventh Ray								•					•										•								•						•													
Twelfth Ray																																																			

Column headings (top matrix):

Khat · Koenign Van Daenmark · Lavender (French) · Lemon · Lilac · Live Forever · Loosestrife · Loquat · Lotus · Luffa · Macartney Rose · Madia · Mango · Manzanita · Marigold (French) · Morning Glory · Mugwort · Mullein · Nasturtium · Nectarine · Onion · Orange · Pansy · Papaya · Passion Flower · Paw Paw (American) · Peach · Pear · Pennyroyal · Petunia · Pimpernel · Pomegranate · Prickly Pear Cactus · Queen Anne's Lace · Redwood · Rosa Webbiana · Rosemary · Sage · Saguaro · St. John's Wort · Self Heal · Shooting Star · Skullcap · Snapdragon · Spice Bush · Spiderwort · Spruce · Squash · Star Tulip · Stinging Nettle · Sugar Beet · Sunflower · Sweet Flag · Sweet Pea · Tuberose · Watermelon · Wood Betony · Wisteria (Chinese) · Yarrow · Yerba Mate · Yerba Santa · Zinnia

Column headings (bottom matrix):

Lilac · Live Forever · Loosestrife · Loquat · Lotus · Luffa · Macartney Rose · Madia · Mallow · Mango · Manzanita · Maple (Sugar) · Marigold (French) · Morning Glory · Mugwort · Mullein · Nasturtium · Nectarine · Onion · Orange · Pansy · Papaya · Passion Flower · Paw Paw (American) · Peach · Pear · Pennyroyal · Petunia · Pimpernel · Pomegranate · Prickly Pear Cactus · Queen Anne's Lace · Redwood · Rosa Webbiana · Rosemary · Sage · Saguaro · St. John's Wort · Self Heal · Shooting Star · Skullcap · Spice Bush · Spiderwort · Spruce · Squash · Star Tulip · Stinging Nettle · Sugar Beet · Sunflower · Sweet Flag · Sweet Pea · Thyme · Tuberose · Watermelon · Wisteria (Chinese) · Wood Betony · Yarrow · Yerba Mate · Yerba Santa · Zinnia

Full List of Flower Essences by Their Common Name

Almond
Aloe Vera
Amaranthus
Angelica
Apricot
Avocado
Banana
Bells of Ireland
Blackberry
Bleeding Heart
Bloodroot
Blue Flag-Iris
Bo
Borage
Bottlebrush
California Poppy
Camphor
Carob
  (St. John's Bread)
Cedar
Celandine
Centuary Agave
Chamomile (German)
Chaparral
Clover (Red)
Coffee
Comfrey
Corn (Sweet)
Cosmos
Cotton
Daffodil
Daisy
Dandelion
Date Palm
Dill
Eucalyptus
Fig
Forget Me Not
Four Leaf Clover
  (Shamrock)
Garlic

Ginseng
Grapefruit
Green Rose
Harvest Brodiaea
Hawthorne (English)
Helleborus (Black)
Henna
Hops
Hyssop
Jasmine
Khat
Koenign Van
  (Daenmark)
Lavender (French)
Lemon
Lilac
Live Forever
Loosestrife
Loquat
Lotus
Luffa
Macartney Rose
Madia
Mallow
Mango
Manzanita
Maple (Sugar)
Marigold (French)
Morning Glory
Mugwort
Mullein
Nasturtium
Nectarine
Onion
Orange
Pansy
Papaya
Passion Flower
Paw Paw
  (American)

Peach
Pear
Pennyroyal
Petunia
Pimpernel
  (Scarlet or Red)
Pomegranate
Prickly Pear Cactus
Queen Anne's Lace
Redwood
Rosa Webbiana
Rosemary
Sage
Saguaro
St. John's Wort
Self Heal
Shooting Star
Skullcap
Snapdragon
Spice Bush
Spiderwort
Spruce
  (Colorado or Blue)
Squash
Star Jasmine
Star Tulip
Stinging Nettle
Sugar Beet
Sunflower
Sweet Flag
Sweet Pea
Thyme
Tuberose
Watermelon
Wisteria (Chinese)
Wood Betony
Yarrow
Yerba Mate
Yerba Santa
Zinnia

Full List of Flower Essences by Their Latin Name

Acer Saccharum
Achillea Millefolium
Acorus Calamus
Agave Americana
Allium Cepa
Allium Sativum
Aloe Vera
Amaranthus Hypochondriacus
Anagallis Arvensis
Anethum Graveolens
Angelica Archangelica
Antirrhinum Majus
Arctostaphlyos Manzanita
Artemisia Vulgaris
Asimina Triloba
Bellis Perennis
Beta Vulgaris
Borago Officinalis
Brodiaea Elegans
Callistemon Viminalis
Calochortus Tolmei
Calycanthus Occidentallis
Carica Papaya
Carnegiea Gigantea
Catha Edulis
Ceratonia Siliqua
Chaparro Amargosa
Celidonium Majus
Chrysanthemum Maximum
Cinnamomum Camphora
Cistus Sinensis
Citrus Limon
Citrullus Vulgaris
Citrus Paradisi
Coffea Arabica
Cosmos Bipinnatus
Crataegus Oxyacantha
Cucurbita Marima
Cucurbita Moschata
Cucurbita Pepo
Daucus Carota
Dicentra Chrysantha
Dodecatheon Media
Dudleya Farinosa

Eribotrya Japonica
Eriodictyon Californicum
Eschscholzia California
Eucalyptus Globulus
Ficus Carica
Ficus Religiosa
Gossypium Arboreum
Gossypium Hirustum Var. Punctatum
Hedeoma Pulegioides
Helianthus Annus
Helleborus Niger
Humulus Lupulus
Hypericum Perforatum
Hyssopus Officinalis
Ilex Paraguariensis
Ipomoea Purpurea
Iris Hartwegii
Iris Versicolor
Jasmine Officinalis
Lathyrus Latifolus
Lavendula Officinalis
Lawsonia Inerinis
Luffa Aegyptiaca
Lythrum Salicaria
Madia Elegans
Malluccella Laevis
Malva Rotundifolia
Malva Sylvestris
Mangifera Indica
Matricaria Chamomilla
Musa Paradisiaca
Myosotis Sylvatica
Narcissus Ajax
Nelumbo Nucifera
Opuntia Vulgaris
Panax Quinquefolius
Passiflora Incarnata
Persea Americana
Petunia Hybrid
Phoenix Dactylifera
Picea Pungens
Polianthes Tuberosa
Prunella Vulgaris
Prunus Amygdalus

Prunus Armeniaca
Prunus Persica
Prunus Persica Var. Nectarina
Punica Granatum
Pyrus Communis
Rosa Chinensis Viridiflora
Rosa Macrantha
Rosa Webbiana
Rosmarinus Officinalis
Rubus Villosus
Salvia Officinalis
Sanguinaria Canadensis
Scuttellaria Lateriflora
Sequoia Sempervirens
Stachys Officinalis
Symphytum Officinale

Syringa Vulgaris
Tagetes Patula
Taraxacum Officinale
Thuja Occidentalis
Thymus Vulgaris
Trachelosperumum Jasminoides
Tradescanthia Virginica
Trapaeolum Majus
Trifolium Dubium
Trifolium Pratense
Urtica Dioica
Verbascum Thapsus
Viola Tricolor
Wisteria Sinensis
Zea Mays
Zinnia Elegans

Flower Essences That Can Be Used Externally

Almond
Aloe Vera
Apricot
Banana
Bleeding Heart
Bloodroot
California Poppy
Camphor
Cedar
Chamomile (German)
Chaparral
Clover (Red)
Comfrey
Corn (Sweet)
Cotton
Daffodil
Daisy
Dandelion
Eucalyptus
Fig
Four Leaf Clover
Garlic

Ginseng
Grapefruit
Green Rose
Harvest Brodiaea
Helleborus (Black)
Henna
Hyssop
Jasmine
Lemon
Lilac
Live Forever
Lotus
Luffa
Macartney Rose
Mallow
Mango
Manzanita
Maple (Sugar)
Morning Glory
Onion
Passion Flower
Peach

Pennyroyal
Petunia
Pimpernel
Pomegranate
Prickly Pear Cactus
Redwood
Rosemary
Saguaro
St. John's Wort
Self Heal
Skullcap
Snapdragon
Spice Bush
Spruce
Star Tulip
Stinging Nettle
Sunflower
Thyme
Wisteria (Chinese)
Yarrow
Yerba Mate
Yerba Santa

APPENDIX I

Principles of Trance Channeling

Through the ages and into the present, political, economic, social, and spiritual leaders have drawn guidance and technological information from channeled sources. While it is not easy to prove this, information is available concerning this process.

Among the early nature cultures, the Mayans, Aztecs, and Hopi benefited from channeled wisdom. Even those organized into city-states received such guidance, particularly the Persians, Sumerians, Greeks, and Romans. Continuing into modern times, evidence of channeling occurs in such movements as mesmerism, spiritualism, theosophy, and the exploration into altered states of consciousness, such as isolation tank therapies, hypnosis, and the examination of what has come to be known as the 'living death' experience.[1] In ancient times, perhaps the most famous and noted example of trance channeling was the Delphic oracle. For many hundreds of years these teachings were attributed to a portion of the mythos, but references to channeling through oracles have been made by Plato,[2] Aristotle, and Socrates. Each, at times, specifically referred to a small, still voice that was not from their own functioning consciousness, but was an independent consciousness from which they not only received ideas or even inspiration but entire theses and discourses. These teachings have become the basis of western principles and laws.[3]

There are also Hebrew texts in which the prophets of old spoke of falling into trance-like or dream-like states and of receiving information.[4] Trance channeling was fairly common among the ancient Israelis, especially the Essenes, the Jewish sect into which Jesus was born. There are literally dozens of examples in the Bible in which the trance state is discussed. One has only to check in a Bible concordance[5] for words like: dead, dream, fell, gifts of the spirit, sleep, trance, and vision. For instance, in Acts of the Apostles 10:10 "He fell into a trance."; 11:05 "...and in a trance I saw a vision."; 22:17 "...even while I prayed in the temple, I was in a trance..."; Revelations 1:17 "...and when I saw him, I fell at his feet as dead."; and in Corinthians 2:14 "But the natural man receiveth not the things (gifts) of the spirit of God, for they are foolishness unto him: neither can he know them because they are spiritually discerned." Heads of state such as the Pharaoh and Joseph's interpretation of the Pharaoh's dream and its prognostic qualities were from altered states of consciousness similar to trance channeling. The destinies of nations were and still are influenced by such bodies of information.

In this age, when millions of people draw inspiration from the channeled teachings of Edgar Cayce, Alice Bailey, Jane Roberts, *The Urantia Book, The Course in Miracles*, and the many teachings of theosophy,[6] there is a growing understanding that spiritual truths and advanced technological information can be manifested in this fashion. Channeled teaching is part of our spiritual heritage.

Individuals such as Thomas Edison, Abraham Lincoln, Sir William Crookes, Sir Henry Cabot Lodge, and John D. Rockefeller attributed their inspiration and, at times, their scientific correlations to channeled sources. In the 20th century such influences are found with: Franklin D. Roosevelt, the Kennedys, Richard Nixon, Lyndon Johnson, and Pierre Trudeau. These individuals were counseled by the following trance channels: Andrew Jackson Davis, Daniel Douglas Home, Leonara Piper, Edgar Cayce, Rudolf Steiner, Madame Blavatsky, Arthur Ford, and Jeane Dixon. Several of these individuals channeled information while conscious rather than in the trance state.

Not only did President Lincoln invite Andrew Jackson Davis to the White House so that he could receive channeled information,[7] but channeled information inspired him to sign the Emancipation Proclamation to end slavery. When Lincoln visited New York City, he frequently visited Andrew Jackson Davis and other channels.

Andrew Jackson Davis was one of the best known and most respected mystics and psychics in the United States during the latter part of the 1800's until his death in 1911. Some of his approximately thirty books appeared in forty-five editions. His spiritual writings comprised many topics including the seven planes of existence, mental and physical health, philosophy, physics, and the structure of a proper educational system. Like Edgar Cayce, he made statements that were later validated by orthodox science. To illustrate, in March, 1846, he described the existence of Neptune and Pluto, correctly naming the approximate mass of Neptune. This was several months before Neptune was actually discovered and many years before Pluto was observed for the first time in 1930.[8]

Winston Churchill and the British government relied on several psychics and astrologers during World War II.[9] This was partly because Churchill realized that Hitler utilized such information, so the British wanted to understand the nature of the information Hitler received, but Churchill also had a personal belief in this field.[10]

Before his death in 1945, Edgar Cayce did trance readings for Franklin D. Roosevelt in the White House and for other politicians in Washington. Arthur Ford and Jeane Dixon have given readings to various members of the Kennedy family, Presidents Johnson and Nixon, and to Prime Minister Trudeau of Canada. The United States government, along with other nations, has quietly worked with channels to assist certain research projects.[11] Newspaper columnist Jack Anderson several years ago stated that for years the United States government has quietly spent millions of dollars on parapsychological research.

Other individuals weaving the tapestry of a knowledge yet to be wholly integrated into the mainstream of society are members of the Findhorn community, channeled information through Uri Geller, Paolo Soleri,[12] Buckminster Fuller, and Ram Dass. All these individuals experience altered states of consciousness during which they receive inspiration and higher teaching. In these years, channeled teachings will expand beyond the scientific and social fields into areas that will create the spiritual transformation of society. Alice Bailey, Jane Roberts, and Edgar Cayce represent this trend.

Many important inventions have been channeled over the years. Thomas Edison received the light bulb, phonograph, and motion pictures from channeled information. The individual considered to have invented the mechanical linotype received inspiration from the teachings of Andrew Jackson Davis.[13] Others received inspiration from Andrew Jackson Davis on improved concepts in the internal combustion engine. Inventions credited to Eli Whitney, including the cotton gin and the development of a process to mass produce musket balls, were received from channeled sources. The same is true with the development of the Winchester rifle by Oliver Winchester. Andrew Carnegie developed formulations for certain steel alloys from channeled guidance.

Thomas Edison's keen interest in working with trance channels to support his inventions is fairly well known. For many years he attempted to develop a machine to communicate with souls on other planes of existence.[14] In 1920, toward the end of his career, he openly discussed in an interview his interest in this field, stating that he had experimented with telepathy, clairvoyance, and interplane communication.[15] Today numerous scientists, especially in medicine, study Edgar Cayce's trance channeled information to gain new insights. Several thousand physicians use the various remedies recommended by Edgar Cayce while he was in trance.

Channeled information is neither positive nor negative, for in truth there is neither positive nor negative. Channeling is a tool that is applied according to social formats, standards, and needs of the day. The acceptance or application of these teachings by incarnate individuals helps determine the pattern or karmic activity on this plane.

The cotton gin, for example, was used to remove seeds from cotton fibers. Its introduction placed pressure on southern institutions to end slavery, because this particular device made it economically infeasible. This, however, was an impersonal force entering into the experiential lives of individuals and the social and economic structures of the day. The key element, to use the device for its benefits, was applied by choice. Nevertheless, it added strength to the argument that slavery should be abolished for humanitarian reasons.

Another choice regarding the instrumentality of channeled knowledge was the Winchester rifle. Again, this device was a tool of neither positive nor negative nature. In the time period that it was presented, the dominant portion of the population, particularly the American Indian, were hunters who existed in a state of balance with nature, partaking of that which nature procreated. Since most were meat eaters, the rifle was but a more humane way to supply the needs of many in those days. This particular instrument, however, was by choice used against humanity rather than to promote balance.

The cotton gin and winchester rifle produced activity that created an understanding and relevancy to the karmic patterns of the day. It is our free will and choice as incarnate souls to determine how any new principles and devices are used or abused. Such choice is really a test of our conscious growth.

Trance channeling is the total setting aside of the consciousness of the self to allow for guidance from discarnate souls who have an identical social, karmic, spiritual, intellectual, and ethical path in coordination and agreement with certain living individuals. In this process, complete bodies of information, often independent of the knowledge of the waking or functioning consciousness of the channel, come through. Individuals are often impressed by this phenomenon, as though it offers greater validation of the information, but this is not necessarily the case.

In contrast, inspired channeling works through the conscious outpourings of the individual. These channelings may be just as pure, in the sense that the inspiration merely correlates with the individual's conscious functioning attitudes. If the person calms himself and does not seek to imprint or interpret the information, then such information has similar degrees of clarity and validity. A person does trance channeling or inspirational channeling according to the lessons he needs to learn.

There are several structures of information that may be received from various discarnate souls in a channeling relationship. There is usually a close karmic connection in the relationship between incarnate and discarnate beings, so generally, discarnate souls also serve as the spirit guides for the incarnate individual. Some of these guides provide this information as part of their own karmic growth experience, while other more evolved souls do this work to serve humanity. Many times entities who present information through trance channeling provide complex material based on teachings from former advanced cultures. This data has great relevancy for our present culture.

Usually, a trance channel has three to six guides. The number varies according to individual human needs. Greater areas of guidance or the personality itself may require a greater number of guides. But in some cases the individual's personality is so integrated that only one guide is needed.

The full spectrum of human dynamics is often represented in a channel's guides. Sometimes those who give guidance are archetypal symbols necessary for the channel's growth. That which represents the Divine is often referred to as the individual's master teacher. The master teacher is not playing the role of leader so much as he or she integrates the necessary levels of energy to produce a coordinated pattern of personal development for the individuals involved in the process. The context of leadership is not very much present in the concepts of the spirit. There are also joy guides that represent the individual's humor. In addition, there are guides to develop the practical elements of the personality. It can also be said that a guide represents a force coordinated with one of the main chakras, for the human personality can be divided according to the levels of the various chakras.

Some guides stay in the background without actually speaking through a trance channel. This may be for several reasons: they cannot properly synchronize with the channel's physical body, there is not sufficient time because the physical body can be in trance for only limited time periods, or there is not the proper context or format for their information to be well received. These guides, therefore, rather than being a direct focalization of information, act more as a contributing factor.

Depending on the type of questions, in certain complex research topics, other discarnate souls may step forward to give advice when the subject is one in which they have special expertise. Or such extra contributions may take place because of a past life relationship between the inquirer or the channel and the visiting discarnate soul. These contributions can, at times, make the process easier, and allow other souls the opportunity to serve.

Often the person asking questions has had past life connections with the channel and his spirit guides, particularly if the channelings continue for some time. At such times there tends to be a syntheses of information from the higher self of the channel and the inquirer. The inquirer acts as editor or focalizer by the nature of his or her questions. In this process, it is wise for the inquirer to have some technical background and knowledge in the areas of inquiry.

There is also the higher self which, while not the akashic records, is a gathering of all the higher principles and experiences from past lives. These sources of information may be contacted and correlated to generate talents and keener insights into the individual's current karmic experiences. The higher self is distinct from the soul in that it is still a product of consciousness and mind relative to the earth plane. Thus, the higher self is not the true self in the sense that the soul identity in its own right is the true self. When one extends to the levels of the higher self, either in the trance state or in semi-conscious altered states, the individual actually manifests all the higher capacities they can activate on this plane, independent of the total merger with the soul itself.

The akashic records focus all records, all past deeds, and all things which are yet to be. These records are the central systems of knowledge and experience throughout all the universes. They are, in part, the collective consciousness and focus of the higher self and baser self resulting from activities in this plane. The ability to do evolved trance or inspirational channeling means activating one's memory to the level of the superconsciousness, which then has access to the akashic records.

You can tell if someone is channeling information from his or her higher or lower self by examining how you feel during and after the channeling. Study the karma of the individual, above all his or her growth, to determine if the information may be considered self-serving or if it is altruistic in nature and in harmony with the self. If it is entirely of a self-serving nature, then this comes from the baser self or the subconscious mind forces. If it comes from the higher self, it is altruistic. The subconscious mind contains both positive and negative or suppressed experiences, while the superconscious level, although having aspects and knowledge of that which is considered past negative experiences, holds only higher spiritual principles.

Usually, the higher self, in more advanced forms of trance channeling, acts as the trance medium's controller and is the screen through which the entities communicate. This is why it is not really necessary for such trance channels to have other forms of psychic protection. When channeling from the higher self, one does not have to worry about lower astral plane entities or wrong information. Edgar Cayce was such a channel. In other forms of trance channeling, it would be wise for the individual to surround himself with pure light and the Christ principle.

Just because someone has discarnate souls speaking through them does not automatically mean they have access to universal wisdom from the higher planes. Sometimes channeled information can come from mischievous souls on the lower astral planes or from the lower subconscious mind of the channel. One should exercise normal precautions in this form of parapsychology, as in all matters. Carefully examine what you experience as to the quality of the channeled information, and the level of consciousness the channel seems to manifest.

Even when the channel and guides are highly evolved, caution must be taken, for sometimes the advice is not sufficiently practical in terms of earthly physical realities. This is mainly because time on the higher planes is different from earth plane physical time. Thus, it is relatively easy to give accurate and specific research information, while projected time-dependent events *may* actually take place at a time slightly different from that suggested.

Some feel trance channels are emotionally unstable people because of their involvement in an unusual field. To the casual observer their behavior *may* appear imbalanced. Some prominent scientists also appear unstable because they are likewise involved in an unusual field. Social and religious criticisms and prejudices also may cause the medium to display greater states of anxiety. If the channel is emotionally stable, there is less likelihood that his or her personality will interfere with the channeled information. Channels should exercise normal discrimination for their physical health and emotional stability.

The inquirer and channel should never declare the information received to be absolute, as though they have a unique source of information. In these days, many channels present valuable and valid information. There is no one source of information or truth. One type of channeling is not superior to another. The various types of channeling merely allow individuals to learn different lessons and demonstrate different states of consciousness.

1 Raymond Moody, *Life After Life* (New York: Bantam Books, 1981).

2 Jeff Mishlove, *The Roots of Consciousness* (New York: Randam House, 1980), p. 22-23.

3 Ibid, p. 24-25.

4 Moses Hull, *Encyclopedia of Biblical Spiritualism* (Amherst, WI: Amherst Press, 1895).

5 James Strong, *Strong's Exhaustive Concordance of the Bible* (Nashville: Abington Press, 1980).

6 John Koffend, "The Gospel According to Helen," *Psychology Today*, XXVII (September, 1980), 74-90.

7 Nat Freedland, *The Occult Explosion* (East Rutherford, NJ: G. P. Putnam's Sons, 1972), p. 67.

8 Andrew Jackson Davis, *The Principles of Nature*, 1847, p. 159-168.

9 Clifford Linedecker, *Psychic Spy: The Story of An Astounding Man* (Garden City, NY: Doubleday & Co., 1976).

10 Trevor Ravenscroft, *The Spear of Destiny* (York Beach, ME: Samuel Weiser, Inc., 1982).

11 Sheila Ostrander, Lynn Schroeder, *Psychic Discoveries Behind the Iron Curtain* (New York: Bantam Books, 1976).

12 Paolo Soleri has established Arcosanti, a community in Arizona to help solve the problems of overpopulation, food shortages, and pollution, and to develop solar energy.
Paolo Soleri, *The Omega Seed: An Eschatological Hypotheses* (Garden City, NY: Anchor Press, 1981).

13 The mechanical linotype was invented by Ottman Mergenthaler in the latter 1800's. With this machine it was possible to reproduce printed matter such as newspapers much more quickly and cheaply than could be done by hand typesetting.

14 Nat Freedland, *The Occult Explosion* (East Rutherford, NJ: G. P. Putnam's Sons, 1972), p. 79.

15 George Meek, *From Enigma to Science* (York Beach, ME: Samuel Weiser, Inc., 1973), p. 103-104.

APPENDIX II

New Information on Homeopathy

Several times in this text there have been references to neutral homeopathic potencies. This important concept is not yet understood among homeopaths. These potencies include: mother tincture to 6x, 6c, 12x, 12c, 200x, 200c, and 10MM.

The energy released by a vibrational remedy flows in waves that affect the physical and subtle bodies. The height of a wave is its amplitude. The 10MM neutral potency is at the top of the wave, and all other neutral potencies occur at or near the bottom of the wave.

crest—10MM

amplitude

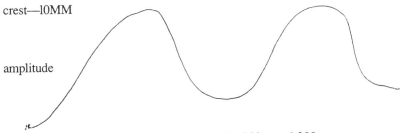

bottom—mother tincture to 6x, 6c, 12x, 12c, 200x, and 200c

This principle is one reason why low homeopathic potencies can often be prescribed for several weeks without any problems developing. The generally recommended dosage for neutral potencies is as follows: mother tincture to 3x or 3c—up to thirty days once or twice a day; 6x and 6c—for two weeks once or twice a day; 12x, 12c, 200x, and 200c—for about one week once or twice a day; and 10MM—for one or two months once or twice a day. These potencies, except for 10MM, are already commonly used in homeopathy.

Most homeopaths would question prescribing a remedy at 10MM more than once, if at all. However, I and several associates have done this well over 100 times, with no disruptions in health or sharp aggravations, and the improvement in health was often quite noticeable.

In traditional homeopathic literature, it is generally stated that a sharp aggravation is often a positive healing crisis and a sign that the remedy is working—the remedy's life force is releasing toxicity from the body by activating the life force in a person. While this pattern does occur, it is also understood that health can be restored through homeopathy without sharp healing crises happening. There are very rarely sharp aggravations when these vibrational remedies are prescribed correctly in neutral potencies. A well chosen remedy given at the exactly correct potency can often greatly improve health with little or no healing crisis occurring. At these neutral potencies it is easier for the system to assimilate the life force of a vibrational remedy.

The 10MM neutral potency is used to alter the consciousness that may, for instance, be causing stress in the physical body. Lower neutral potencies are prescribed when a person needs to assimilate the physical properties of the remedy, and when blocks in consciousness are not causing the problems. For example, when stress results in the body being stripped of calcium, a low neutral potency would help restore calcium to the body, but not necessarily deal with the cause of the stress. The high neutral potency would help restore calcium to the body by working upon the cause of the problem. Flower essences, in these neutral potencies, are almost always prescribed at only 10MM. As previously stated, this is because they work on realms of consciousness.

There are many other concepts concerning neutral potencies, and they will be discussed in the future. For instance, 200x and 200c have several unique features when they are used as neutral potencies; moreover, except for 10MM, these potencies are not necessarily prescribed only as neutral potencies.

APPENDIX III

Statement of John's Purpose

I once asked John what his main purpose is in speaking through Ryerson, because he is Ryerson's main guide.

"The purpose of the channel speaking is to bring as clarity, new insight, and authority to the activities of the *Book of Revelation* as a work of transformational accord so as to draw individuals into a personal and closer relationship to the principles of the Christ within themselves, and to draw them closer unto that pattern which the man Jesus represented in same. That transformation of self is but to restore the personal relationship with the one force that is God which is love through this particular instrumentality."

Q How would you relate that to all the specific teachings that you give forth with such technical detail?

"This is, in part, information that is a by-product on the part of the inquiring mind. The inquiring mind is as the scribe and the intellectual student that eventually must be as spiritualized in same. As individuals ask various questions, eventually selected individuals are as drawn unto the truer resources and desire the transformation and the completion of coming unto the Christ within themselves and completely surrender themselves unto the nature of Divine Love. It is not that the channel speaking must as be that point of transformation. That transformation must come from within people; that as sons and daughters of man, then, in turn, they may also be as accepted within the accord of being as sons and daughters of God. For no one may come unto the Father except by the Son. It is by their own acceptance of their Divine nature and above all fusing these things upon this plane and transforming mind, body, and spirit to serve as a whole unit in same. The channel speaking may seek to inspire individuals to that path so as to have and to receive these things. If the inquiring mind brings forth questions, then the channel speaking would as give forth answers, but also the activities of the channel speaking are as to seek to draw them into the light. For in all things that are interlaced with the channel speaking, there is never the divergency from the point of view that there must be the aspect of the manifestation of God's true love. For in closing on these things all these affairs are but as tools to bring harmony which is an expression of God's love. But it is only love itself that is God."

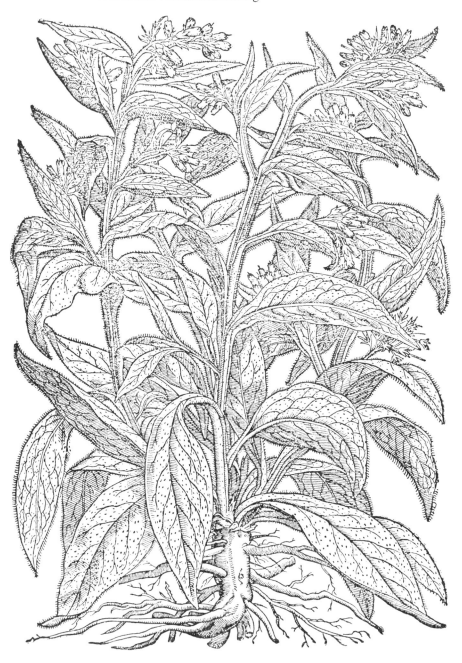

Comfrey

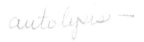 *autolysis —*

GLOSSARY

Akashic records: Cosmic records of all human deeds, thoughts, and events from the past, present, and future. They may be consulted by those with a proper spiritual evolution.

Alchemy: The art of transmuting metals and other substances into silver or gold, generally to produce a healing elixir called the Philosopher's Stone. In its highest form, alchemy involves transforming the self.

Allopathy: A term used especially in homeopathy to describe orthodox medical practice.

Androgyny: The actual physical state of being joined together into one sex—male and female.

Apportation: The movement of an object through the ethers from one location to another. This is usually accomplished by stabilizing the interior molecular dynamics of the object to be moved within the ethers.

Astral body: One of the subtle bodies surrounding the physical body.

Astral projection: Also known as an out-of-body experience. The astral body temporarily separates from the physical body. This usually occurs when asleep, but can also occur when awake.

Atlantis: An ancient civilization covering what is now the Atlantic Ocean.

Aura: An invisible, luminous radiation or halo that surrounds the physical body. It varies widely in size, density, and color depending on the evolution of each person, and it exists around all life forms. Some psychic or sensitive individuals see it.

Biofeedback: The ability of the mind to control involuntary body functions.

Biomagnetic: The patterns of magnetic energy that are generated as a by-product of molecular activity. The released energy becomes part of the aura.

Biomolecular: Refers to the chemical activity in the subatomic level within each cell.

Causal body: An ethereal body that exists around the physical body.

Cellular level: At the level of each individual cell.

Chakra: A spiritual energy center just outside, but connected to, the physical body.

Clairaudience: The ability to hear sounds from other dimensions.

Clairvoyance: A general term signifying many psychic gifts such as the ability to see things miles away.

Collective consciousness: The combined thoughts or feelings of large groups of people.

Creative visualization: The use of the mind to create a mental image.

Doctrine of signature: The principles that there is a relationship between the anatomy of people and the color, odor, shape, taste and texture of gemstones and plants. In this relationship lie many clues as to how gemstones and plants can be used in healing and conscious growth.

Emotional body: A subtle body that exists around the physical body.

Ethereal fluidium: Part of the etheric body that is connected to each cell.

Etheric: Refers to the formative forces that exist vibrationally in relation to all life on earth.

Etheric body: A subtle body that exists just outside and around the physical body.

Ethers: Seven or more dimensional states that vibrate faster than the speed of light.

Gem elixir: The placement of a mineral specimen in pure water for several hours under the sun to transfer the mineral's vibration into the water. The diluted liquid is ingested for healing and conscious growth.

Hara: An energy center in the human body located near the navel.

Higher self: The location where all higher principles and experiences from past lives are stored in the person.

Integrated spiritual body: This, and the term spiritual body, signify the combination of the spiritual properties of the subtle and physical bodies.

Karma: A Sanskrit word meaning the sum total of a person's actions in their many lives. These past life traits are carried over into each new life with continuing opportunities for growth.

Kundalini: A powerful spiritual energy normally lying dormant in the physical body at the base of the spine. Once carefully awakened, spiritual growth ensues.

Lemuria: An ancient civilization covering what is now the Pacific Ocean.

Mental body: A subtle body existing around the physical body.

Meridians: Ethereal patterns of energy that carry the life force into the physical body.

Miasms: Various subtle imbalances residing in the cells and subtle bodies that are activated to cause numerous diseases when karmic patterns prevail.

Molecular: Refers to the chemical activity in the subatomic level within each cell.

Nadis: An extensive ethereal nervous system just outside the physical body, and directly connected to the nervous system.

Nosodes: Biological toxins that are prepared into homeopathic remedies.

Pendulum: A small item attached to a thread and used to analyze or diagnose.

Philosopher's stone: An alchemical term traditionally meaning a powerful elixir that will transmute base metals into gold or silver. It can also be used to treat ill people and to stimulate spiritual illumination.

Prana: A Hindu or yogic term used to describe the life force.

Radionics: The use of an instrument and operator for sending vibrations to, and receiving vibrations from, a person miles away. It has been used as a modality in healing and in agriculture for many years.

Soul body: A very ethereal subtle body that exists around the physical body.

Spirit guides: Individual souls existing in other dimensions who assist people on the earth plane. They may speak through someone in trance.

Subtle bodies: A general term referring to all the bodies that exist just outside and around the physical body.

Telepathy: The transmission of thoughts between two people over any distance. This communication takes place without the senses as normally understood .

Thermal body: A heat field existing just outside the physical body near the etheric body.

Thought forms: Semi-materialized ethereal forms or shapes that the mind builds.

Tissue regeneration: The complete rebuilding of parts of the body to full health.

Trance: A state of intense concentration and sleep-like condition in which the mind and body are overshadowed by the higher self or spirit guides from other dimensions.

Bibliography

Androgeny
O'Flaherty, Wendy D. *Women, Androgynes and Other Mythical Beasts*. Chicago: University of Chicago Press, 1980.
Singer, June. *Androgyny: Toward A New Theory of Sexuality*. New York: Doubleday & Co., 1976.
Zolla, Elemire. *The Androgyne, Reconciliation of Male and Female*. New York: Crossroad/Continuim, 1981.

Alice A. Bailey
Bailey, Alice A. *A Compilation on Sex*. New York: Lucis Publishing Co., 1980.
_____. *The Consciousness of the Atom*. New York: Lucis Publishing Co., 1974.
_____. *Esoteric Healing*. New York: Lucis Publishing Co., 1980.
_____. *Esoteric Psychology*, Vol. II. New York: Lucis Publishing Co., 1975.
_____. *Letters on Occult Meditation*. New York: Lucis Publishing Co., 1973.
_____. *Ponder on This*. New York: Lucis Publishing Co., 1980.
_____. *The Soul and Its Mechanism*. New York: Lucis Publishing Co., 1981.
_____. *Telepathy and the Etheric Vehicle*. New York: Lucis Publishing Co., 1980.
_____. *A Treatise on Cosmic Fire*. New York: Lucis Publishing Co., 1977.
Master Index of the Tibetan and Alice Bailey Books. Sedona, AZ: Aquarian Educational Group, 1974.

Bath Therapies
Barber, Bernard. *Sensual Water: A Celebration of Bathing*. Chicago: Contemporary Books, Inc., 1978.
Buchman, Dian D. *The Complete Book of Water Therapy, 500 Ways to Use Our Oldest and Safest Medicine*. New York: E. P. Dutton, 1979.
Cerney, J. *Modern Magic of Natural Healing With Water Therapy*. San Diego: Reward Books, 1977.
Finnerty, Gertrude, and Theodore Corbitt. *Hypnotherapy*. New York: Frederick Ungar Publishing Co., 1960.
Fleder, Helen. *Shower Power: Wet, Warm and Wonderful Exercises for the Shower and Bath*. New York: M. Evans and Co., Inc., 1978.
Frazier, Gregory, and Beverly Frazier. *The Bath Book*. San Francisco: Troubador Press, 1973.
Lust, John. *Kneipp's My Water Cure*. Greenwich, CT: Benedict Lust Publishing, 1978.
Ramachakara, Yogi. *Hindu-Yogi Practical Water Cure*. Jacksonville, FL: Yoga Publication Society, n.d.
Szekely, Edmond Bordeaux. *Healing Waters*. San Diego: Academy Books, 1973.

Botanical Reference Material

Bailey, L. H. *The Standard Cyclopedia of Horticulture.* New York: MacMilliam Publishing Co., 1935.

Daydon, Jackson. *A Glossary of Botanic Terms.* New York: Hofner Publishing Co., 1965.

Hortus. New York: MacMilliam Publishing Co., 1976.

Nickells, J. M. *Botanical Ready Reference.* Beaumont, CA: CSA Press, 1976.

Perry, Frances, ed. *Complete Guide to Plants and Flowers.* New York: Simon & Schuster, 1974.

Schuler, Stanley, ed. *Guide to Trees.* New York: Simon & Schuster, 1978.

Chakras

Chinmoy, Sri. *Kundalini: The Mother Power.* Jamaica, NY: Agni Press, 1974.

Colton, Ann Ree. *Kundalini West.* Glendale, CA: ARC Publishing Co., 1978.

Leadbeater, C. W. *The Chakras.* Wheaton, IL: The Theosophical Publishing House, 1972.

Madhusudandasji, Dhyanyogi Shri. *Shakti Hidden Treasure of Power*, Vol. I. Pasadena, CA: Dhyanyoga Centers, Inc., 1979.

Mookerjee, Ajit. *Kundalini: The Arousal of the Inner Energy.* New York: Destiny Books, 1982.

Motoyama, Dr. Hiroshi, and Rande Brown. *Science and the Evolution of Consciousness-Chakras, Ki and Psi.* Brookline, MA: Autumn Press, Inc., 1978.

Motoyama, Dr. Hiroshi. *Theories of the Chakras: Bridge to Higher Consciousness.* Wheaton, IL: The Theosophical Publishing House, 1981.

Rieker, Hans-Ulrich. *The Yoga of Light.* Los Angeles: The Dawn Horse Press, 1977.

Schwarz, Jack. *Voluntary Controls: Exercises for Creative Meditation and For Activating the Potential of the Chakras.* New York: E. P. Dutton, 1978.

Sanford, Ray. *The Spirit Unto the Churches.* Austin, TX: Association For the Understanding of Man, 1977.

Tirtha, Swami Vishnu. *Devatma Shakti: Kundalini Divine Power.* Rishikesh, India: Sadhan Granthmala Prakashan Samiti, 1962.

Vyas, Dev Ji, Swami. *Science of Soul (Atma-Viynana).* Rishikesh, India: Yoga Niketan Trust, 1972.

Creation Myths

Asimov, Issac. *In The Beginning.* New York: Crown Publishing, 1981.

Blavatsky, Helena, P. *The Secret Doctrine.* Wheaton, IL: The Theosophical Publishing House, 1980.

Farmer, Antonio. *Beginnings: Creation Myths of the World.* New York: Atheneum Publishing Co., 1979.

Gribbin, John. *Genesis: The Origins of Man and the Universe.* New York: Dial/Delacorte, 1981.

Maclagan, David. *Creation Myths.* New York: Thames and Hudson, 1977.

Peacocke, A. R. *Creation and the World of Science.* New York: Oxford University Press, 1979.

Preston, E. W. *The Story of Creation.* Wheaton, IL: The Theosophical Publishing House, 1947.

Van Over, Raymond, ed. *Sun Songs: Creation Myths From Around the World.* Bergenfield, NJ: New American Library, 1980.

Andrew Jackson Davis
Davis, Andrew Jackson. *The Great Harmonia,* Vol. I, *The Physician.* Mokelumne Hill, CA: Health Research, 1973.
_____. *The Harbinger of Health,* Mokelumne Hill, CA, Health Research, 1971.
_____. *The Temple: Diseases of the Brain and Nerves.* Mokelumne Hill, CA: Health Research, 1972.
_____. *The Principles of Nature.* 1847.

Flowers and Flower Essences
Bach, Dr. Edward. *The Bach Flower Remedies.* New Canaan, CT: Keats Publishing, Inc., 1979.
_____. *Heal Thyself.* Saffron Walden, Essex, England: The C. W. Daniel Company Ltd., 1974.
_____. *The Twelve Healers and Other Remedies.* Saffron Walden, Essex, England: The C. W. Daniel Co. Ltd., 1975.
Chancellor, Philip. *Handbook of the Bach Flower Remedies.* Saffron Walden, Essex, England: The C. W. Daniel Co. Ltd., 1974.
Clements, Julie. *Treasury of Rose Arrangements and Recipes.* Nashville: Hearthside Press, 1959.
Coats, Alice F. *Flowers and Their Histories.* New York: McGraw-Hill Book Co., 1971.
Coats, Peter. *Flowers in History.* New York: Viking Press, 1970.
Evans, Jane. *Introduction to the Benefits of the Bach Flower Remedies.* Saffron Walden, Essex, England: The C. W. Daniel Co. Ltd., 1980.
Grossman, Karl. "Sacrificial Spiderwort." *Mother Jones,* IV (December, 1979), 14.
Heline, Corinne. *Magic Gardens.* Marina del Rey, CA: DeVorss & Company, 1980.
Hilarion. *Wildflowers.* Toronto: Marcus Books,1982.
Jones, T. W. Hyne. *Dictionary of the Bach Flower Remedies.* Barnstead, Surrey, England: T. M. Jones, 1977.
Kull, A. Stoddard. *Secrets of Flowers.* Brattleboro, VT: The Stephen Greene Press, 1966.
Lehner, Frank & Johanna. *Folklore and Symbolism of Flowers, Plants and Trees.* New York: Tudor Publishing Co., 1960.
The Mother. *Flowers and Fragrance,* Part I and II. Pondicherry, India: Sri Aurobindo Society, 1979.
_____. *Flowers and Their Messages.* Pondicherry, India: Sri Aurobindo Ashram, 1979.
Nash, Elizabeth. *One Hundred and One Legends of Flowers.* New York: Gordon Press Publications, 1977.
Powell, Claire. *The Meaning of Flowers.* Boulder, CO: Shambhala Publications, 1979.
Rohde, Eleanor. *Rose Recipes.* Danby, PA: Arden Library, 1979.
Tergit, Gabriele. *Flowers Through the Ages.* Philadelphia: Dufour Editions, 1962.

Weeks, Nora, and Victor Bullen. *The Bach Flower Remedies: Illustrations and Method of Preparation.* Saffron Walden, Essex, England: The C. W. Daniel Co. Ltd., 1976.

Weeks, Nora. *The Medical Discoveries of Edward Bach, Physician.* Saffron Walden, Essex, England: The C. W. Daniel Co. Ltd., 1976.

Wheeler, F. J. *The Bach Remedies Repertory.* Saffron Walden, Essex, England: The C. W. Daniel Co. Ltd., 1974.

Wielkopolska, Elizabeth Bellhouse. *Vita Florum and the Master Science.* Taunton, Somerset, England: The Vita Florum Trust, 1977.

Gemstones

Chadbourne, Robert, and Ruth Wright. *Gems and Minerals of the Bible.* New Canaan, CT: Keats Publishing, Inc., 1970.

Fernie, Dr. William T. *The Occult and Curative Powers of Precious Stones.* New York: Harper & Row Publishers, 1981.

Glick, Joel and Julia Lorusso. *Healing Stoned: The Therapeutic Use of Gems and Minerals.* Albuquerque, NM: Brotherhood of Life, 1979.

Gurudas. *Gem Elixirs and Vibrational Healing*, Vol I. San Rafael, CA: Cassandra Press, 1985.

Gurudas. *Gem Elixirs and Vibrational Healing*, Vol II. San Rafael, CA: Cassandra Press, 1986.

Kozminski, Isidore. *The Magic and Science of Jewels and Stones*, Vol I. San Rafael, CA: Cassandra Press, 1988.

Kozminski, Isidore. *The Magic and Science of Jewels and Stones*, Vol II. San Rafael, CA: Cassandra Press, 1988.

Kunz, George. *The Curious Lore of Precious Stones.* New York: Dover Publications, Inc., 1971.

Pelikan, Wilhelm. *The Secrets of Metals.* Spring Valley, NY: Anthroposophic Press, Inc., 1973.

Health and Vibrational Healing

Aero, Rita. *The Complete Book of Longevity.* East Rutherford, NJ: G. P. Putnam's Sons, 1980.

Ballard, Juliet Brooke. *The Hidden Laws of Earth.* Virginia Beach, VA: ARE Press, 1979.

Besant, Annie, and C. W Leadbeater. *Thought Forms.* Wheaton, IL: The Theosophical Publishing House, 1969.

Brooks, Wiley. *"Breatharianism."* Arvada, CO: Breatharianism International, Inc., 1982.

Burkardt, Titus. *Alchemy.* Baltimore: Penguin Books, 1971.

Burne, Jerome."The Intimate Frontier." *Science Digest*, LXXXIX (March, 1981), 82-85.

Burr, Harold. *Blueprint for Immortality.* Sudbury, Suffolk, England: Neville Spearman Ltd., 1972.

Butler, Francine. *Biofeedback: A Survey of the Literature.* New York: Plenum Publishers, 1978.

Cousens, M.D., Gabriel. *Spiritual Nutrition and the Rainbow Diet.* San Rafael, CA: Cassandra Press, 1986.

Cousins, Norman. *Anatomy of An Illness As Perceived by the Patient*. Los Angeles: Cancer House, 1979.

Cunningham, Donna. *Astrology and Vibrational Healing*. San Rafael, CA: Cassandra Press, 1988.

David, William. *The Harmonics of Sound, Color and Vibration*. Marina del Rey, CA: DeVorss & Company, 1980.

Day, Langston, and George De La Warr. *Matter in the Making*. London: Vincent Stuart Ltd., 1966.

_____. *New Worlds Beyond the Atom*. London: Vincent Stuart Ltd., 1956.

Diamond, John. *Behavioral Kinesiology*. Los Angeles: Regent House, 1981.

Edmunds and Associates, and H Tudor. *Some Unrecognized Factors in Medicine*. London: The Theosophical Publishing House, 1976.

Gallert, Mark. *New Light on Therapeutic Energy*. London: James Clarke & Co. Ltd., 1966.

Guirdham, M.D., Arthur. *A Theory of Disease*. Sudbury, Suffolk, England: Neville Spearman Ltd., 1957.

_____. *The Psyche in Medicine*. Sudbury, Suffolk, England: Neville Spearman Ltd., 1978.

Hall, Manly P. *Healing: Divine Art*. Los Angeles: Philosophical Research Society, 1971.

Heindel, Max. *Occult Principles of Health and Healing*. Oceanside, CA: The Rosicrucian Fellowship, 1938.

Holland, John. "Slow Inapparent and Recurrent Viruses." *Scientific American*, CCXXX (February, 1974), 32-40.

Hotema, Hilton. *Man's Higher Consciousness*. Mokelumne Hill, CA: Health Research, 1952.

Hunte-Cooper, Le. *The Danger of Food Contamination by Aluminum*. London: John Bale Sons and Danielson Ltd., 1932.

Irion, J. Everett. *Vibrations*. Virginia Beach, VA: ARE Press, 1979.

Jung, Carl. *Man and His Symbols*. New York: Doubleday & Co., 1969.

Krippner, Stanley, and John White, eds. *Future Science*. Garden City, NY: Anchor Books, 1977.

Krishna, Gopi. *The Awakening of Kundalini*. New York: E. P. Dutton, 1975.

_____. *Kundalini, The Evolutionary Energy in Man*. Boulder, CO: Shambhala Publications, 1967.

Lakkovsky, Georges. *The Secret of Life*. Mokelumne Hill, CA: Health Research, 1970.

Mann, John A. *Secrets of Life Extension: How to Halt the Aging Process and Live a Long and Healthy Life*. San Francisco: And/Or Press, 1980.

Medicines for the New Age. Virginia Beach, VA: Heritage Publications, 1977.

Medical Group. *The Mystery of Healing*. London: The Theosophical Publishing House, 1958.

Mendelsohn, M.D., Robert. *Confessions of a Medical Heretic*. New York: Warner Books, 1980.

Milner, Dennis, and Edward Smart. *The Loom of Creation*. New York: Harper & Row Publishers, 1976.

Narayananda, Swami. *The Primal Power in Man or the Kundalini Shakti*. Gylling, Denmark: N.U. Yoga Trust Ashrama, 1979.

Null, Gary. "Aluminum: Friend or Foe?" *Bestways*, X, 60-65.

Oberg, Alcestis, and Daniel Woodward. "Anti-Matter Mind Probes and Other Medical Miracles." *Science Digest*, XC, (April, 1982), 54-62.

Pandit, M. P. *Kundalini Yoga.* Madras, India: Ganesh & Co., 1968.

Playfair, Guy, and Scott Hill. *The Cycles of Heaven-Cosmic Forces and What They are Doing to You.* New York: St. Martin's Press, 1978.

Pykett, Ian L. "NMR Imaging In Medicine." *Scientific American*, CCXLVI (May, 1982), 78-88.

Reichenbach, Baron Karl Von. *The Mysterious Odic Force.* Wellingborough, England: Thorsons Publishers Ltd., 1977.

Rele, Vasant. *The Mysterious Kundalini.* Bombay, India: Taraporevala Sons & Co., 1960.

Russell, Edward. *Report on Radionics.* Sudbury, Suffolk, England: Neville Spearman Publishers Ltd., 1973.

Russell, Walter. *The Secret of Light.* Waynesboro, VA: University of Science and Philosophy, 1947.

Sannella, M.D., Lee. *Kundalini-Psychosis or Transcendence.* San Francisco: Henry S. Dakin, 1976.

Scheer, James F. "Electroacupuncture: New Pathway to Total Health," *Bestways*, X (June, 1982), 40-4719.

Sivananda, Swami. *Kundalini Yoga.* Rishikesh, India: Divine Life Society, 1935.

Soleri, Paolo. *The Omega Seed: An Eschatological Hypotheses.* Garden City, NY: Anchor Press, 1981.

Tansley, D. C., David. *Dimensions of Radionics.* Saffron Walden, Essex, England: Health Science Press, 1977.

Taylor, F. S. *The Alchemists.* St. Albans, England: Paladin, 1976.

Tomlinson, H. *Aluminum Utensils and Disease.* Romfort, England: L. N. Fowler & Co., 1967.

Ulmer, M.D., David. "Toxicity From Aluminum Antacids." *The New England Journal of Medicine*, 294 (January, 1976), 218-219.

Waite, Arthur E., ed. *The Hermetic and Alchemical Writings of Paracelsus.* Boulder, CO: Shambhala Publications, 1976.

Wingerson, Lois. "Training To Heal the Mind." *Discovery*, Vol. 3 no. 5 (May, 1982), 80-85.

Woodroffe, Sir John. *The Serpent Power.* New York: Dover Publications, 1974.

Herbs

Grieve, M. A. *A Modern Herbal.* New York: Dover Publications, 1971.

Gurudas. *The Spiritual Properties of Herbs.* San Rafael, CA: Cassandra Press, 1988.

Kloss, Jethro. *Back to Eden.* Santa Barbara: Woodbridge Press, 1979.

Lust, John. *The Herb Book.* New York: Bantam Books, Inc., 1974.

Messegue, Maurice. *Health Secrets of Plants and Herbs.* West Caldwell, NJ: William Morrow and Co., 1979.

_____. *Way to Natural Health and Beauty.* New York: MacMillan Publishing Co., Inc., 1974.

Stuart, Malcom., ed. *The Encyclopedia of Herbs and Herbalism.* New York: Crescent Books, 1981.

Homeopathy

Bach, M.D., Edward. "A Clinical Comparison Between the Actions of Vaccines and Homeopathic Remedies." *British Homeopathic Journal*, IX (January, 1921), 21-24.

_____."The Relation of Vaccine Therapy to Homeopathy." *British Homeopathic Journal*, X (April, 1920), 67-81.

Boericke, M.D., William. *A Compend of the Principles of Homeopathy.* Mokelumne Hill, CA: Health Research, 1971.

_____. *Materia Medica with Repertory.* New Delhi, India: B. Jain Publishers, 1976.

_____, and Willis DeWey, M.D. *The Twelve Tissue Remedies of Schussler.* New Delhi, India: B. Jain Publishers, 1977.

Blackie, M.D., Margery. *The Patient Not the Cure.* London: Macdonald and Jane's, 1976.

Choudhuri, M.D., N. M. *A Study on Materia Medica.* New Delhi, India: B. Jain Publishers, 1978.

Clarke, M.D., J. H. *A Clinical Repertory to the Dictionary of Materia Medica.* Saffron Walden, Essex, England: Health Science Press, 1971.

_____. *Constitutional Medicine.* New Delhi, India: B. Jain Publishers, 1974.

_____. *Dictionary of Materia Medica.* Saffron Walden, Essex, England: Health Science Press, 1977.

Coulter, Ph.D., Harris. *Divided Legacy: A History of the Schism in Medical Thought*, Vol. III. Washington, D.C.: Wehawken Book Co., 1973.

Farrington, M.D., E. A. *Clinical Materia Medica.* New Delhi, India: B. Jain Publishers, 1975.

Hahnemann, M.D., Samuel. *The Chronic Diseases-Theoretical Part.* New Delhi, India: B. Jain Publishers, 1976.

_____. *Organon of Medicine.* New Delhi, India: B. Jain Publishers, 1977.

Hubbard-Wright, M.D., Elizabeth. *A Brief Study Course in Homeopathy.* St. Louis, MO: Formur, Inc., 1977.

Kent, M.D., James T. *Lectures on Homeopathy Philosophy.* Calcutta, India: Sett Dey & Co., 1967.

_____. *Repertory Materia Medica.* Chicago: Ehrhart and Karl, 1957.

Muzumda, M.D., K. P. *Pharmaceutical Science in Homeopathy and Pharmacodynamics.* New Delhi, India: B. Jain Publishers, 1974.

Nash, M.D., E. B. *Leaders in Homeopathic Therapeutics.* Calcutta, India: Sett Dey & Co., 1959.

Patterson, M.D., John. "The Role of the Bowel Flora in Chronic Disease." *British Homeopathic Journal*, XXXIX (January, 1949), 3-26.

Roberts, M.D., Herbert. *The Principles and Art of Cure by Homeopathy.* Saffron Walden, Essex, England: Health Science Press, 1976.

Ross, M.D., A. C. Gordon. "The Bowel Nosodes." *British Homeopathic Journal*, LXII, 42-44.

Tomlinson, M.D., H. *Aluminum Utensils and Disease.* London: L. N. Fowler & Co., 1967.

Tyler, Dr., M. L. *Homeopathic Drug Pictures.* Saffron Walden, Essex, England: Health Science Press, 1975.

Vithoulkas, George. *The Science of Homeopathy.* New York: Grove Press, Inc., 1980.

Weiner, Michael, and Goss, Kathleen. *The Complete Book of Homeopathy*. New York: Bantam Books, 1982.

Whitmont, M.D., Edward. *Psyche and Substance*. Richmond, CA: North Atlantic Books, 1980.

Lemuria and Atlantis

Berlitz, Charles. *The Mystery of Atlantis*. New York: Avon, 1977.

Cayce, Edgar. *Atlantis: Fact or Fiction*. Virginia Beach: VA, ARE Press, 1962.

Cayce, Hugh., ed. *Edgar Cayce on Atlantis*. New York: Warner Books, 1968.

Cerve, W. S. *Lemuria: The Lost Continent of the Pacific*. San Jose: AMORC, 1977.

Churchward, James. *The Children of Mu*. New York: Warner Books, 1968.

_____. *The Cosmic Forces of Mu*. New York: Warner Books, 1968.

_____. *The Lost Continent of Mu*. New York: Warner Books, 1968.

_____. *The Sacred Symbols of Mu*. New York: Warner Books, 1968.

_____. *The Second Book of the Cosmic Forces of Mu*. New York: Warner Books, 1968.

Donnelly, Ignatius. *Atlantis: The Antediluvian World*. New York: Dover Publications, 1976.

Earll, Tony. *Mu Revealed*. New York: Warner Books, 1970.

Montgomery, Ruth. *The World Before*. New York: Fawcett Book Group, 1977.

Phylos. *A Dweller on Two Planets*. Alhambra, CA: Borden Publishing Co., 1969.

_____. *An Earth Dweller Returns*. Alhambra, CA: Borden Publishing Co., 1969.

Randall-Stevens, H. C. *Atlantis to the Latter Days*. Jersey, England: The Knight Templars of Aquarius, 1966.

Scott-Elliot, W. *The Story of Atlantis and The Lost Lemuria*. London: The Theosophical Publishing House, 1972.

Steiner, Rudolf. *Cosmic Memory: Atlantis and Lemuria*. New York: Harper & Row Publishers, 1981.

Nature Spirits

Briggs, Katherine. *An Encycolpedia of Fairies, Hobgoblins, Brownies, Bogies and Other Supernatural Creatures*. New York: Pantheon, 1978.

_____. *Fairies in Tradition and Literature*. London: Routledge & Kegan Paul Ltd., 1977.

_____. *The Vanishing People: Fairy Lore and Legends*. New York: Pantheon, 1978.

Doyle, Sir Arthur Conan. *The Coming of the Fairies*. York Beach, ME: Samuel Weiser, Inc., 1972.

Hall, Manly P. *Unseen Forces*. Los Angeles: The Philosophical Research Society, 1978.

Hawken, Paul. *The Magic of Findhorn*. New York: Bantam Books, 1974.

Hodson, G. *Fairies at Work and Play*. Wheaton, IL: The Theosophical Publishing House, 1925.

Findhorn Community. *The Findhorn Garden*. New York: Harper & Row Publishers, 1976.

New Physics

Bearden, Thomas. E. *Excalibur Briefing.* San Francisco: Strawberry Hill Press, 1980.

Bentov, Itzhak. *Stalking the Wild Pendelum.* New York: Bantam Books, 1981.

Besant, Annie, and Charles Leadbeater. *Occult Chemistry.* Mokelumne Hill, CA: Health Research, 1967.

Bohm, David. *Wholeness and the Implicate Order.* London: Routledge & Kegan Paul, 1980.

Capra, Fritjof. *The Tao of Physics.* New York: Bantam Books, 1980.

Dossey, Dr. Larry. *Space, Time and Medicine.* Boulder, CO: Shambhala Publications, 1982.

King, Serge. *Mana Physics: The Study of Paraphysical Energy.* New York: Baraka Books, 1978.

Pagels, Heinz. *The Cosmic Code: Quantum Physics as the Language of Nature.* New York: Simon & Schuster, 1982.

Reincourt, Amaury De. *The Eye of Shiva: Eastern Mysticism and Science.* New York: William Morrow & Co., 1981.

Russell, Bertrand. *The ABC of Relativity.* Bergenfield, NJ: New American Library, 1969.

Sergre, Emilo. *From X-Rays to Quarks-Modern Physicists and Their Discoveries.* San Francisco: W. H. Freeman & Co., 1980.

Talbot, Michael. *Mysticism and the New Physics.* New York: Bantam Books, 1981.

Toben, Bob. *Space-Time and Beyond.* New York: E. P. Dutton, 1982.

Trefil, James. "Nothing May Turn Out to Be the Key to the Universe," *Smithsonian,* XII (December, 1981), 143-149.

Wolf, Fred Alan. *Taking the Quantam Leap: The New Physics for Nonscientists.* New York: Harper & Row Publishers, 1981.

Zukav, Gary. *The Dancing Wu Li Masters.* New York: Bantam Books, 1980.

Parapsychology

Beck, Robert. *Extreme Low Frequency Magnetic Fields and EEG Entrainment, A Psychotronic Warfare Capacity?* Los Angeles: Bio-Medical Research Associates, 1978.

Hull, Moses. *Encyclopedia of Biblical Spiritualism.* Amherst, WI: Amherst Press, 1895.

Freedland, Nat. *The Occult Explosion.* East Rutherford, NJ: G. P. Putnam's Sons, 1972.

Linedecker, Clifford. *Psychic Spy: The Story of an Astounding Man.* Garden City, NY: Doubleday & Co., 1976.

Meek, George. *From Enigma to Science.* York Beach, ME: Samuel Weiser, Inc., 1973.

Mishlove, Jeff. *The Roots of Consciousness.* New York: Random House, 1980.

Monroe, Robert. *Journeys Out of the Body.* New York: Anchor Press, 1977.

Moody, Raymond. *Life After Life.* New York: Bantam Books, 1976.

Ostrander, Sheila, and Lynn Schroeder. *Psychic Discoveries Behind the Iron Curtain.* New York: Bantam Books, 1976.

Ravenscroft, Trevor. *The Spear of Destiny.* York Beach: ME. Samuel Weiser, Inc., 1982.

Woodward, Mary Ann., ed. *Edgar Cayce's Story of Karma*. New York: Berkley Books, 1972.

Pendulum
Graves, Tom. *The Diviner's Handbook*. New York: Warner Books, 1977.
Hitching, Francis. *Dowsing the PSI Connection*. New York: Anchor Press, 1978.
Mermet, Abbe. *Principles and Practice of Radiesthesia*. London: Watkins Publishing, 1975.
Reyner, J. H. *Psionic Medicine*. York Beach, ME: Samuel Weiser, Inc., 1974.
Richards, Dr. W. Guyon. *The Chain of Life*. Hustington, Sussex, England: Leslie J. Speight Ltd., 1974.
Tomlinson, Dr., H. *The Divination of Disease: A Study of Radiesthesia*. Saffron Walden, Essex, England: Health Science Press, 1953.
Westlake, Dr. Aubrey. *The Pattern of Health*. Boulder, CO: Shambhala Publications, 1974.
Wethered, Vernon D. *An Introduction to Medical Radesthesia and Radionics*. Saffron Walden, Essex, England: The C. W. Daniel Co. Ltd., 1974.
_____. *The Practice of Medical Radesthesia*. Saffron Walden, Essex, England: The C. W. Daniel Co. Ltd., 1977.

Pyramids
Benavides, Rodolfo. *Dramatic Prophecies of the Great Pyramid*. Mexico: Editores Mexicanos Unidos, S.A., 1974.
Edwards, T. E. *Pyramids of Egypt*. New York: Penguin Books, 1975.
Evans, Humphrey. *The Mystery of the Pyramids*. New York: Funk & Wagnalls, 1979.
Flanagan, Pat. *Pyramid Power*. Marina del Rey, CA: DeVorss & Co., 1976.
Lemesurier, Peter. *The Great Pyramid Decoded*. New York: Avon, 1979.
Nielsen, Greg, and Thoth, Max. *Pyramid Power*. New York: Warner Books, 1976.
Schul, Bill, and Pettit., ed. *Secret Power of Pyramids*. New York: Fawcett Publications, 1977.
_____. *Pyramids and the Second Reality*. New York: Fawcett Publications, 1979.
Tompkins, Peter. *Secrets of the Great Pyramid*. New York: Harper & Row Publishers, 1971.

Religion
Bible, King James Version. New York: Thomas Nelson Publishers, 1972.
Charles, R. H., ed. *The Book of the Secrets of Enoch*. Mokelumne Hill, CA: Health Research, 1964.
Eiselen, F. C., Edwin Lewis, and D. G.Downer., ed. *The Abington Bible Commentary*. Garden City, NY: Doubleday & Co., 1979.
Koffend, John. "The Gospel According to Helen," *Psychology Today*, XXVII (September, 1980), 74-90.
Laurence, Richard, trans. *The Book of Enoch the Prophet*. San Diego: Wizards Bookshelf, 1972.
Robinson, James., ed. *The Nag Hammadi Library*. New York: Harper & Row Publishers, 1977.
Strong, James. *Strong's Exhaustive Concordance of the Bible*. Nashville: Abington Press, 1980.

Rudolf Steiner and Anthroposophical Medicine

Abbot, A. E. *The Art of Healing.* London: Emerson Press, 1963.

Bott, M.D., Victor. *Anthroposophical Medicine.* London: Rudolf Steiner Press, 1978.

Davy, John., ed. *Medicine-Extending the Art of Healing.* London: Rudolf Steiner Press, 1975.

Glas, Norbert. *How to Look At Illness.* London: New Knowledge Books, 1951.

Kirchner-Bockholt, M.D., Margaret. *Fundamentals of Curative Eurythmy.* London: Rudolf Steiner Press, 1978.

Leroi, M.D., Rita. *An Anthroposophical Approach to Cancer.* Spring Valley, NY: Mercury Press, 1973.

Sayers, William. *Body, Soul, and Blood.* Troy, MI: Asclepiad Publications, Inc., 1980.

Steiner, Rudolf. *An Occult Physiology.* London: Rudolf Steiner Press, 1951.

_____. *An Outline of Anthroposophical Medical Research.* London: British Weleda Co., 1925.

_____. *Anthroposophical Approach to Medicine.* London: Anthroposophical Publishing Co., 1951.

_____. *Curative Education.* Spring Valley, NY: The Anthroposophical Press, 1982.

_____. *The Etherisation of the Blood.* London: Rudolf Steiner Press, 1971.

_____, and Ita Wegman, M.D. *Fundamentals of Therapy.* London: Rudolf Steiner Press, 1967.

_____. *Geographic Medicine and the Mystery of the Double.* Spring Valley, NY: Mercury Press, n.d.

_____. *Health and Illness*, Vol. I. Spring Valley, NY: The Anthroposophical Press, 1981.

_____. *Invisible Man Within Us: Pathology Underlying Therapy.* Spring Valley, NY: Mercury Press, n.d.

_____. *Karmic Relationships*, Vol. I. Spring Valley, NY: The Anthroposophic Press, 1981.

_____. *Man-Hieroglyph of the Universe.* London: Rudolf Steiner Press, 1972.

_____. *The Occult Significance of Blood.* London: Rudolf Steiner Press, 1967.

_____. *Overcoming Nervousness.* Spring Valley, NY: The Anthroposophic Press, 1973.

_____. *Reincarnation and Immortality.* New York: Harper & Row Publishers, 1980.

_____. *Spiritual Science and the Art of Healing.* London: Anthroposophical Publishing Co., 1950.

_____. *Spiritual Science and Medicine.* London: Rudolf Steiner Press, 1975.

_____. *Study of Man.* London: Rudolf Steiner Press, 1975.

_____. *Supersensible Man.* London: Anthroposophical Press, 1943.

_____. *What Can the Art of Healing Gain Through Spiritual Science.* Spring Valley, NY: Mercury Press, n.d.

_____. *The World of the Senses and the World of the Spirit.* North Vancouver, Canada: Steiner Book Centre, Inc., 1979.

Wachsmuth, Dr. Guenther. *Etheric Formative Forces in Cosmos, Earth and Man.* Spring Valley, NY: Anthroposophical Press, 1932.

Wegman, M.D., Ita. *Anthroposophical Principles of the Art of Healing.* London: British Weleda Co., 1928.

_____. *Rudolf Steiner's Work for an Extension of the Art of Healing.* London: British Weleda Co., 1928.

Wolff, Otto. *Anthroposophical Orientated Medicine and Its Remedies.* Arlesheim, Switzerland: Weleda, AG, 1977.

Many out of print Steiner and Anthroposophy books can be ordered from:
Rudolf Steiner Farm School & Library
Harlemville, R.D. 2,
Ghent, NY 12075

Subtle Bodies

Bagnall, Oscar. *The Origin and Properties of the Human Aura.* York Beach, ME: Samuel Weiser, Inc., 1975.

Besant, Annie. *A Study in Consciousness.* Madras, India: The Theosophical Publishing House, 1975.

_____. *Man & His Bodies.* Wheaton, IL: The Theosophical Publishing House, 1967.

Bendit, Laurence, and Phoebe Bendit. *The Etheric Body of Man.* Wheaton, IL: The Theosophical Publishing House, 1977.

Hall, Manly P. *The Occult Anatomy of Man.* Los Angeles: Philosophical Research Society, 1957.

Heindel, Max. *The Vital Body.* Oceanside, CA: The Rosicrucian Fellowship, 1950.

Heline, Corinne. *Occult Anatomy and the Bible.* La Canada, CA: New Age Press, 1981.

Kilner, Walter J. *The Human Aura.* York Beach, ME: Samuel Weiser, Inc., 1978.

Leadbeater, C. W. *Man Visible and Invisible.* Wheaton, IL: The Theosophical Publishing House, 1980.

Mead, G. R. S. *The Doctrine of the Subtle Body.* Wheaton, IL: The Theosophical Publishing House, 1967.

Powell, A. E. *The Astral Body.* Wheaton, IL: The Theosophical Publishing House, 1978.

_____. *The Causal Body.* Wheaton, IL: The Theosophical Publishing House, 1972.

_____. *The Etheric Double.* Wheaton, IL: The Theosophical Publishing House, 1969.

_____. *The Mental Body.* Wheaton, IL: The Theosophical Publishing House, 1975.

Rubin, Daniel, and Stanley Krippner. *The Kirlian Aura.* New York: Doubleday & Co., 1974.

Tansley, D.C., David. *Radionics and the Subtle Anatomy of Man.* Saffron Walden, Essex: Health Science Press, 1972.

_____. *Subtle Body: Essence and Shadow.* London: Thames & Hudson, 1977.

Walker, Benjamin. *Beyond the Body.* Boston: Routledge & Kegan Paul, 1974.

Index

For information on this continuing research, please contact:

Gurudas
P.O. Box 868
San Rafael, Ca. 94915

For information on purchasing the flower essences and gem elixirs
described in this book, please contact:

Pegasus Products, Inc.
P.O. Box 228
Boulder, Co. 80306
800-527-6104

29 – STINGING NETTLES – ... DIVORCE – ANIMALS +
   RAISE NEW+ POSITIVE THOUGHT: ...–? PLANTS

RMDD – RADULAS ...